EPIDEMIC CITY

EPIDEMIC CITY

THE POLITICS OF PUBLIC HEALTH IN NEW YORK

JAMES COLGROVE

Russell Sage Foundation • New York

The Russell Sage Foundation

The Russell Sage Foundation, one of the oldest of America's general purpose foundations, was established in 1907 by Mrs. Margaret Olivia Sage for "the improvement of social and living conditions in the United States." The Foundation seeks to fulfill this mandate by fostering the development and dissemination of knowledge about the country's political, social, and economic problems. While the Foundation endeavors to assure the accuracy and objectivity of each book it publishes, the conclusions and interpretations in Russell Sage Foundation publications are those of the authors and not of the Foundation, its Trustees, or its staff. Publication by Russell Sage, therefore, does not imply Foundation endorsement.

Library of Congress Cataloging-in-Publication Data

Colgrove, James Keith.
   Epidemic city : the politics of public health in New York / James Colgrove.
     p. cm.
Includes bibliographical references and index.
   ISBN 978-0-87154-497-1 (hardcover : alk. paper)   ISBN 978-087154-063-8
(pbk. : alk. paper)   ISBN 978-1-61044-708-9 (e-book hardcover)   ISBN
978-1-61044-745-4 (e-book pbk.)
   1. Medical policy—New York (State)—New York.   2. Public Health—New
York (State)—New York.   I. Title.
   RA395.A4N732 2005
   362.10974'1—dc22   2010052211

Text design by Suzanne Nichols.

The opinions expressed are those of the authors and may not represent those of the institutions they represent.

RUSSELL SAGE FOUNDATION
112 East 64th Street, New York, New York 10065
10 9 8 7 6 5 4 3 2 1

Contents

Acknowledgments

The generous support of several funders made this book possible. I am grateful to the Russell Sage Foundation, the National Library of Medicine (grant number 5G13LM9159-2), the Greenwall Foundation Faculty Scholars in Bioethics Program, and the Milbank Memorial Fund for sustaining my research and writing over five years.

This book draws extensively on interviews with some four dozen people (listed with the references) who collectively possess an incalculable amount of knowledge and expertise in public health. I owe them an enormous debt. Their patience and candor in answering my questions added critical details to the stories told here.

I benefited from the diligent assistance of numerous archivists. The New York City Department of Records and Information Services holds a wealth of information about the city's history, especially its public health system; I thank Leonora Gidlund, Kenneth Cobb, Tobi Adler, Steven Barto, and Michael Lorenzini for their efforts on my behalf over the years. I also thank Douglas Di Carlo at the La Guardia and Wagner Archives, La Guardia Community College, City University of New York, and Mary Marshall Clark and the staff of the Oral History Research Office at Columbia University.

I am fortunate to be part of a unique research and teaching environment, the Center for the History and Ethics of Public Health at Columbia University's Mailman School of Public Health. My colleagues in the center have been and continue to be unfailingly thoughtful, supportive, and generous with their time, and it is a pleasure to have yet another opportunity to thank them: Ronald Bayer, Amy Fairchild, Janlori Goldman, Barron Lerner, Nitanya Nedd, Gerald Oppenheimer, David Rosner, and Kavita Sivaramakrishnan. I thank Linda Fried, dean of the Mailman School of Public Health, for her enthusiastic support of the center.

In addition to my fellow faculty members in the Center for the History and Ethics of Public Health, several colleagues read some or all of the manuscript and offered detailed and thoughtful feedback. I am indebted to Jennifer Hirsch, Kim Hopper, Sylvia Law, Gerald Markowitz,

James Mohr, and Constance Nathanson. Thomas Frieden provided critical assistance at various stages of the research and many valuable comments on the manuscript. Conversations with Cynthia Connolly, Bob Harvey, Sheena Morrison, and Michael Yudell gave me key insights.

Lela Cooper did a superb job of transcribing interviews. Alison Bateman-House and Laura Bothwell provided expert research assistance. Leslie Laurence helped in the final review of the manuscript and assisted with securing images. At the Russell Sage Foundation, Suzanne Nichols was an exceptionally patient and helpful editor, and April Rondeau guided the book smoothly through production. I thank two anonymous referees who gave cogent suggestions for improving the manuscript.

Portions of chapter 1 originally appeared in altered form in the *Journal of Policy History* and are reprinted here with permission.

I could not have accomplished this work without the support of friends and loved ones. David Dunbar, as always, was an unfailing source of insight and humor. Naomi Schegloff and Vanessa Vichitvadakan provided encouraging words on occasions too numerous to mention. Carole Cooper, William Fisher, James Holmes, Marni Sommer, and Darla Villani provided companionship and good cheer.

Lastly and most significantly, I thank Robert Sember for reminding me what is important.

About the Author

James Colgrove is associate professor in the Center for the History and Ethics of Public Health at Columbia University's Mailman School of Public Health.

Introduction

Public Health and the American City

THE NAMES of great scientists and healers are carved on the facade of 125 Worth Street in lower Manhattan, a frieze of the familiar, the vaguely remembered, and the forgotten: Hippocrates, Pasteur, Jenner, Lister, Koch, Nightingale, Shattuck. Bronze medallions depicting allegories of health adorn the exterior walls of the imposing ten-story structure, built in art deco style with New Deal funds during the Great Depression. The building occupies an entire block on Foley Square, a short walk north of Wall Street, City Hall, and the site of the former World Trade Center. It houses the headquarters of the New York City Department of Health.[1] Its placidly monumental appearance belies the heated clashes that have taken place over the years in front of and within its walls: a protest in 1970 at which twin rows of marchers, pro and con, faced off over health code regulations that would prevent abortion—legalized in New York State only a few months earlier—from being performed in the offices of private physicians; a public hearing five years later where, as the city collapsed into insolvency, citizens angrily demanded the ouster of the commissioner because of his proposed cutbacks to community health services; a raucous piece of street theater on the building's front steps in 1991 where AIDS activists chanted and shook canisters of used syringes like giant maracas to protest the city's failure to support needle exchange programs.

This book is about public health in New York City in the last decades of the twentieth century. It tells the story of how the nation's first and in many ways preeminent local health agency sought to limit death and disease and promote the well-being of city residents. The department's employees—several thousand professionals from diverse backgrounds serving a city of some eight million residents—are the central figures in this story. They are surrounded by a supporting cast of individuals and groups who influenced public health in the city: elected officials at the

1

local, state, and national levels; nongovernmental organizations devoted to health and social welfare causes; community activists; doctors in private and hospital practice; researchers and academics; business leaders; employees of other city agencies; and journalists.

New York, like most large American cities, has confronted a remarkably complex array of health threats in recent decades: new and reemerging contagions such as HIV, tuberculosis, and West Nile virus; chronic conditions such as obesity and tobacco-related illness; unhealthy consequences of the built environment such as lead poisoning and asthma; and problems symptomatic of social deprivation and inequality such as violence, homelessness, and illicit drug use. Public health professionals draw upon diverse technical bases to tackle these problems, including epidemiology, statistics, medicine, nursing, law, and the social and behavioral sciences. Good public health practice depends on the appropriate application of methods derived from these disciplines. But intervening to prevent disease also raises questions that transcend technical expertise and involves issues of ethics, values, and priorities. Whether— to take an example from later in this book—a program to identify and notify the sexual and drug-sharing partners of HIV-infected people represents an unacceptable violation of the privacy of stigmatized groups is a question that cannot be answered (adequately) by referring to an "evidence base." Further, public health often involves moving ahead in the face of incomplete or conflicting scientific information, and the consequences of a course of action cannot always be accurately predicted when it is undertaken.

The questions that run through this book have to do with how public health programs were created and implemented in New York City during these years: What social and political factors influenced policies and practices? How were goals determined, and what forces were barriers or facilitators to meeting them? Which actors were most influential, and what strategies did they use to advance their interests? What were the major challenges to achieving a healthy city?

The answers to these questions are not as straightforward as might be assumed. A central premise of this book is that public health practices are not just the result of initiative from within the profession, nor are they solely determined by dispassionate evaluation of empirical data. To begin with, a problem must be defined as falling within the purview of public health (as opposed to being, for example, an issue of individual responsibility, the marketplace, or criminal justice). Public health professionals—influenced by the diverse constituencies described earlier— then make a series of decisions, not always explicitly acknowledged, about how resources of money, time, and effort should be allocated. Of problems thought to be appropriate targets, not all are deemed significant or urgent; some solutions are seen as realistic and feasible, others not. Funding for city public health programs, which comes from local taxes, state and federal aid, and external grants, rises and falls from year to year. Because health is woven into so many aspects of the city's life, the potential reactions of affected communities must be taken into account, and even relatively small-bore interventions may have unintended or unwanted consequences.

This book posits that public health issues do not have fixed or self-evident meanings. Rather, interest groups and individuals shape and define the significance of diseases and risks by selecting relevant facts to emphasize and publicize, assigning blame and accountability, and designating authority for solving the problem.[2] Popular perceptions of threats to the public health are influenced—and often distorted—by the anxieties, misapprehensions, and psychological biases people bring to the task of assessing risks. Rare or exotic risks such as tropical illnesses seem more alarming than quotidian or banal ones such as automobile accidents, for example; risks that are involuntary are more disturbing than those willingly taken.[3]

An additional premise of the book is that the shaping of a city's public health agenda, like government policymaking more generally, is a fluid, manipulable process in which varied actors may be influential at different moments. The health commissioner and his or her top deputies may drive the agenda, but so may people outside the department with different priorities and goals. These actors select from an array of potential policy approaches—the public health "tool kit" ranging from persuasive measures such as mass media education and social marketing to more coercive interventions such as quarantine or regulation of property or commerce. People involved in these processes take advantage of windows of opportunity, such as a perceived state of epidemiological, fiscal, or moral crisis, to advance a particular course of action.[4]

In sum, public health practice, while rooted in science, is an inherently and necessarily political enterprise. To be sure, views about public health do not map neatly onto liberal or conservative ideologies. But to the extent that public health entails collective rather than individual responses to illness, its activities inevitably raise questions about how government should act on behalf of citizens. The field's nineteenth-century pioneers in the United States and Europe embraced the idea that improving the health of populations was a political, social, and economic undertaking as much as a medical one.[5]

This account is not an institutional history, although it is concerned with internal processes of decisionmaking, program development, and implementation; nor is it an exhaustive chronicle of all the Health Department's activities, which are far too varied and extensive to be cataloged in a single volume. Rather, this book highlights a series of critical episodes over four decades that illustrate the varied factors shaping public health actions and outcomes.

Defining Local Public Health

Local health departments play a critical—though often invisible—role in the life of American cities. They are the linchpin of the public health system in the United States, limiting disease and promoting well-being in the city or county they serve and conveying critical information to their counterparts at the state and federal levels.

Ask a cross-section of big-city residents about public health, and most will give vague expressions of approval without a precise understanding of what they are supporting. Many laypeople equate public health with free clinics for the poor.[6] This perception is ironic, since providing clinical services represents only a small part of the field's mission, and many within the profession have long argued that it should not be in the business of curative medicine at all. Public health is distinct from what is generally thought of as "health care" in two key respects: its focus on the prevention of illness rather than cure, and its intervention at the level of populations rather than individual patients. While government agencies play a lead role, public health also comprises various research and service activities carried out by private philanthropies, nonprofit community-based organizations, and academic institutions. "What we, as a society, do collectively to assure conditions in which people can be healthy" is how the Institute of Medicine, which published comprehensive reports on the subject in 1988 and 2003, defined the field.[7] Given this expansive—indeed, potentially unlimited—scope of work, it is not surprising that the profession is poorly understood and has been criticized for lacking a coherent vision.[8] Jonathan Mann, a pioneer in linking medicine with human rights, memorably described public health as "a little bit of everything and not enough of anything."[9]

This diffuse mission has its roots in the mid-nineteenth century, when physicians, housing reformers, advocates for the poor, and scientists trained in new techniques of chemistry and civil engineering came together to fight problems growing out of urbanization and industrialization. The first public health crusaders, working with local and state governments, established regulations over such diverse aspects of civic life as the production and distribution of meat and milk, tenement construction, garbage collection, private and public privies, "noxious trades" like slaughterhouses and tanneries, and reservoirs and water supplies.[10] Local health departments at the level of village, town, city, or county were first established in this country in the urban Northeast, where these problems arose most urgently. New York, Boston, Providence, Philadelphia, Baltimore, and New Haven developed early and activist health departments with dynamic leadership. Laws and regulations were important tools for limiting threats to the common welfare.[11]

The unlikely professional alliance that gave rise to public health soon splintered, with profound consequences for the subsequent evolution of the field. Especially significant was the break, in the early twentieth century, between doctors in private or hospital practice and those working in government. The former, represented by their increasingly powerful lobby, the American Medical Association (AMA), claimed authority over the domain of patient care and vehemently opposed any initiative to provide clinical services in the public sector.[12] The notable exception was care for expectant mothers and their infants, an area where public health doctors had established a strong base of expertise. Local health departments were also left with responsibility for a few necessary but unglamorous categories of care that the medical profession disdained to provide: services for the indigent, treatment of sexually transmitted diseases, and control of once-epidemic but rapidly dwindling contagions such as tuberculosis and smallpox.[13]

As preventive practices such as routine physicals became common in the 1920s, public health officials clashed with doctors in private practice over who should deliver these services. Ambitious health departments in several cities, including Milwaukee, Cincinnati, Pittsburgh, and New Haven, sought to create networks of community-based health centers that would provide government-supported care for their poor populations. Opposition from local medical societies, combined with a lack of support at the level of city government, scuttled most of these experiments in what critics labeled "socialized medicine."[14]

It was during these years that the dichotomies that have defined American health care ever since would take shape: curing illness was emphasized over preventing it; the individual rather than society was seen as the proper focus of intervention; and the private marketplace had primacy over the public sector. The heterogeneous public health workforce of doctors, nurses, epidemiologists, and educators claimed a more enlightened, sociologically informed view than the narrow focus of biomedicine, and some of the profession's activist members sought to advance an environmentally focused approach that gave greater responsibility to the government. But their lack of political influence constrained their ability to shape the institutional landscape of health.[15] Meanwhile, some of the sanitary activities for which health departments had been responsible, such as garbage collection, air pollution control, and noise abatement, were pulled under the aegis of other professions and government agencies.[16]

In 1940 the American Public Health Association (APHA) passed a resolution codifying the standard repertoire of services that a local health department should provide—what became known as the "basic six." Health departments were responsible for collecting vital statistics, including birth and death rates and the incidence and prevalence of significant diseases. They were to control communicable diseases with methods such as outbreak investigations, contact tracing, partner notification, and (rarely) isolation and quarantine. They were charged with ensuring environmental sanitation in areas such as the municipal water supply (though, as noted earlier, these duties were sometimes housed in units of government other than health). They had responsibility for providing the laboratory services needed for the diagnosis of illnesses by private doctors, hospitals, and other clinicians. They were charged with providing maternal, infant, and child health services, such as education of expectant parents, prenatal checkups, immunizations, and well-baby screening. Finally, they were to provide education, through brochures, posters, pamphlets, and other mass media, to promote healthy behaviors.[17]

Although services were to some extent standardized along these lines, there was interstate variation—as in so many aspects of policy and politics in the United States, what local health departments actually did depended on the vagaries of state and local statutes and funding streams. Some departments offered a more limited range of programs, while others took a role in issues, such as housing, that lay outside the basic six.[18] Jurisdictional arrangements varied widely, with local health departments being responsible for a single city, a county, a region, multiple cities or counties, or some combination of these. State-level authority differed as well: some state departments provided no direct services, instead delegating all such work to local units, while others had highly centralized systems largely controlled in the capital.[19] On the whole, the growth of local public health was halting and uneven: as late as World War II, one-third of the U.S. population lived in an area that was not served by a full-time health official.[20]

The primacy of local and state responsibility for public health was partly a function of the U.S. constitutional system, which delegates authority to states, and partly the result of long-standing antipathy to federal power. The U.S. Public Health Service, which originated to police the nation's ports against imported contagions, had evolved little since the early republic, while the Surgeon General, ostensibly the nation's chief health officer, had scant authority (though a few of those who held the position used the office's bully pulpit effectively). The first national board of health was created in 1879 in response to an epidemic of yellow fever in the Tennessee Valley, but it proved politically unsustainable and soon fell victim to sectional power struggles.[21] An ill-fated effort by reformers to reestablish a national board in 1913, at the height of Progressive Era faith in rational government, united in successful opposition an unlikely congeries of anti-statist activists and medical liberty groups.[22]

When it was finally cobbled together in 1953 from a disparate assortment of federal agencies, the Department of Health, Education, and Welfare (DHEW) embodied political expediency more than any coherent vision of a healthy nation.[23] The DHEW, subsequently renamed the Department of Health and Human Services (DHHS), came to play an increasingly important role in local health through grants to states and cities. So did the Center (later Centers) for Disease Control and Prevention (CDC) in Atlanta, the nation's chief public health authority, established in 1946 as an outpost of the nation's malaria eradication effort in the South.[24] Nevertheless, local health departments occupied a critical niche on the front lines of the battle—as their work was often conceptualized—for healthy communities.

Eight Million Lives

The New York City Health Department, like the metropolis it serves, has always been paradoxical: it is at once prototypical and unique. On the one hand, its history encapsulates virtually all of the major epidemiological challenges faced by its peer agencies around the country. It has established pioneering programs in many areas, including health education, public health nursing, well-child care, and infectious disease control, which have served as models for other cities and states.

At the same time, New York City's size, diversity, and status as a global crossroads set it apart. In the decades after World War II, the city's population ranged between seven million and eight million—greater than the population of all but a handful of states. The city encompasses extremes of wealth and poverty, with some of the richest and poorest census tracts in the country. Overall it is politically liberal, but it includes swaths of relative conservatism, including largely residential areas of Queens, Brooklyn, and Staten Island, where residents often look with suspicion on the political and financial elites of Manhattan. Its racial, ethnic, linguistic, and cultural heterogeneity outstrip any other big city in the nation.

As a result of this complexity, "doing public health" in New York City has always presented exceptional challenges and opportunities. The Health Department operates with unusual autonomy from the rest of the state, enforcing a health code that supersedes state regulations in many areas; state health commissioners in Albany have often cast envious eyes down the Hudson River at the powers wielded at 125 Worth Street. Just as New York City, which holds some 40 percent of the state's population, has always overshadowed "upstate" in the political arena, so has its Health Department been the tail that wagged the dog.

New York City's—and the nation's—first permanent Board of Health was created by the state legislature in 1866, largely in response to cholera, a recurrent scourge of nineteenth-century urban centers.[25] The board had nine members, including the mayor, the chief health officer, and—reflecting the strong regulatory character of the era's public health—the four police commissioners. In 1870, as part of a sweeping reform of the city charter, the Department of Health was created as one of ten new units of city government. The department's work was divided among four bureaus: Sanitary Inspection, Street Cleaning, Records and Inspection, and Sanitary Permits. (Street Cleaning was transferred to the Police Department in 1873 and placed in a newly created Department of Sanitation in 1881.[26]) The nine-member Board of Health remained responsible for overseeing the department's activities and the content of the sanitary code; in a victory for home rule, the four members previously appointed by the governor were now to be mayoral choices.[27]

While cholera provided the spur for the creation of the new agency, the problems it faced were multifarious. What had been in 1800 a town of 60,000 residents concentrated on the southern tip of Manhattan had become by the 1860s a sprawling metropolis of more than 800,000. As new arrivals jammed into slums, filth and contagion spread, resulting in the human misery famously documented by reformers such as Jacob Riis. Dead horses, human and animal excrement, and every type of refuse clogged the city's streets. While much of the department's sanitary work disproportionately benefited the poor, it visibly, often dramatically, improved the quality of life in the city for all classes.

These efforts were not without skeptics. Many business owners bristled at being forced to abide by sanitary regulations. Citizens who doubted the safety and efficacy of smallpox immunization often fled when the squad of vaccinators descended—with police accompaniment—on their neighborhood. Muckraking reporters charged, sometimes legitimately, that Tammany Hall was packing the department with patronage appointments. But the public and politicians alike came to accept both the new department and the broader principle it represented: that preventing illness was an acceptable rationale for government to intrude on commerce and private behavior.

During the bacteriological revolution of the late nineteenth century, the department became a national leader in translating breakthroughs in the understanding of disease etiology into interventions that benefited the people. The emblematic success story of this era was the department's campaign to save children from diphtheria. The department's Division of Pathology, Bacteriology, and Disinfection, newly established in 1892 with a staff of twenty-five working out of two small laboratories, gained swift renown for manufacturing the first antitoxin to treat the ravages of the disease. Department physicians then fanned out across the city to get the antitoxin from the laboratory into the arms of sick children. When city aldermen were slow to appropriate money for the campaign, department leaders secured private funding and then partnered with reporters at the *Herald* on a series of human interest articles to dramatize the problem and its solution.[28] The diphtheria effort was a model of the skillful deployment of science in the community.

The driving force behind that effort was Hermann Biggs, the first head of the bacteriology laboratory. Biggs went on to even greater success leading the department's multipronged attack against the era's greatest killer, tuberculosis. His efforts showcased the range of instruments in the public health tool kit: compulsory reporting of cases by physicians to a central registry; free bacterial diagnosis of sputum samples; hospitalization of the sick; and home visits by sanitary inspectors to ensure healthy conditions and instruct patients and their families on how to prevent the spread of the disease.

Biggs, though he never served as commissioner, was a towering figure in the department's early history. He successfully advanced an openly paternalistic vision of public health authority, and while he preferred to achieve his goals through suasion, he had no qualms about invoking government's coercive hand against "recalcitrant" patients or uncooperative physicians. "The government of the United States is democratic," Biggs wrote in 1897, "but the sanitary measures adopted are sometimes autocratic, and the functions performed by sanitary authorities paternal in character. We are prepared to introduce and enforce measures which might seem radical and arbitrary, if they were not plainly designed for the public good, and evidently beneficent in their effects."[29]

In 1905 Biggs originated the axiom that soon became the unofficial motto of local and state health departments around the country: "Public health is purchasable. Within natural limitations a community can determine its own death rate." Yet generations of public health professionals would discover, to their frustration, that feckless communities often preferred to spend their money on other things.

During the Progressive Era, the porous boundaries between medicine, public health, and social welfare led to protracted debates in New York City (as elsewhere) about the role of the Health Department. Healthy babies were a preoccupation of the era's reformers, and the special value that children held in the nation's future well-being enabled the department to carve out a niche in the care of infants, children, and expectant mothers. What began as outposts providing pure milk quickly expanded into a network of child health stations offering a range of well-baby services; in 1908 the department established the Division of Child Hygiene—the nation's first—under the leadership of S. Josephine Baker, a formidable physician and social reformer. Baker hired a corps of dozens of nurses who made home visits to poor mothers to instruct them in proper methods of care.

Efforts to provide a broader range of clinical care for the general population, however, met with less success. Two commissioners during the 1910s, S. S. Goldwater and Haven Emerson, drew up far-reaching plans to establish community clinics that would bring medical and social services, housed under one roof, to the city's poorest neighborhoods. An initial district was established on the Lower East Side, the notoriously crowded slum with some of the city's worst health statistics; additional demonstration projects were started in other poor neighborhoods over the next two decades, often backed by support from private philanthropies. But a full-fledged expansion of publicly funded care for the poor remained blocked by the opposition of private doctors and the inertia of city government. When Mayor James J. Walker created the city's Department of Hospitals in 1929, uniting under one umbrella eighteen public institutions that had previously been run by the Department of Health and other city agencies, including the Department of Public Welfare, the move both reflected and reinforced the growing institutional separation of prevention from treatment.[30] It also enshrined the inpatient stay rather than ambulatory services as the dominant form of health care.

Although the well-being of many New Yorkers suffered during the financial and material hardships of the Depression, the city's health infrastructure improved during the decade, owing to Mayor Fiorello La Guardia's enthusiasm for public health and his skill at steering New Deal relief money into the city.[31] Millions of dollars from federal programs such as the Public Works Administration (PWA) and the Works Progress Administration (WPA) funded expansions of programs ranging from air quality improvement to mosquito control. The Health Department's major building program under La Guardia resulted, by 1940, in the new headquarters at 125 Worth Street (see figure I.1) along with fifteen new district health centers and nine new baby health stations.[32]

It was during this period that plans originated years earlier by Goldwater and Emerson to create "health districts" came to partial fruition. By dividing the city into thirty areas of about 200,000 residents each, the department could tailor services to the needs of particular neighborhoods, which varied widely in the socioeconomic status and (not coincidentally) the health outcomes of residents (see figure I.2). The health centers that served each district had doctors and nurses on staff, but they were not clinics in the traditional sense: beyond treatment for tuberculosis and venereal disease, they did not provide medical care. Instead, they were centers for education, prevention, and data gathering. The staff counseled district residents about health issues, offered screening and limited diagnosis, and collected statistics about the district. The centers served as a base for nurses who made home visits in the district and for physicians who worked in the area's schools; many of the buildings also made space available for community-based welfare and social service organizations serving the neighborhood.[33] Anyone found to have a med-

Figure I.1   Headquarters for Health

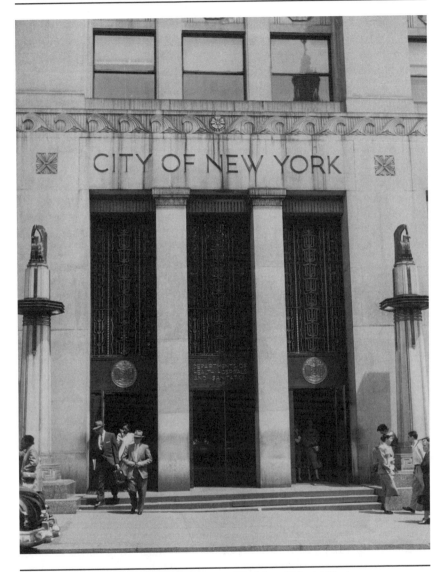

Source: Courtesy New York City Department of Health and Mental Hygiene.
Note: The Health Department headquarters at 125 Worth Street, a few blocks north of City Hall in lower Manhattan. The building was constructed with New Deal funds during the Depression and also housed the city's departments of hospitals and sanitation.

ical condition requiring treatment was referred elsewhere: those who were able to pay were sent to private physicians; those unable to pay were sent to the outpatient departments of the city's public hospitals.

By midcentury, the city's population had peaked at just under eight million, and the department's staff had grown to some 4,800. From four divisions in 1866, it had expanded to encompass a wide range of specialized functions and technical approaches. The department's five divisions and twenty bureaus handled everything from blood drives to restaurant inspections, from prenatal care to cardiovascular screening for the elderly. Its leadership had become far less confrontational than it had been in the era of Biggs; it accommodated powerful interests while excelling within the relatively narrow sphere of the basic six functions. It created a special ambulance service to speed premature babies to the nearest well-equipped care facility, established a poison control hotline, created the Bureau of Nutrition in recognition of the increasing importance of non-infectious sources of illness, and set up a research arm to investigate emerging epidemiological problems.

Programs such as these flourished under the dynamic leadership of Leona Baumgartner, whose savvy networking among the city's political, medical, and business elites made her the model of a modern health commissioner. Baumgartner maintained close rapport with Mayor Robert Wagner and never missed an opportunity to remind him of the many ways in which Health Department programs benefited city residents. She had a keen eye for photo opportunities and provided good copy for the local papers, whether giving Elvis Presley a polio shot or heaving a shovel of dirt at the groundbreaking for a new health center.

By the time Baumgartner stepped down in 1962, the department had come to be known within the profession as the "gold standard" among local health agencies nationwide. Some of this vaunted reputation can be attributed to skillful mythmaking on the part of an organization that always recognized the importance of good public relations and did much to celebrate its achievements in its publications and through the local media. But this reputation cannot be dismissed as mere puffery. The department had had more than its share of commissioners and senior staffer members—Biggs, Baker, Goldwater, Emerson, Baumgartner, and many others—who were innovators of national importance; its peer agencies around the country looked to New York City for guidance and inspiration.

It is important, however, to keep the department's very real successes and storied history in perspective. In terms of funding and prestige, public health remained a distinctly second-tier activity within the American health care system, receiving far less government support and popular recognition than clinical medicine. This was as true in New York City as anywhere else. The city had a vast and complicated health sector

Figure I.2   Health Districts

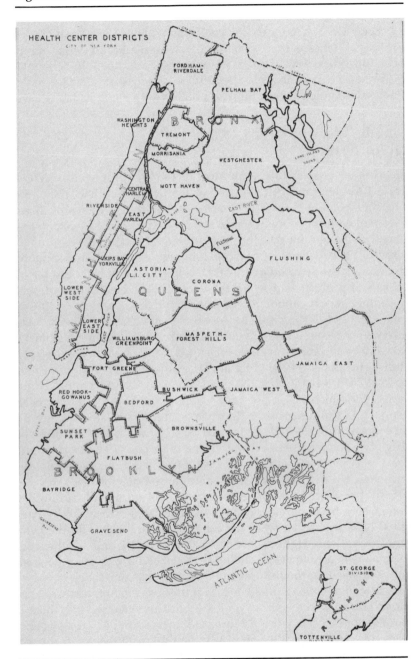

Source: Courtesy New York City Municipal Archives.
Note: In the 1930s, the Health Department divided the city's five boroughs into thirty health districts of about 200,000 residents each for purposes of data gathering and analysis, planning, and program delivery.

that included the largest public hospital system in the country, academic medical centers for research and teaching, and wealthy private institutions for patient care. In this environment, even a health department as successful and well regarded as New York's could not help being overshadowed. The position of the department within this web of power and influence had much to do with how public health got done in the city.

From the War on Poverty to the War on Terror

The years covered in this book—the 1960s through the early 2000s—were a turbulent and difficult period for public health in the United States and in New York City in particular. Shifting patterns of disease dovetailed with transformations in society and politics to create unprecedented challenges for the city's Department of Health.

By the 1960s, advances in vaccination and environmental sanitation had dramatically reduced many of the contagions that had been the major focus of public health work for decades. The Health Department's 1962 annual report confidently declared that the nation was "at the end of the great era of the battle against infectious disease." The hubris of this statement was soon evident: contagious diseases were far from banished and would return with a vengeance in forms both familiar (tuberculosis) and novel (HIV). More accurate was the department's prediction that "we are entering the great era of cold war against chronic diseases for which we do not have biologic cures." But as public health attempted to shift its focus to "lifestyle" conditions related to consumption—morbidities attributable to diet, exercise, and use of licit and illicit substances, among others—it would find these conditions to be far more intractable, and the methods for preventing them far less straightforward, than had been the case with controlling contagions.

At the same time, the social turmoil of this era upended traditional relationships between citizens and the elite professional and governmental institutions that were supposed to serve them. With the rise of feminism, patients' rights, consumer activism, and the many other social movements that followed in the wake of the civil rights struggle, members of affected communities began assertively, sometimes bitterly, to contest the decisions of public health professionals. Activists mobilized around issues of race, gender, and sexuality and charged that those responsible for protecting the public's health were complicit in a system of oppression fundamentally inimical to health. In the years during and after the Vietnam War and Watergate, public trust in institutions and authorities—the government, the military, the education system—plummeted, and the health professions were not spared.[34]

Coinciding with these social transformations were changes in the national political scene. The federal government grew dramatically beginning in the 1960s, carving out new roles in the regulation of commerce and industry and creating vast new entitlements involving health and social welfare spending.[35] Beginning with the legislative "big bang" of the Johnson administration that brought forth Medicaid, Medicare, community mental health centers, and a host of other programs, the health care arena was transformed. While new sources of funding made possible the expansion of some public health initiatives, they were hardly an unalloyed benefit for the profession: increasing federal expenditures on hospital care and medical technologies reinforced the paradigm of curative medicine and further overshadowed the role of prevention. The accretion of power in Washington, D.C., also laid the groundwork for the backlash of the Reagan revolution and a new era of fiscal austerity and small-government ideology.

These were difficult years for local health departments around the country. In 1977 a survey found "an unevenly operative public infrastructure of community and personal health services—understaffed, underfunded, and widely ignored."[36] Eleven years later, when the Institute of Medicine examined the state of the nation's public health infrastructure, its report was a grim catalog of inadequacy: "disorganization, weak and unstable leadership . . . hostility to public health concepts and approaches, outdated statutes, inadequate financial support for public health activities . . . gaps in the data gathering and analysis . . . lack of effective links between the public and private sectors."[37]

New York City's Department of Health faced acute problems during these years. The city's fiscal travails were the most notorious and paradigmatic of the "urban crisis" that gripped many large cities around the country, especially in the Rust Belt and the Northeast.[38] Beginning in the administration of Mayor Lindsay, the city's economic position deteriorated amid increasing social unrest and racial and ethnic polarization.[39] These economic woes culminated in the city's infamous insolvency in 1975. With layoffs in the thousands, the city's public health infrastructure was especially hard hit, and the budget slashing undertaken in these years had consequences that were still being felt decades later. At the same time, the city continued to be disproportionately affected by severe and intractable health issues. Epidemiological, social, political, and economic forces—extending far beyond the walls of 125 Worth Street—created the public health challenges that are the subject of this book.

At the beginning of the twenty-first century, public health was given high priority in the city under the new mayor, Michael Bloomberg, who hired an innovative and sharp-elbowed health commissioner, Thomas Frieden. The ambitious policies and programs in recent years, coming after more than three decades in which the Health Department struggled to overcome severe constraints, might be seen as a renewal of sorts. But casting the events in this book as a teleological narrative of "decline and rebirth" is an oversimplification that obscures as much as it explains. Rather, events since 1965 provide illuminating examples of both successes and failures—however variously these events may have been defined by the many individuals and groups concerned with public health in New York City.

This book is a work of narrative history—a story, or collection of stories, that seeks to convey the texture and detail of what it was like to address public health issues in a particular place and time and to understand why specific actors made the choices they did. Although it is informed by theoretical constructs drawn from the social sciences related to the definition of public problems and the setting of policy agendas, it remains grounded in the particularity of history. Whatever this approach may sacrifice in terms of generalizability to other jurisdictions and other eras, my hope is that a richer understanding of an individual case will compensate for this limitation.

Chapter 1

To Provide or Protect

I
N THE midst of a boisterous three-way mayoral race in the fall of 1965, the Health Department submitted a statement to the City Council explaining a deceptively modest element of its capital budget: a proposal to convert two of the nineteen district health centers to full-service outpatient clinics. "Health prevention and promotion on the one hand and diagnostic and curative services on the other," the document argued, "must be brought together into a more comprehensive, non-fragmented, easily available package for the consuming public."[1] The plan represented the first steps in an ambitious and far-reaching effort to fulfill a dream from a half century before, when the centers had first been envisioned as under-one-roof outposts for the health needs of the city's poor.

Although John Lindsay, the Republican candidate, called the city's public hospital system "an unmitigated disgrace," health did not figure prominently in the mayoral contest.[2] Police brutality, rising crime, and racial and ethnic polarization all presented more urgent and dramatic challenges. As soon as Lindsay emerged victorious, however, health services surged to the forefront of the political agenda amid a stream of dire reports about the city's medical infrastructure. Lindsay proposed a massive overhaul that would merge the Health Department with three related agencies; a farrago of disconnected, often redundant services would—so the plan went—be rationalized and coordinated, resulting in better care and greater efficiency and cost-effectiveness. At first blush, Lindsay's reorganization seemed to dovetail with the initiative that the Health Department was proposing. But things did not work out that way. Five years later, plans for the new clinics had barely gotten off the drawing board, and instead the department had taken on a very different role in ambulatory care, not as a provider but as a "watchdog."

In the 1960s, there were numerous efforts inside and outside of 125 Worth Street to break down the institutional walls that for decades had separated prevention from treatment. If there was any moment that seemed propitious for such an attempt, it was at the height of Great

Society liberalism, as a reformist mayor who had great faith in the power of government took the city's helm and a new federal entitlement program promised a steady funding stream for new programs. The events of this period provide an object lesson in the sometimes counterintuitive ways that political developments at the local, state, and national levels could influence—or swamp—plans originated by Health Department employees.

An Old Debate, Revived

To appreciate how the Health Department came to make its proposal, it is helpful to understand the broad climate of opinion within the field of public health about providing clinical services. In November 1963, as Congress began debating the legislation that would eventually result in Medicaid and Medicare, Surgeon General Luther Terry told an audience at the annual meeting of the American Public Health Association (APHA) that, after skirting the issue for decades, "we have decided we belong in the field of medical care."[3] Terry acknowledged uncertainty about what the new involvement would entail. "It seems quite evident," he conceded, "that neither the health officer nor the Health Department nor the public health movement as a whole is going to 'take over' the field of medical care. Nor are we likely, except within certain specific limits, to have the mantle of over-all direction and leadership thrust upon us."[4] Instead, Terry suggested, the field should parlay its strengths, such as collecting and analyzing population-level health information and statistics, into a stronger role in guiding services and research.

Terry's subtly conflicted message—calling simultaneously for change and accommodation—symbolized the disagreement within the profession on this issue. On the one hand, liberals in the APHA who had long urged greater involvement in medical care were becoming more vocal. Members of the association's Medical Care Section, a progressive stronghold, convinced the editors of the *American Journal of Public Health* to publish a three-volume collection of the journal's articles on innovative models of health care.[5] At the same time, however, many in the rank and file looked askance at the idea of taking on new curative responsibilities. They believed that the separation of prevention from treatment was appropriate; each represented very different orientations and skill sets, in their view, and this division of labor allowed each specialized discipline to do what it did best. Others had more pragmatic concerns: taking on curative services would require cutting back existing programs, or it might make their work more difficult by antagonizing private doctors, whose cooperation they needed.[6]

The new prominence of this old debate could not have been predicted just a few years before. During the Depression, the APHA's progressives, who favored a unified system of prevention and treatment, had faced off against conservatives who believed that public health professionals should stick to preventive programs and narrowly defined categories of care.[7] In the postwar years, however, the issue had faded into the background. The growth of the biomedical research enterprise, exemplified by the dramatic rise in federal funding for the National Institutes of Health (NIH) and the proliferation of new hospitals fueled by the Hill-Burton legislation of 1946,[8] eclipsed the role of prevention and reinforced the paradigm that illness was to be fought at the physiological rather than the societal level. Medical care remained firmly entrenched in a fee-for-service model, especially after the ignominious defeat in 1948 of Harry Truman's proposal for national health insurance at the hands of the American Medical Association (AMA).[9] The AMA's strategy of hanging the label of "socialism" on any proposal for publicly funded health care successfully defused such initiatives amid the Cold War paranoia of the 1950s.[10]

The emergence of poverty as a political issue in the Kennedy administration reopened the subject, and the heady days following Lyndon Johnson's election in 1964 seemed filled with promise. Questions that had long stirred the field's progressive wing were on the table once again: How should medical care be linked not just with prevention but with housing, education, employment, and other aspects of welfare broadly conceived? What was the role of the public sector in providing these services? Health was at the top of Johnson's first legislative agenda after the State of the Union address in January 1965 in which he conjured the Great Society; new programs premised on sociological and economic theories about the roots of poverty and inequality soon began pouring money into communities around the country.[11] Over the next several years, Congress would pass approximately fifty pieces of legislation related to health, providing funds that flowed through units of the federal government, including the Office of Economic Opportunity (OEO), the Children's Bureau, and the U.S. Public Health Service. Annual federal spending on health grew from $3 billion in 1959 to 1960 to $21 billion in 1970 to 1971.[12]

The neighborhood health centers—the emblematic Great Society initiative—were demonstration projects designed to provide integrated screening, diagnosis, and treatment closely linked with ancillary services, such as job training, that would improve patients' life prospects. The centers' guiding principles included involvement of community members as advisers and lay workers; by explicitly seeking to foster the political empowerment of patients, the centers were intended to serve not merely as sites for care but as engines of social change.[13] In 1965 and 1966, the first round of eight centers opened, followed by another thirty in 1967 and 1968.[14]

The Great Society opened a window of opportunity for public health professionals to argue that their field, by virtue of its unique perspective and experience, should play a leading role in health care reform. It was far from clear, however, that the new federal involvement and funding would strengthen the institutional position of public health, at least in its traditional bastion of state and local health departments. Johnson's poverty warriors generally bypassed government agencies in their grant-making in favor of private or quasi-public agencies, believing that local health departments were too reluctant to challenge entrenched interests and move beyond their traditional categorical functions.[15]

Tellingly, the neighborhood health centers were not a product of the federal public health establishment. Jack Geiger and Count Gibson, the Tufts University physicians who were architects of the model, originally asked the U.S. Public Health Service to serve as a home for the program, but the agency, long reluctant to antagonize the medical lobby by treading on its professional turf, referred the two men to the Office of Economic Opportunity.[16] The OEO made most grants for neighborhood health centers to medical schools and hospitals, on the grounds that they were best positioned in terms of facilities, equipment, and clinical expertise to get the clinics up and running quickly. As a result, some public health officials saw the centers as undermining their position as the group best qualified to care for the poor.[17] In addition, the availability of health-related funding to nonprofit community-based organizations and other lay providers threatened to further splinter the field of public health and dilute its already limited political influence by adding to the diversity of the people addressing the connections between health, poverty, and social conditions.[18]

The status quo was also under attack from the left. The dominant models of medical care were sharply criticized by radical groups such as the Student Health Organizations (SHOs), chapters of medical students who rejected the conservative politics of the American Medical Association as they undertook outreach in poor communities around the country, and the Health Policy Advisory Center (Health/PAC), an organization of progressive doctors, journalists, and academics that would take on the hospital industry in the 1970 polemic *The American Health Empire*.[19] Robb Burlage, who had been a member of Students for a Democratic Society (SDS) and was a cofounder of Health/PAC, had high hopes that public health professionals might be a force for radical change when he wrote that the new federal funds flowing into New York City "provide the opportunity for public health officials to move beyond their traditionally residual and narrow responsibilities to induce and coordinate the entire pattern of health services."[20] It soon became apparent to Burlage and his colleagues that such a vision was unrealistic, however, and in subsequent years Health/PAC members increasingly found themselves at odds with Health Department employees, whom they viewed as entrenched bureaucrats unwilling to advocate for social justice.

Much was in flux in the new environment, and it was far from certain what role public health professionals would play in the reforms that seemed to be taking shape.

The Neighborhood Family Care Centers

In the years leading up to its proposal to expand its clinical services, the Health Department had tested the waters by providing ambulatory care for two specific populations: geriatric and pediatric. In 1961, supported by a grant from the U.S. Public Health Service, the department had opened a "health maintenance clinic" in the Queensbridge Housing Project in the neighborhood of Astoria, Queens. The apartment complex had a large elderly population at high risk for health problems requiring inpatient stays, and it was in an isolated industrial area more than an hour's bus ride from the nearest medical facility. The clinic was a demonstration project to see if offering ambulatory care could prevent hospitalization of the elderly residents. The city's Housing Authority offered the space for the clinic rent-free; physicians from the nearest hospital, Elmhurst, gave specialty, emergency, and inpatient care.[21] Several community-based social welfare organizations provided services there. The program was the brainchild of Irving Starin and Nicetas Kuo, two Health Department veterans with a longtime interest in delivering services in nontraditional community settings. (Starin had once set up an X-ray booth in the lobby of a Bronx post office to screen for tuberculosis.)

Shortly after the Queensbridge project opened, the department added a full range of pediatric treatment services to the Bedford district health center. The expansion was sparked by a crisis at nearby Kings County Hospital, which had experienced exploding use of its pediatric emergency room in recent years. Families spilled out into dingy, congested hallways, where parents stood for hours holding their crying and coughing children. Most of the children were from poor African American families, many of them having recently arrived from the South and settled into the dilapidated, overcrowded tenement housing of Bedford-Stuyvesant. After being alerted to the dire situation by the hospital's director of pediatrics, Leona Baumgartner had convinced Mayor Robert Wagner to approve an emergency appropriation that would allow the Bedford center to begin offering comprehensive care on site. The center was soon providing medical, laboratory, and social work services to some 2,600 children per month.[22]

The success of the Queensbridge project and the Bedford pediatric treatment clinic, along with the increasing prominence of new models of care and federal funding from Great Society initiatives, spurred the

Health Department to set its sights on transforming the district health centers into full-service ambulatory care facilities. Employees who worked in the centers had long been frustrated at having to refer patients elsewhere for care, knowing that follow-through was unlikely because of the notoriously poor conditions in the outpatient departments of the city's public hospitals.[23]

Unlike many of the proponents of the OEO's neighborhood health centers, Health Department employees tended to be liberal but not radical. Career public servants, they were motivated by a newly prominent discourse of justice and rights that meshed with the ideas about comprehensive care they had formed during their years on the front lines working with low-income populations. Theirs was a moderate, incremental vision of reform, borne of the realism that came from working in the city's civil service. They sought primarily to move beyond their traditional preventive activities to include ambulatory care, and secondarily to involve community members in the planning of services. But they did not see these changes as the gateway to radical social change or patients' political empowerment.

The department's most forceful advocate for expanding its provision of ambulatory care was Mary McLaughlin, an assistant commissioner (figure 1.1). A physician who had risen through the department ranks during two decades of service in poor neighborhoods, she had worked with Starin and Kuo on the Queensbridge project. McLaughlin was a tough and methodical bureaucrat skilled at maneuvering within the constraints of city government. Her soft-spoken manner belied a tenacity that had enabled her to succeed in an era when few women forged careers as doctors. In early 1965, McLaughlin and her colleagues developed plans to expand the services of the district health centers beyond what they had traditionally offered to include a full range of outpatient care.

The first sites chosen for expansion would be in two of the city's most economically depressed neighborhoods with the worst health profiles, Bedford and Brownsville in north-central Brooklyn. Each center would cover a patient base of 10,000 to 20,000 people. Like the Queensbridge service, the plan was collaborative and designed to leverage existing resources: each center would partner with a nearby hospital that would furnish the clinicians and equipment. Still, extensive funds were needed for the physical renovation of the centers, which lacked many needed structural elements, such as rooms for examinations, consultations, X-rays, and equipment storage. While the partner hospitals would provide most of the clinical staff, the department would have to cover additional personnel needs, including clerical and janitorial staff, to handle the expanded patient load.[24]

Because of the stigma that clung to free clinics for the poor, the new facilities would be named neighborhood family care centers. "The term 'clinic' is scrupulously avoided in speaking of this program," McLaugh-

Figure 1.1   Mary McLaughlin

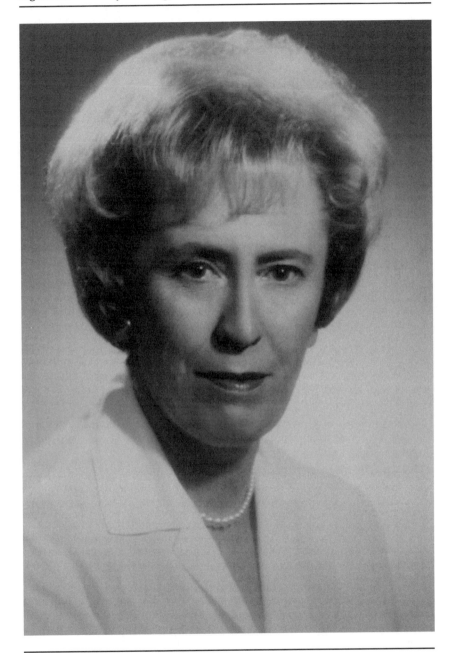

Source: Courtesy New York City Municipal Archives.
Note: Mary McLaughlin, a department veteran who championed the expansion of outpatient care in poor neighborhoods, first proposed the transformation of district health centers into full-service clinics in 1965.

lin explained in a subsequent report. Each center would "operate on an appointment basis and we hope to pattern it on the type of care given in a private physician's office or a good group practice unit. The usual clinic appearance of benches, crowding, and lack of regard for patients' comfort, is a thing of the past."[25]

The budget request that the department submitted to the City Council reflected both the ideals and the rhetoric of the Great Society. It argued that "health and medical care programming must become very closely involved with social and welfare activities, public assistance programs and public housing, these in recognition that socio-economic factors are major determinants of health status."[26] In referring to potential patients as "the consuming public," the request also showed the influence of the nascent patients' rights movement, which advanced the idea that health care was a commodity with which its purchasers had a right to be satisfied.[27]

In explaining its proposed partnership with hospitals to provide clinical services, the department contended that there was "an awakening and growing awareness by hospitals that their programs cannot remain parochial and unresponsive to the total health needs of their surrounding communities, and that they must be equal partners with the Health Department in the shaping of comprehensive health services for local communities."[28] Such an "awakening" was more aspiration than fact. The city's hospitals—especially those in poor neighborhoods—had shown scant interest in the needs of their surrounding communities. While they had cooperated with some Health Department initiatives, such as the ambulance service for premature newborns, they hardly viewed the Health Department as an "equal partner" in their work. To the extent that hospital administrators were aware of the department at all, most viewed it as a civil service backwater far removed from the important business of patient care.

Not all Health Department employees were enthusiastic about transforming the district health centers. The clinical staff of the centers that were slated for expansion included many physicians with a more traditional orientation toward the appropriate spheres of public health and medicine.[29] Because the new neighborhood family care centers were to be operated in partnership with an affiliated hospital, many Health Department doctors feared that they would be subordinated in their work to better-trained hospital-based practitioners, or worse, that they might be moved onto the hospital payroll and lose the seniority they had gained within the city's civil service system.[30]

Nevertheless, the stars seemed aligned for the undertaking, with a new professional philosophy ascendant and new monies to make it a reality. But when the Lindsay administration took office, the Health Department suddenly and unexpectedly faced a series of new challenges that threatened its ability to bring the plans to fruition. When the widely respected health commissioner, George James, resigned to become dean of the Mount Sinai School of Medicine during the 1965 campaign, Mayor Robert Wagner, who was not seeking reelection, put the department under the temporary charge of an acting commissioner, anticipating that the incoming mayor would want to make his own choice for the position. Once Lindsay took office, however, it appeared that the commissioner's job might be eliminated and the Health Department itself might cease to exist as an independent city agency.

Good Government, Good Health

John Lindsay took office as New York City's 103rd mayor in a traditional City Hall ceremony at midnight on December 31, 1965. A charismatic liberal Republican and rising star on the national political scene, Lindsay promised to reform what he characterized as twelve years of corruption and complacency under Wagner and the city's Democratic machine. He brought with him a cadre of "good government" planners armed with the latest ideas in municipal reform.[31] As part of their efforts to revitalize and streamline city bureaucracy, Lindsay's team swiftly moved to consolidate some fifty departments and agencies into ten "superagencies" that would unite related functions of government under broad rubrics such as finance, housing, and transportation.[32]

One of these was to be a new entity called the Health Services Administration (HSA), which would join the Department of Health and Department of Hospitals under the same administrative umbrella along with two other health-related agencies, the Community Mental Health Board and the Office of the Chief Medical Examiner. "Good government" principles of efficient administration, not an ideological commitment to any particular vision of health care delivery, provided the impetus for the new structure. The proposed consolidation was nonetheless consistent with the Health Department's plans to integrate preventive and curative health services and seemed to augur well for the neighborhood family care centers.

By any measure, the city's health sector was ripe for reform. Health-related expenses accounted for about 15 percent of the city's $4 billion annual budget in 1965; almost one in five of the city's 42,500 employees worked in either the Department of Health or the Department of Hospitals. For inpatient and ambulatory care, the Hospitals Department ran nineteen institutions with some 18,500 beds. The city's Department of Welfare also ran seven clinics especially for welfare recipients.[33] The Health Department complemented these by providing prevention and screening at its nineteen district health centers and ninety-four child health stations. There was an apparent abundance of services, but for those seeking care in this bewildering maze, more was less. The Department of Welfare operated dental clinics for its clients only, for example, while the Health Department ran dental clinics for children only, and the Department of Hospitals performed tooth extractions only.[34]

When Lindsay took office, this agglomeration of services had few champions and many critics. The first months of the new administration saw a steady stream of highly critical reports by task forces and expert panels that found inefficiency, duplication of effort, and gaps in care.[35] The city's public hospitals drew the harshest criticism, in part because they presented the largest target. The Department of Hospitals dwarfed all the other health-related agencies; in 1966 its annual budget of $266 million was more than ten times that of the Health Department.[36] The public hospitals had long been plagued by chronic staff shortages, deteriorating physical plants, and accusations of substandard care.[37] Investigators found rampant administrative inefficiency, wide disparities in the quality and quantity of preventive and curative services given to people of differing socioeconomic backgrounds, an unwillingness to adapt services to the needs of a racially and ethnically diverse patient population, and a lack of outpatient care facilities.[38]

Demands on the system were growing, and its patient population was changing. Between 1950 and 1970, the city's white population declined by about 1.3 million, while its population of African Americans and Puerto Ricans increased by about the same number.[39] Many of these new arrivals were concentrated in slum neighborhoods, and their de facto primary care providers were the understaffed and overcrowded emergency rooms and outpatient departments of the city's hospitals. Emergency room visits to city hospitals doubled between 1960 and 1966.[40] Close to one-third of the city's population, about 2.5 million people, were medically indigent.[41]

Lindsay had virtually no knowledge of the health sector, but he cared passionately about improving the lot of the poor and increasing the efficiency of government, and the plan for the Health Services Administration seemed to serve both these ends. "It's been idiotic," Lindsay told *The New Yorker*, "to have lived so long with things the way they used to be—all the separate sections, with separate budgets, with overlapping functions, with nobody in charge of the whole picture."[42] According to his vision, the hospitals would be hubs and small neighborhood health centers would be spokes in a system of accessible, integrated care throughout the city.

At least superficially, the plan to bring the Departments of Health and Hospitals closer administratively seemed to be a rational way to coordinate preventive and curative care. (Several big cities, including Boston, Denver, Los Angeles, and Philadelphia, announced similar reorganization plans around this time.[43]) The move was also politically and economically strategic: the city would be better positioned to win federal grants for new programs if the varied components of its health sector worked harmoniously.[44] But many observers quickly realized that yoking the Health Department to its much larger and very troubled sister agency promised as many drawbacks as advantages. "Public health people fear that their preventive programs will be lost in the daily crises of providing hospital care for large numbers of patients," noted Alonzo Yerby, a leading figure in preventive medicine, after the proposal was unveiled. Yerby spoke from experience: he had led the city's Department of Hospitals before taking a professorship at Harvard. "Administrators of public hospitals," he said, "feel too hard-pressed by obsolete facilities, personnel shortages, strikes and work stoppages, and ever-mounting demands for services to consider the special needs of a program of prevention."[45] Cecil Sheps, a hospital administrator and adviser to Lindsay, put it more succinctly: "When there's blood to stop flowing, and bones to mend, public health can get lost."[46]

As plans for the HSA were drawn up in the summer and fall of 1966, one of the most contentious questions was whether all organizational borders between the four health-related agencies would be dissolved or whether separate departments would be retained, with a new layer of bureaucracy overlaid to coordinate their diverse functions. Arthur Bushel, a Health Department veteran whom Lindsay had named as acting commissioner during the reorganization, warned the mayor's budget director that the merger "might well turn out to be a 'submerger'— that we and our preventive approach are in danger of virtual extinction."[47]

The extent of anxiety about the mayor's plans was revealed by the unusual step that Health Department physicians took in the summer of 1966. Alarmed by the absence of a strong leader to serve as their advocate (Arthur Bushel was serving in a temporary capacity only), they sought the assistance of former commissioner Leona Baumgartner, who remained an influential figure on the local health scene. "We feel that [creation of the Health Services Administration] will lead inevitably to a complete takeover of our department's functions by voluntary hospitals whose experience, goals and capabilities do not encompass the public health field at all," the doctors warned. "The end result of subordinating the Health Department's functions to those of hospitals will, we believe, result in a sharp curtailment or elimination of important preventive programs, a complete breakdown of department morale, and a resultant serious threat to the public health."[48]

Members of the Board of Health shared such concerns and insisted to Lindsay that public health had to retain its independent status.[49] The board's plea carried far more weight than Bushel's. With its five-member body responsible for the content of the city's health code, the board was made up of elite physicians and lawyers and was led by Louis Loeb, a partner in the white-shoe law firm of Lord, Day & Lord. Loeb was the former president of the city's bar association and the general counsel to the *New York Times* who had defended the paper in a landmark 1964 libel case before the Supreme Court. He also had Lindsay's ear as the chair of the mayor's screening committee for judges. Though Lindsay had initially stated that all organizational boundaries would have to be erased for the plan to succeed, he eventually backpedaled and promised the board members that the reorganization legislation would provide for a separate and independent Health Department.[50]

The assurance from Lindsay provided a much-needed measure of stability, but at this critical juncture, there were serious questions about the department's ability to maintain its traditional functions, let alone undertake an expansion into a major new programmatic area, especially one as expensive and politically sensitive as ambulatory care.

The most critical challenge facing the department was staffing. At a time when many new physicians needed to be recruited, the decades-old gap in prestige and remuneration between public health and medicine made it difficult to attract qualified medical personnel. The starting annual pay for an assistant commissioner in the Department of Health, a position that required a medical degree, was $25,000, compared to $27,500 for a master's-level non-physician administrator in the Department of Hospitals.[51] The charismatic leadership of Leona Baumgartner and her successor George James had gone a long way in retaining staff, but following James's departure in 1965, middle- and upper-level managers had begun to leave the Health Department in large numbers.

A freeze on filling vacancies in city agencies enacted early in the Lindsay administration made it even more difficult to attract top-flight professionals to the department's ranks. It was especially difficult to recruit the physicians who were paid an hourly rate to staff the district health centers.[52] When the centers had begun operating during the Depression, the promise of steady income offered by a civil service position attracted many physicians worried about supporting themselves through private practice.[53] But much had changed in the subsequent decades: the medical profession boomed in the postwar years, and salaries in the private sector climbed sharply as high-paying specialties multiplied. Relatively few doctors were attracted to public health, least of all to settings where their work would consist primarily of mundane tasks such as routine screening.

While the lack of doctors was the most acute need, shortages extended to all categories of workers: nurses, nutritionists, physical therapists, and social workers were handing in their notices in alarming numbers during Lindsay's first months in office.[54] "Years ago," wrote one health official, "the dynamic programming of the department with opportunity to do public health research as well as the desire of physicians to live in 'fun city' was sufficient to attract and keep staff. This is no longer true. Many now desire to leave the City where the problems sometimes seem insoluble and City living is no longer attractive."[55]

Staffing problems were especially severe among public health nurses, the department's "most scarce and valuable category of personnel," according to Bushel. The nurses, who made home visits in the city's poorest neighborhoods, provided the department's human face in the community. They worked in difficult conditions; after the attempted rape of a visiting nurse in the South Bronx, a new policy required the nurses to go out into the field in pairs, essentially halving the services available.[56] They were highly trained, yet they earned less than their hospital-based peers. When understaffing of nurses at the district health centers forced the cancellation of some programs, such as immunization clinics for low-income children, Bushel pleaded with Lindsay to exempt the nurses from the hiring freeze.[57] After bad publicity about the canceled services embarrassed the mayor, the hiring freeze was lifted, but the nurses continued to be dissatisfied with low salaries, especially after their counterparts in hospitals won a pay raise.

In May 1966, almost all of the department's three hundred nurses staged a walkout, the first such mass job action the department had ever faced; during the three-day walkout, almost all of the ninety-four child health stations closed for the first time in the department's history.[58] The action was not technically a strike, since the nurses were not unionized. Three years later, they would vote to join District Council 37 of the American Federation of State, County, and Municipal Employees (AFSCME), which had won the hospital nurses their wage increase and which aggressively and successfully courted city workers during the 1960s.[59]

Low salaries were the most pressing budget challenge for the Health Department, but not the only one. The department's computer systems were "totally inadequate," while the situation in vital records, the unit responsible for furnishing thousands of birth and death certificates each year, was "disgraceful."[60] Outmoded X-ray equipment for tuberculosis screening exposed patients to more radiation than was acceptable under current standards.[61] Most worrisome, given the department's plans to begin providing outpatient medical care on a wide scale, was upkeep of the district health centers, which after years of deferred maintenance "[were] dingy and unattractive" and "badly need painting and new lighting."[62] There was a widespread sense in the department that Lindsay's budget staff did not adequately understand public health and that Lindsay was insufficiently attentive to the needs of the department (which was undoubtedly true, given the myriad crises involving not just the hospitals but transit workers, police officers, and other municipal services that plagued the mayor's first months in office).

These deficits made the prospect of creating new ambulatory services seem more daunting but did not dampen enthusiasm for the task. During 1966, the plans expanded from the two initial centers in Brownsville and Bedford to six additional conversions; in 1967 the department requested $4.8 million—close to one-quarter of its total budget—for the renovations of eight centers at a cost of some $600,000 each. At the end of Lindsay's first year in office, acting commissioner Arthur Bushel remained optimistic. "During the coming year," Bushel told Lindsay's staff, "we believe we will be able to convert eight of our existing district health centers into full-scale ambulatory care facilities."[63]

The prospects for the centers seemed to improve when Lindsay filled two key leadership posts. To serve as the city's first health services administrator, who would be charged with fostering close relationships between departments that had operated with distinctly different missions and professional cultures, Lindsay's search committee chose Howard J. Brown after a five-month search. An experienced program planner and manager as well as a physician, Brown had gained a strong reputation locally and nationally by designing an innovative outpatient clinic that served low-income residents of the city's Lower East Side and provided one of the models for the neighborhood health center program. He went on to serve as the OEO's chief medical adviser and helped establish similar facilities in rural Mississippi, in Watts, California, and in several other cities.[64]

The choice of Brown provided a direct link between New York City's health care system and the reform initiatives and funding that were emerging from the OEO. Brown was firmly in the camp of the Health Department's progressives who sought to expand their ambulatory services, and his appointment augured well for these efforts. As Brown explained to Louis Craco, the young lawyer who chaired the Mayor's Task Force on Reorganization of the Government, shortly after accepting his new post: "There is a general consensus among modern public health and medical care professionals that the clinical, preventive and mental health services now fragmented should be united into coherent programs."[65] Preparing a statement that Lindsay would read in testimony before the U.S. Congress on the health challenges facing the country's large urban areas, Brown identified the two most pressing problems as rebuilding deteriorating hospitals and financing and organizing medical care for "ghetto" areas.[66]

Brown was not just committed to retaining an independent Department of Health within the HSA; he foresaw that it would be first among equals in the new bureaucracy. "The major planning, coordination, surveillance and evaluation responsibility of the total health programs in New York City" would rest with public health professionals, Brown asserted. The other units would have "more specialized functions, major as they will be, as compared to this broad charge of the Health Department."[67] The Department of Hospitals, he believed, would be limited to "bricks and mortar considerations." The Health Department's charge would not be "to do all that is necessary to protect and promote the city's health, but to make sure it is done" through standard-setting, surveillance, research, and demonstrations. In Brown's vision, the public health workforce should return to its social medicine roots of the nineteenth century, when reformers such as Rudolph Virchow and Lemuel Shattuck led the field. The public health leaders of the future, Brown predicted, would be "board certified public health physicians with training and skills in community medicine—medical sociologists, health urbanists—whatever they might be called . . . with one foot in the technical field of the science of medicine and the other in community dynamics."[68]

At the end of 1966, Lindsay also filled the post of health commissioner, who would report to Brown (see figure 1.2). Edward O'Rourke, a Harvard graduate and the former health commissioner of Cambridge, had worked overseas with the U.S. Agency for International Development (USAID). He had come to the city from Washington, D.C., where he was a midlevel official in the U.S. Public Health Service. Like Lindsay, O'Rourke had an outgoing manner and patrician grace that inspired confidence in those around him; unlike the mayor, he was a skilled administrator. O'Rourke shared Brown's commitment to new models of care that united prevention with treatment and integrated public- and private-sector services.[69] Indeed, O'Rourke embraced the idea of expanding ambulatory care with even more enthusiasm than either Bushel or McLaughlin had. Just a few months after his appointment, O'Rourke confidently announced to an audience at the New York Academy of Medicine the department's plan to open thirty neighborhood family care centers—eighteen in rehabilitated facilities and twelve in newly built ones.[70]

With the hiring of Brown and O'Rourke, Lindsay moved ahead with a series of meetings to plan the transition to the new superagency. In subsequent months, however, it became apparent that it would take more than shuffling the boxes in the municipal organization chart to change how the city conceived and delivered medical care. Although everyone paid lip service to such anodyne propositions as "reducing fragmentation" and "increasing coordination," the cold reality was that all parties—the Health Department no less than others—were centrally concerned with protecting their own interests and ensuring that their own facilities, programs, and personnel were maintained.[71] At a time when so much new federal money was pouring into the health sector, ceding control meant possibly losing out on some of this largesse. In proposing the Health Services Administration, Lindsay and his team not only misjudged the complexity of the vast network of health-related entities in

Figure 1.2   A New Commissioner

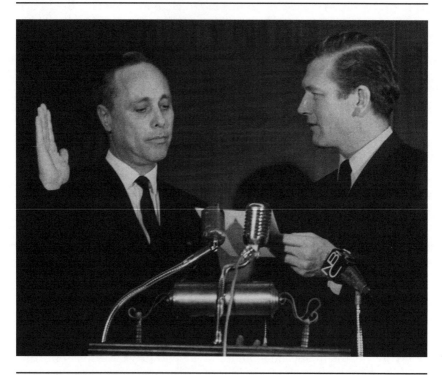

Source: Courtesy New York City Municipal Archives.
Note: When Mayor John Lindsay (right) swore in Edward O'Rourke as health commissioner in February 1967, the department had been without a permanent, full-time leader for more than a year, during which time its status as an independent agency was in doubt.

both the public and private sectors but underestimated the intransigence of large bureaucracies and the commitment of government officials to maintaining control of their fiefdoms.

Almost immediately, turf battles broke out among the four constituent agencies that had publicly supported their consolidation into the Health Services Administration superagency. The four commissioners resented not having direct access to the mayor and clashed with Brown over having to go through him.[72] Brown's every move as health services administrator represented an intrusion on someone's territory. When he appointed an administrator to oversee all narcotic services in the city, for example, the chief of the Community Mental Health Board, which had its own drug programs, went over Brown's head to complain to Lindsay that Brown had overstepped his authority.[73] Mary McLaughlin, an early proponent and prime mover for the creation of family care centers, angrily accused Brown of shutting her out of the planning process for the centers once the capital budgets had been approved.[74]

Brown also underestimated the recalcitrance of the city's doctors in private and academic settings, who were unwilling to embrace his understanding of "community dynamics." His increasingly blunt public criticisms of his fellow physicians—in one speech he contended that they organized care based on "their own need for professional distinction" rather than concern for patients—cost him critical support among what should have been a core constituency.[75]

Brown lasted less than eighteen months on the job. By the end of 1967, he had grown disillusioned with what he saw as Lindsay's failure to understand the complexities of city government.[76] There was another, more personal reason for his departure. In December, while Brown was recovering in the hospital from a bout of hepatitis, his brother-in-law, a *New York Times* reporter, gave him bad news: the investigative journalist Drew Pearson, who had recently written an exposé of homosexuals working for California governor Ronald Reagan, was planning a similar article about the Lindsay administration. Brown, a gay man whom the *Times* had coyly identified as a forty-two-year-old bachelor who lived in a Greenwich Village townhouse when it announced his appointment, believed that the public destruction of his reputation would cost him his ability to function effectively in the job.[77] He submitted his letter of resignation to Lindsay the next day, before the City Council had even given its official approval to the creation of the Health Services Administration.

Brown's successor was Bernard Bucove, the health commissioner for Washington State, which had a population less than half that of New York City. Bucove was named after a protracted search that made clear how thankless the position was. (Contacted by reporters when his appointment was announced, Bucove quipped, "Are you amazed that somebody finally took the job?"[78]) Like Brown, Bucove championed the concept of the family care centers and advocated for increased capital expenditures for them. Also like Brown, he was frustrated by the recalcitrance of the city bureaucracy and abruptly left after less than two years on the job.[79]

From Provider to "Protector"

From the time of the first capital request in 1965, the Health Department's plans to transform its district health centers into full-service clinics steadily expanded in scope. The two conversions proposed initially had grown to nine the following year and to thirty by the end of 1967, when Edward O'Rourke took the helm. Those closely connected with the plans, including O'Rourke, Mary McLaughlin, and Arthur Bushel, talked up their vision of expanded ambulatory care in memos to colleagues in city government, addresses to professional groups, and statements to the press. But progress was scant, and the confident public face the department was putting forth concealed how fraught with uncertainty and delays the plans were.

The critical issue was money. Although city tax levy would fund the capital expansions, the neighborhood family care centers would be heavily dependent on support from Washington, D.C., and Albany in the form of grants and Medicaid reimbursement, and on that front the picture was cloudy at best. Many other institutions in the city were vying for the health-related funds the federal government was disbursing. The HSA superagency having failed to produce anything like coordination, several hospitals, both public and private, were in competition with the Health Department (and each other) for the same pots of money to pay for their own expansions of ambulatory care.[80] And the funds were shrinking: by the end of 1966, the OEO's budget was already being cramped by the escalating costs of the war in Vietnam, and the office took a large hit in 1968 congressional appropriations.[81]

The biggest wild card was Medicaid, which Lyndon Johnson had signed into law in the summer of 1965. Enacted as Title XIX of the Social Security Act, Medicaid provided federal money matched by states to reimburse health care providers who cared for low-income patients. The poor, according to proponents, would no longer be dependent on charity care but would be able to purchase medical services wherever they wanted (from among those doctors who chose to participate in the program, of course). Reimbursements from Medicaid were expected to cover a major portion of the costs of the clinical services that the Health Department's family care centers would offer.[82] But the state's Medicaid program had been in disarray virtually from its inception in 1966, owing to unexpectedly high costs that had blindsided even knowledgeable insiders. Within two years, New York City accounted for one-quarter of the country's total Medicaid enrollment and one-fifth of the national expenditure on the program. Some 2.5 million residents—more than 30 percent of the city's population—had enrolled.[83]

In response to the upwardly spiraling costs, the state legislature made drastic cutbacks in eligibility in June 1968, throwing almost 1.8 million adults and children off of the rolls. ("As a result of the confusion and despair regarding eligibility for medical benefits," cautioned a Health Department report that summer, "we may one day very soon witness the first demonstrations for the right to health care in the United States."[84]) Although some of these individuals were subsequently re-enrolled, the overall rolls dropped by close to one million recipients.[85] In this volatile environment, it was impossible to predict from one month to the next what level of funding would be available for the new ambulatory care services. McLaughlin described the program's financing as "quicksand."[86]

As the family care centers lurched forward amid questions about their fiscal viability, the Health Department was carving out a new role for itself in ambulatory care: not as a provider of services, as had originally been envisioned, but as a watchdog of the services provided by private doctors and paid for by Medicaid. This new role was made possible by a combination of legal and administrative authority in the federal Title XIX legislation and New York State's Medicaid law.[87] These provisions empowered the Health Department to set guidelines for the quality of care given through Medicaid and to ensure that participating doctors adhered to those standards.

In 1967 Howard Brown hired Lowell Bellin, an official with the Health Insurance Plan of Greater New York, to serve as the executive medical director of the city's Medicaid program in the Health Department, with responsibility for standard-setting and auditing of doctors who accepted Medicaid payments. Bellin was ideally suited to this watchdog role. Several years earlier, he had left a private internal medicine practice to serve as the commissioner of health of Springfield, Massachusetts, after becoming convinced that public health rather than clinical care was where he could have the greatest impact. A Brooklyn native with a combative personality, he did not shrink from—indeed, he relished—confrontation over matters of principle. An Orthodox Jew whose religious beliefs powerfully informed his professional ethics, he had a highly developed (critics would say overdeveloped) sense of right and wrong and an unshakeable conviction that he was on the side of the angels.

Bellin threw himself with gusto into the role of "medical cop." First, he and his staff held a series of consultations with committees of medical experts to codify the standard components of various types of patient visits, the time needed for services, the appropriate fees to charge, and the necessary qualifications for providers.[88] Then, with his team of physician-auditors, he set about ensuring that these guidelines were met. The auditors turned up in the offices of Medicaid physicians to look through patient charts for signs of unnecessary procedures, reviewed invoices for evidence of overcharging or duplicate billing, and reexamined patients to confirm diagnoses. They uncovered abuses among some 5 percent of participating doctors. One general practitioner was found to be routinely giving injections of iron for anemic patients when cheaper oral doses were recommended; another was billing for house calls for non-emergency situations such as hypertension or insomnia. An internist was referring his patients for liver and brain scans of questionable necessity; a podiatry practice routinely and unnecessarily X-rayed both feet of all their patients, resulting in overutilization of about 60 percent. Suspect physicians were summoned to an administrative hearing to discuss the irregularities. In cases where errant conduct was determined to be the result of misunderstanding by the physician, the department provided advice on remediation, but Bellin's unit did not hesitate to penalize cases found to be malfeasant. They could recover overbilled fees, suspend providers from participating in Medicaid, and in extreme cases refer the physician to the district attorney or state medical licensing board.[89]

It was no surprise that local physicians resisted Bellin's efforts. The right to self-police was one of the most fiercely guarded professional prerogatives of American medicine, and the city's doctors were not about to submit passively to regulation by a civil servant, even one who held a medical degree. "Quality medical care," insisted one of the local doctors' organizations, "can no more be legislated than any Congress or Assembly or Senate can legislate honesty or integrity or tolerance."[90] Another local society passed a resolution declaring itself "unalterably opposed to . . . any governmental agency evaluating the quality of medical care."[91] But Bellin was not one to be intimidated. "His idea of a fair fight," a colleague later recalled, "was six hundred angry private practicing physicians attacking him. He could take those guys on and he knew it."[92]

In his willingness to confront the medical establishment, Bellin was a throwback to Hermann Biggs, the city's most aggressive health official in the early twentieth century. Just as Biggs had sought to convince physicians to report cases of tuberculosis by claiming the disease was comparable to the other contagions traditionally tracked by the department, Bellin drew a comparison between Medicaid monitoring and well-accepted regulatory functions such as inspecting food service establishments. The Health Department "furnishes a restaurant a license, which confers privileges," he argued.

> It can always withdraw the license together with the privileges for due cause, that is, a cause in the interest of the public health. The analogy is obvious. The provision of foodstuffs to the public bears a potential hazard to the public health and therefore falls within the official purview of the local Health Department. Similarly, the provision of personal health services to the public bears potential hazard to the public health and therefore should fall within the official purview of the local Health Department.[93]

The Health Department's standard-setting program was one of its most successful reform efforts. It was sustained in large measure by the sheer force of Bellin's dogged personality. Commissioner Edward O'Rourke let Bellin run the program as he saw fit; Mayor Lindsay was preoccupied with a series of crises involving racial tensions, unions, poverty, and police abuses and had little direct involvement with any of the department's initiatives in this period. In 1968 the Medicaid auditing unit, which cost just under $700,000 annually to operate, saved the city an estimated $27 million—a forty-one-to-one return on investment,

Bellin proudly noted in a journal article on the program. The following year, rulings were handed down in three lawsuits challenging the department's authority to regulate tax-supported private medical care, and in each case, the department's position prevailed.[94]

Hospitals, Communities, and the Politics of Control

Around the same time that the court rulings confirmed the Health Department's right to audit Medicaid services, it was unexpectedly able to seize an additional set of regulatory powers: overseeing the outpatient departments of almost two dozen of the city's private hospitals. This unlikely turn of events capped a yearlong tale of politics, money, and unintended consequences. The story began when employees in the state Department of Health in Albany asked the New York legislature to do something about the shortage of medical care available to the poor in urban and rural slum areas. In the summer of 1968, two bills were introduced amending the state public health law to allow local health departments to provide clinical services and to receive reimbursement from the state for 50 percent of their costs, the same proportion they received for their traditional categorical programs related to tuberculosis and venereal disease. The new funding stream was nicknamed "ghetto medicine" in order to make clear that this was a poverty program and to head off the opposition of the medical establishment, which was ever-vigilant against the incursions of "socialized health care." The bills slipped under the radar and passed the legislature late in the session without debate.[95]

"Ghetto medicine" funding initially looked like a promising source of support for the Health Department's family care centers. Mary McLaughlin submitted several applications to the program, three of which were funded. Within a year, however, the program was unexpectedly redirected. After millions of New Yorkers were thrown off the Medicaid rolls in mid-1968, many of New York City's private hospitals faced fiscal crises because of the sudden loss of revenue they had anticipated from Medicaid. The hospital lobby, which enjoyed close access to Governor Nelson Rockefeller, sent representatives to Albany in the midst of the crisis to say that they faced ruinous losses that could force the closure of some of their outpatient services.[96] Rockefeller in turn pressured the state health department to allow "ghetto medicine" funding to be used to keep the private hospitals' ambulatory care services from going bankrupt. Thus, money that had originally been intended to allow local health departments to create new outpatient services was instead diverted to propping up existing services in private institutions.

Progressive health advocacy and civic organizations were dismayed. They dubbed the plan "Operation Bailout" and insisted that private hospitals with abysmal track records in caring for the poor should not receive public funds.[97] But faced with a more skilled and better connected lobby, public health was outflanked. A critical analysis by a member of the Citizens Committee for Children charged that public health "did not wish to take on the voluntary hospital establishment or else did not know how to do it. Public health leadership was invisible, seemingly unable or unwilling to compete in the political arena."[98]

The diversion of "ghetto medicine" money from health departments to hospitals was another blow to the fiscal prospects of the family care centers. But the move did open another, unexpected window through which the department could expand the watchdog role it had taken on for Medicaid providers. To be eligible for state aid, the private hospitals had to become quasi-public institutions. Their ambulatory care services were therefore "municipalized"—placed under the aegis of the city Health Department.[99] This arrangement provided the Health Department with a wedge it could use to improve the care in private institutions. As Bellin explained in a subsequent report, the "ghetto medicine" program allowed the department to use its "newly acquired fiscal leverage to accelerate socially desirable policies and administrative changes in voluntary hospitals historically insulated from Health Department dissatisfactions and restiveness."[100]

In December 1969, the Health Department entered into contracts with the twenty-two private hospitals in the city that had accepted "ghetto medicine" funding, began formal monitoring of their outpatient services, and established a new Bureau of Ambulatory Care to oversee the work.[101] Hospital outpatient departments—a low-status, low-paying area of medicine that failed to attract top-flight physicians or administrators—had long been seen as a black hole in the city's health care system where patients faced interminable waits and indifferent care. Armed with new contracts, the Health Department attempted to effect sweeping reforms. Among many other changes, each hospital was required to hire a director specifically responsible for outpatient care, develop lists of available services, create an appointment system, provide interpreters for patients, and convene regular public hearings on matters of hospital policy.

In theory these were far-reaching changes, but in fact it was unclear how much the care in the hospitals actually improved. Subsequent evaluations by the Bureau of Ambulatory Care found that many of the old problems persisted in spite of the new oversight. Part of the problem was relatively limited enforcement. There were just twenty-four staff in the bureau, compared to forty-five in the Medicaid auditing unit, and the frequency of site visits to the hospitals was just over once a year.[102]

In assuming an oversight role in hospitals' outpatient services, the Health Department stepped into the midst of rancorous debates about "community control" over medical care. In return for receiving state aid, each hospital receiving state funds was required to create an advisory board having 51 percent of its members from the community it served.[103] This provision had been added in response to pressure from advocacy groups, including Health/PAC and the Citizens' Committee for Children. The Health Department was supposed to work closely with community members, serving as a kind of mediator between their interests and perspectives and those of the hospitals. But the degree of authority these advisory bodies would have over hospitals' decisionmaking, and indeed the precise nature of their mission, was ambiguous. According to the official guidelines promulgated by the city, the groups "should neither be interpreted as having 'community control' nor as performing a perfunctory role. The committee should be viewed as a mechanism to facilitate both delivery and community utilization of ambulatory services."[104] In the radicalized environment of the late 1960s, however, members of poor communities increasingly sought to challenge powerful institutions, and when they were rebuffed, they often responded with protests and lawsuits. In 1969 and 1970, Gouverneur Health Center on the Lower East Side of Manhattan and Lincoln Hospital in the Bronx were both sites of demonstrations and sit-ins as neighborhood residents and community groups battled hospital administrators over issues such as staffing and service delivery.[105]

No matter how much they claimed to represent the "health rights" of the poor, the career civil servants in the Health Department were not natural allies of community organizations: in their background, training, and temperament, they had more in common with the hospitals than with the poor. The advisory committees varied widely in their knowledge of the health care sector and their skill at dealing with the byzantine operations of hospitals. Said one representative of a community group, "Some knowledgeable consumers did attempt to make some change, but they were quickly reminded that they were only in an advisory position."[106] The relationships between the community advisory boards and the hospitals often degenerated into mutual mistrust and hostility; one committee filed suit against both the hospital and Mary McLaughlin, claiming that they deliberately withheld needed information.[107]

These conflicts illustrated the increasingly bitter and polarized atmosphere surrounding the right of communities to control health services. As will be seen in the next chapter, the rise of citizen mobilizations and protest movements, growing out of the struggles over civil rights and the Vietnam War, would greatly complicate the work of the New York City Health Department.

By the time the department created the Bureau of Ambulatory Care to monitor the "ghetto medicine" contracts at the end of 1969, the ambitious predictions that all of the district health centers would soon provide a full range of preventive and treatment services had largely ceased. The Bedford District Health Center, with the support of grants from the OEO and the Children's Bureau, had begun offering ambulatory care in 1967, and over the next two years the district health centers in Jamaica, Brownsville, and Sunset Park, in partnership with nearby hospitals, had added some outpatient care to their traditional preventive activities.[108] But these were tiny figures on the health care landscape, dwarfed by hospital programs. Combined visits to all free-standing clinics in the city amounted to less than 7 percent of the number of visits to the outpatient departments of municipal, nonprofit, and private hospitals.[109] Instead of becoming a major provider of services, the Health Department had shifted its focus to serving as a "protector."

This shift was signaled by an address that Mary McLaughlin gave at the annual meeting of the American Public Health Association in 1970. The department had been "transmuted," she said, into the "protector of consumer health services." The experience of the department as watchdog under Medicaid and the monitoring of hospital outpatient care under the "ghetto medicine" program "presage[d] a new era for the development and enforcement of standards and consumer protection."[110] Indeed, McLaughlin predicted that all the Health Department's direct care services—not just the neighborhood family care centers, but the child health stations and the categorical programs for tuberculosis and venereal disease as well—would eventually be transferred to the Health and Hospitals Corporation, a newly created quasi-public entity that had replaced the city's old Department of Hospitals. The Health Department would be responsible only for testing demonstration projects for new models of care, McLaughlin believed. Her crystal ball turned out to be cloudy, however. The department would not divest itself of all treatment services, as she predicted; it would, on the other hand, end up ceding its watchdog functions to the state in the next decade as New York City sank into insolvency.

A long distance had been traveled from the optimistic summer of 1965, when the plans for the transformation of the district health centers had taken shape. What had seemed, just a few years earlier, like an unstoppable wave of social change that would sweep away old barriers and enable the creation of new models of care for the poor turned out to be far more ephemeral. The deeply entrenched economic and political interests of the city's health sector proved too refractory, and the department's champions of ambulatory care lacked sufficient political strength and backing to effect change. They might have accomplished more with vigorous and consistent support from Mayor Lindsay or his top deputies, but the mayor's office was preoccupied with too many other pressing issues to make the ambitious experiment of the Health Services Administration a success.

Recognizing the limits of what they would be able to accomplish with their own ambulatory care program, Mary McLaughlin, Lowell Bellin, and others in the Health Department took up a "watchdog" role as an alternate way of helping the city's poor and medically underserved to receive better outpatient care. This was the kind of pragmatic, incremental reform at which public health had excelled for decades. In the late 1960s, however, as health "consumers" made new demands, the role of protector turned out to be unexpectedly difficult to fulfill. The relationships among the Health Department, the city's public hospitals, the private medical establishment, and the community members they all served would continue to be complicated and fraught with tension. The dream of creating new models of care that brought together prevention and treatment would remain a dream deferred.

Chapter 2

Public Health and the People

IN LATE 1967, a few months after a confrontation in Tompkins Square Park between hippies and the police had escalated into a near-riot, the Health Department turned its attention to the youth counterculture. Illnesses prevalent among hippies included malnutrition, tuberculosis, syphilis, gonorrhea, and drug abuse (especially LSD and marijuana). Meeting the population's needs would require understanding this new lifestyle and its orientation toward health. "The Hippie is dissatisfied with the values of present day society and is making an attempt at self-evaluation as a first step in understanding others," an internal report noted. "Characteristic dress including beads, flowers or bells is often present. There is an acceptance and practice of communal sharing of food and shelter."[1] While existing clinical facilities could meet hippies' needs, the report concluded, special outreach was called for.

The "hippie health" issue exemplified the challenges that public health professionals faced amid the social upheavals of the 1960s. The struggle for African American civil rights and the identity-based activist movements that followed in its wake; the rise of militant protests over issues such as the Vietnam War and urban poverty; plummeting popular faith in the benevolence of professions and institutions; jurisprudence that carved out new territory related to privacy, civil liberties, and the rights of marginalized groups—all of these trends had profound and lasting implications for public health work. As the Health Department tried to find ways to improve clinical care for the city's impoverished residents, it also sought to address the health problems that were bound up with inflammatory social issues. In so doing, it confronted an altered relationship between those inside and outside of 125 Worth Street.

One way the department sought to adapt to this unsettled environment was to integrate community members into service delivery. Involvement of the public was a cornerstone of the Great Society's health programs. It was codified in federal legislation such as the Community Mental Health Centers Act of 1963, which mandated the creation of community advisory boards, and it was later strengthened by the Office of Economic Opportunity's requirement for "maximum feasible participation" of poor communities in the neighborhood health centers.[2] Service recipients, according to the vision of Lyndon Johnson's poverty warriors, would play major roles in developing and delivering the programs from which they would benefit. The sociological research that informed Great Society programs advanced the concept of "indigenous nonprofessionals"—freshly trained lay health workers fanning out through their neighborhoods to promote programs such as nutrition and vaccination.[3]

By 1970, the Health Department had used federal and state grants to hire more than one hundred part-time and almost three dozen full-time "health guides," residents of poor communities who conducted outreach and education among their neighbors.[4] Efforts to integrate lay workers into public health activities did not always go smoothly, however. In 1971 New York State enacted the Work Relief Employment Program, which required welfare recipients to work as a condition of receiving their assistance. Some three hundred participants in the program took jobs as aides in the department's school health program, performing routine tasks that required no medical or nursing expertise, such as vision tests, height and weight measurement, and clerical work.[5] The workers were a boon to the Bureau of School Health, which had been plagued by shortages of nurses for years.[6] But the program drew the wrath of both the American Civil Liberties Union (ACLU), which denounced it as "a resurrection of slavery," and District Council 37, which saw it as barely concealed union-busting that undermined the civil service system.[7]

Many department employees welcomed greater lay involvement in their programs. "The growth of active citizen organizations at the local level will facilitate the decentralization of the services of the department," the director of health education predicted in 1967. "It will help get the services to the people and the people to the services. It will help break down the lack of understanding of what our services will do for the people, and overcome the lethargy that keeps people from using our services."[8] This prediction—too sanguine by half—failed to take into account the growth of radical protest movements. Ironically, even as the department was seeking to elicit the input and support of the public, many community members were coming to view the department as part of an oppressive social structure.

As the language of rights came to dominate political discourse and people began to assert themselves as "consumers" of health services, the interactions between public health professionals and the many constituencies they served grew more contentious.[9] Health Department employees saw "represent[ing] the public as their advocate in achieving their health 'rights'" as part of their changing mission.[10] At the same time, however, community members increasingly asserted their right to challenge—and override—decisions made on their behalf by health professionals.

Mary McLaughlin, who dealt with community groups while planning the neighborhood family care centers, later recalled the 1960s as the time when things became "hot"—relationships grew tense, and representatives of the Health Department were viewed with suspicion.[11] During the planning for the family care centers, several neighborhood associations complained to Lindsay that the Health Department had failed to get their input on centers to be opened in Harlem and Jamaica, Queens.[12] The Citywide Health and Mental Health Council accused health officials of displaying "a colossal disregard for community concern, dissent, and recommendation."[13] McLaughlin recalled that during a meeting in Brooklyn about the location of a proposed family care center, the attitude of the neighborhood residents was: "Just put the money on the table and get out."[14] Acceptance of the Health Department as a benevolent, paternalistic force for betterment was replaced by demands for control; as the political scientist Herbert Kaufman wrote in 1969, neighborhood groups "no longer want just to *tell* the government what to do; they want to *be* the government that does it."[15]

The involvement of civic groups in public health was not a new phenomenon. Since the nineteenth century, New York City had had a well-developed charitable and philanthropic sector of service organizations devoted to fighting illness. The "health voluntaries," as they were known, had been critical adjuncts of the department on issues such as tuberculosis and infant mortality.[16] These groups tended to represent members of the city's white Protestant and Jewish elite; upper-class reformers, they accomplished their goals by cultivating relationships with key opinion leaders and decisionmakers in government, business, and the media.

What changed in the 1960s was the array of organizations and individuals advancing claims, the tone of their advocacy, and the readiness of some to use protest, civil disobedience, and other forms of direct action.[17] In contrast to more-established groups, this new breed of community activist rejected compromise and incrementalism. "Frustration, confrontation, and overt conflict are more and more becoming the modes of problem-centered action by those interested enough to get involved," noted an analysis by a sociologist in 1969. "In the past, service projects were not cooperative ventures; they were imposed—albeit in a charitable way—from the one side, and the clients were at least expected to be happy with what they got. Today that is impossible. The new identity and increased self-esteem of the 'other America' has rejected the supplicant's role and demands more than charity."[18]

An episode involving the Young Lords, a group of Puerto Rican radi-

cals, was illustrative. The Young Lords first made a mark in 1969 by collecting garbage from the sidewalks of East Harlem and piling it in the
middle of the streets, forcing the Department of Sanitation to remove it
so that traffic could flow. The garbage dumpings escalated over the summer into demonstrations in which the Lords barricaded neighborhood
streets and clashed with police. In the fall, the group issued a "10-point
health program" that included demands for "total self-determination of
all health services in East Harlem" and "free publicly supported health
care for treatment and prevention." The plan clearly revealed the extent
to which they viewed poor health as inseparable from other forms of
social injustice: one of the ten points demanded "education programs for
all the people to expose health problems—sanitation, rats, poor housing,
malnutrition, police brutality, pollution, and other forms of oppression."[19]

In the summer of 1970, the Young Lords "liberated" a tuberculosis
screening van parked at 116th Street and Lexington Avenue in East Harlem. They drove the van six blocks and parked it across the street from
the group's headquarters, draped a Puerto Rican flag over it, and re-
christened it the Ramón Emeterio Betances Health Truck, in honor of the
nineteenth-century Puerto Rican doctor and antislavery revolutionary.
The X-ray technicians inside continued to perform their duties as crowds
milled around outside, television crews parked at the scene, and a heavy
police presence gathered, including officers stationed on the roofs of ad-
joining buildings.[20] After several hours of tense negotiations involving
the Young Lords, the health officer in charge of East Harlem, and department officials downtown, an agreement was reached stipulating that the
truck would be free to travel "anywhere in the metropolitan area as
deemed necessary by the Young Lords party for the best health care for
our poor and oppressed people."[21]

These challenges to authority took place within an increasingly dis-
cordant public sphere. New York City in the late 1960s was riven along
lines of race and class; bitter political clashes following one upon another gave a sense that the city's social fabric was unraveling. Student
demonstrations at Columbia turned violent after the university administration brought the heavy hand of the police down on protesters who
had occupied buildings on campus. Riots and looting shook slum neighborhoods. All the while, municipal services seemed to deteriorate, with
sanitation and transit worker strikes and accusations of police brutality
and corruption.[22] The most divisive battles over "community control"
broke out in the New York City school system. In the Brooklyn neighborhoods of Ocean Hill and Brownsville, African American parents increasingly came to believe that their children were being victimized by a racist bureaucracy that was more concerned about protecting teachers' job
security than educating children. Much of their criticism came to focus
on the United Federation of Teachers; for months, tensions escalated as

militant activists and galvanized parents clashed with education officials and school personnel.[23] The school system was ultimately divided
into thirty-two semi-autonomous "community school boards" that gave
a measure of control to parents over how their children were taught.

The Health Department's district health centers, as outposts of municipal government in the most economically and socially deprived
parts of the city, occupied a difficult position in this environment. The
district health officer in Bedford wrote in the summer of 1970 that "legitimate grievances . . . tend to erupt suddenly, because of frustrations
over jobs, housing, racism, and so forth." The situation was similar, he
said, to

> guerilla warfare tactics, where the "outs" call the shots or ambushes, while
> the "ins" try to guess what will happen next. Thus one can see a sniping
> incident one day and a looting incident another day, followed by a sit-in
> demonstration a third day.. . . These problems are also related to housing
> and environmental protection services in the minds of the community res-
> idents; so that a problem in any one area could "escalate" into a problem in
> the others.[24]

Senior managers in the Health Services Administration were on high
alert during the summer months; the city "had to equip at least two of
our ghetto hospitals as though they were awaiting a wartime siege,"
Howard Brown wrote.[25]

It was in this context that the Health Department sought to implement
programs freighted with symbolic meanings around power, inequity, and
social disorder. Three such initiatives—on lead paint poisoning, heroin
addiction, and abortion—were launched almost simultaneously in 1970.
These programs were the culmination of years of conflict arising from the
social changes of the 1960s, and all three illustrated the volatile nature of
the era's public health. In all three cases, initiative from within the department was mediated by external political pressures that shaped the
responses that were ultimately adopted.

Children, Lead, and Poverty

American public health had its roots in housing reform. Nineteenth-
century activists saw squalid living conditions as critical determinants
of moral and physical well-being, and laws prescribing adequate light
and space in tenement buildings were among the first great achievements of the sanitary movement. During the twentieth century, however, housing issues had drifted out of the public health ambit.[26] Some in
the profession called attention to the ill effects of substandard housing,
but remedying conditions such as overcrowding, lack of heating and

ventilation, and inadequate toilet facilities was not among the "basic six" health department functions.[27] One of the most pernicious of all the problems related to poor housing was the slow poisoning of children exposed to flaking chips of lead-based paint, and the failure of municipal health officials to act aggressively against the problem became a point of bitter controversy in the newly radicalized climate of the 1960s.

Human exposure to lead toxicity was a problem dating from antiquity, though its harmful effects were not fully recognized until the nineteenth century. Lead was an ingredient in pottery, ceramics, plumbing, paint, and other implements in households and workplaces. Lead ingestion could cause headache, nausea, abdominal pain, vomiting, cramps, hyperactivity or lethargy, or convulsions; high levels of lead in the bloodstream could result in brain damage and death. Lead poisoning was often asymptomatic, so that irreparable harm could be done before the cause was known. The problem was initially one of industry, especially among painters. In the late nineteenth century, medical journals began to note cases of poisoned children. Young people were especially vulnerable to lead exposure because of their propensity to put things in their mouths, such as toys decorated with lead paint, foil candy wrappers, and flaking wall paint. (One physician described the taste of lead paint chips as "surprisingly good . . . a sweet taste kind of like a cordial candy."[28])

Confronted with evidence that their products threatened children, manufacturers of lead-containing goods, represented by their trade group, the Lead Industries Association, mounted a decades-long and largely successful public relations campaign to reframe the poisoning as a consequence of pica, an abnormal craving for non-edible substances. According to this narrative, the unnatural urges of a subset of children, not toxins widespread in the built environment, lay at the root of the problem.[29]

In the 1950s, some health departments in cities with large quantities of deteriorating housing stock, notably Baltimore and Chicago, mounted outreach programs to uncover cases of lead poisoning among poor children.[30] In New York City, two of the Health Department's most senior physicians—Morris Greenberg, director of the Bureau of Preventable Diseases, and Harold Jacobziner of the Bureau of Child Health—conducted pioneering studies. They mapped the epidemiology of childhood lead poisoning and identified the city's "lead belt"—poor neighborhoods with high concentrations of old and dilapidated buildings, including Bedford, Bushwick, Brownsville, Red Hook, and Fort Greene in Brooklyn; Central and East Harlem; and the South Bronx.[31] The department undertook several measures in response to these studies. It began a physician education campaign throughout the city so that pediatric clinicians would be on the alert for signs of lead poisoning. Doctors in the department's child health stations asked about a history of pica in all checkups and offered screening of blood lead levels. When high lead levels were diagnosed, a sanitarian visited the apartment to take paint samples from the walls and other interior surfaces to be tested for lead, and a public health nurse visited to discuss the situation with the family and urge testing of other children in the household. Poisoned children were given intravenous chelating agents, a treatment that required up to a week of hospitalization.

Many in the department ruefully noted that remediating the problem after a child had been poisoned was hardly an optimal approach. "A real attack on lead poisoning in children," said a staff member in the Bureau of Preventable Diseases, "can only be mounted through an attack on slum housing."[32] But in a city with a vacancy rate of roughly 2 percent and almost half a million housing units dating from the prewar period, when paint with high lead content was common, a truly preventive strategy—removing the toxin from all home environments—seemed a course of almost unimaginable cost and complexity. Lead paint abatement was expensive and time-consuming because it often required removing the plaster behind the paint. The fiscal burden of carrying it out on a massive scale would have to be borne at least in part by the city. Even assuming that a financial solution could be found, there remained the problem of where to relocate families while their apartments were being renovated. Members of the Board of Health who inquired about the feasibility of large-scale renovations were told by colleagues in city government that housing reform "was not a real health problem, not the business of the department."[33]

The closest thing to an environmental approach came by way of the regulatory powers that the Board of Health wielded. Under the revised health code of 1959, use of lead paint on interior surfaces was banned, and the Health Department was empowered to order the cleanup of an apartment after lead poisoning had been diagnosed in a child. Landlords were given five days' notice to remove the paint; in cases of noncompliance, the department could ask the city's Department of Rent and Housing Maintenance to send an emergency team to make the repairs and bill the landlord.[34] But with no bureau in the Health Department dedicated to housing or lead poisoning control—responsibility for the issue was dispersed among several bureaus, including Nursing, Poison Control, Laboratories, Environmental Health, Preventable Diseases, and Child Health—enforcement of the law was scattershot. There were, moreover, loopholes in the department's procedures. When families were relocated to temporary apartments while their homes were being repainted, the temporary shelter was not investigated, so that children were sometimes placed in an environment as risky as the one they had left. Further, when the child returned to the old home, the problems that had led to the original peeling and chipping of paint, such as water leaks, often remained. These flaws in the program drew complaints from physicians at hospitals in the Bronx and Brooklyn, where large numbers of lead-poisoned children were diagnosed.[35]

As a result of expanded case finding efforts, diagnosed cases of higher-than-acceptable levels of blood lead in children more than tripled in the city between 1962 and 1965, from 137 to 496. At the same time, the proportion of cases with encephalopathy and deaths from lead poisoning declined significantly, indicating that early screening and removal of the child from the problem environment were having at least some success.[36] The diagnosed cases represented just a small fraction of those thought to be at risk, however. Approximately 120,000 children were estimated to live in contaminated home environments. It was becoming axiomatic, based on epidemiological studies and the experience of health departments in cities that undertook case-finding programs, that the more one looked for lead poisoning in children, the more one found. As the apparent scope of the problem expanded, the Health Department's efforts came under increasing fire from activists.

In late 1967, the New York Scientists' Committee for Public Information, a group of about one hundred mostly young liberal academics advocating on issues as diverse as nuclear disarmament and environmental degradation, took up the cause of lead poisoning. They began to pressure the Health Department to test more children and to aggressively enforce the health code provisions requiring cleanup of contaminated units. New York City's efforts looked anemic compared to the vigorous attacks on the problem being mounted in other cities. In 1968, Chicago, which had less than half the population of New York, tested about five times as many children.[37] Representatives of the Scientists' Committee met with Donald Conwell, an assistant commissioner in the Bureau of Preventable Diseases, who explained that expanding the department's case-finding efforts would be difficult at a time of acute staffing shortages and fiscal uncertainty, when even the department's ability to maintain its existing programs was in doubt.[38]

Following the meeting with the Scientists' Committee, a departmental task force was formed to coordinate the efforts that were dispersed among several bureaus and to reach out to other city agencies with responsibility for the problem. This initiative did nothing, however, to increase the scope of case-finding or apartment repair. Conwell suggested that the activists put pressure on City Hall: if Lindsay's advisers could be convinced to find more money for the problem, then the Health Department would be able to expand its outreach. The group met with Lindsay's aides for both housing and health issues, but the meetings proved fruitless. The Scientists' Committee determined that a concerted strategy to create public awareness—and outrage—was necessary. The group joined forces with other activists concerned about the issue and in early 1968 formed the Citizens to End Lead Poisoning (CELP). Prominent members included Glenn Paulson, an environmental scientist who had chaired the Scientists' Committee, and Paul DuBrul, a community organizer devoted to issues such as labor rights, urban planning, and housing.

Over the next two years, CELP mobilized pressure both at the grass-roots level and among key opinion leaders in government and the media. The group organized a two-day conference at Rockefeller University in the spring of 1969 that attracted prominent scientists, such as the widely respected microbiologist René Dubos, who called lead poisoning in children "a social crime" and claimed that if the problem was not eliminated, "our society deserves all the disasters that have been forecast for it."[39] Local politicians, including U.S. congressional representatives and City Council members, began to pressure the Health Department to do more to combat the problem. Robert Abrams, a reformist state assembly member running for Bronx borough president, held a news conference in June 1969 with the mother of a child who had died of acute lead poisoning to charge that the department's response was "scandalously slow." (Abrams went on to win his race.)[40] The *Times, Post,* and *Daily News* ran human interest stories on the problem.

At the same time that they stirred outrage among elites, CELP members sought to mobilize affected communities. "No progress will be gained in the battle against lead poisoning," the group wrote in a strategy document, "without massive mobilization of the ghetto community."[41] CELP organized outreach programs in which residents in the "lead belt" neighborhoods partnered with workers from federal anti-poverty programs and staff from community-based service organizations to educate their neighbors and encourage blood testing of at-risk children who had shown signs of lead ingestion. In the Brownsville neighborhood, the Black Panthers made lead poisoning part of their platform against racial injustice, charging that health problems related to dilapidated housing constituted "genocide."[42]

Mayor Lindsay had had a poor relationship with health commissioner Edward O'Rourke, and in mid-1969 he replaced O'Rourke with Mary McLaughlin, who had spearheaded the efforts to increase the department's provision of ambulatory care. McLaughlin had a long-standing interest in the issue of lead paint poisoning. As a district health officer in Queens in the 1950s, she had collaborated with Morris Greenberg and Harold Jacobziner on the early epidemiological studies of the lead belt. In the intervening years, however, community expectations of the Health Department had changed, and McLaughlin quickly came under fire for not doing enough about the issue. In a series of articles in the fall of 1969, muckraking columnist Jack Newfield of the radical weekly the *Village Voice* pilloried McLaughlin and Lindsay for what he perceived as deplorable inaction. Newfield wrote that McLaughlin and Lindsay's aide for health, Werner Kamarsky, were "cut off from the dailiness of injustice by their positions and life styles." (He noted snidely that McLaughlin lived not in New York City but in the Long Island suburb of Manhasset.)[43] He accused McLaughlin of lying to the mayor and the press about the extent of the lead paint problem and the department's response.[44]

That McLaughlin, who for fifteen years had been a pioneer in studying and raising awareness of the dangers of lead paint, now found herself attacked for inattention to the problem was both a bitter irony and a barometer of the charged political environment of the 1960s. Activists were no longer willing to wait for the slowly turning gears of city bureaucracy; lack of urgency in attacking health problems rooted in social inequity was increasingly grounds for moral outrage.

Under pressure to act, McLaughlin transferred $150,000 from other department programs to hire fifteen new chemists and sanitarians to increase the capacity to test children and inspect households. At the same time, she promulgated a major change to the health code: the Health Department would be required, rather than simply allowed, to order cleanup of contaminated units. Equally significant, landlords would be allowed to install wallboard to cover lead-painted walls instead of having to remove the paint; this provision would make it much easier for property owners to comply with the law.[45]

The change in the health code fulfilled a key demand of activists, but controversy persisted over the scope of case-finding efforts. One of the main barriers to expanded testing was that the blood draw was invasive and unpleasant for children and required special training for outreach workers. Such efforts also met with resistance from community members. The district health officer for Harlem recalled that some parents in the neighborhood did not want to have their children's blood drawn because they were convinced he was going to sell it.[46] An alternative seemed to be at hand when a method for testing urine for elevated lead levels was developed. The company that made the test, eager to put its product into wide use, donated 40,000 test kits to the Health Department. Evidence about the reliability and validity of the test was mixed, however, and Health Department employees associated with the lead program were reluctant to invest time and energy on widespread deployment of an experimental product. Their failure to use tests that they had been given for free appeared to activists to be further proof of official indifference to the problem.

This inaction drew the attention of the Young Lords, the Puerto Rican radicals who had adopted the health of the residents of "el barrio" as a primary focus of their activism (and who would later commandeer a tuberculosis screening van).[47]

On the morning of November 24, 1969, about thirty of the Young Lords and their supporters entered McLaughlin's office on the third floor of 125 Worth Street and demanded that the department turn over the urine test kits so that they could do the outreach themselves. McLaughlin and Donald Conwell were at an all-day conference across town, but the group insisted that they would not leave the premises without the kits. McLaughlin's secretary was able to reach one of the health commissioner's deputies, David Harris, who rushed to her office to meet with the group. With the demonstrators sitting on the floor and perched on tabletops, Harris brokered a deal to allow the Young Lords to use a limited number of kits in collaboration with Health Department doctors who had expertise in lead screening.[48]

The confrontation in the commissioner's office epitomized the clashing perspectives of health professionals and activists. Where McLaughlin, Conwell, and Harris saw the need to proceed carefully according to scientific evidence so as not to waste scarce resources on measures that might be ineffective or counterproductive, aggrieved community members saw bureaucratic stonewalling. The urine test, it was later confirmed, had a high rate of both false positives and false negatives and was thus unsuitable as a screening tool.[49]

Activists were increasingly successful at shaping public perceptions of the problem. Shortly after the occupation of McLaughlin's office, Paul Cornely, the first African American to serve as president of the American Public Health Association, was quoted in the *Times* claiming that the Health Department's lack of action on the issue was due to the fact that most poisoned children were black or Puerto Rican.[50] Cornely was a firebrand who had often criticized his colleagues for shrinking from political engagement, so his bluntness was not entirely unexpected. Nevertheless, the head of the public health profession's national organization publicly accusing one of the country's premier municipal health agencies of racism was an astonishing spectacle that showed how far the terms of the debate over the connection between poverty and health had shifted.

By 1970, the level of political pressure was such that Lindsay approved a special appropriation of $2.4 million from city funds. In January, the department created a dedicated Bureau of Lead Poisoning Control. McLaughlin placed the bureau under the direction of Vincent Guinee, an energetic young epidemiologist who had joined the department in 1966. Guinee had not been involved with the issue of lead poisoning, but he knew the lead belt well. He had directed the city's measles and rubella vaccination programs in the poor areas of Brooklyn and the Bronx that were hotspots of childhood disease outbreaks and low immunization rates. During that effort, he had proved skillful at partnering with community-based organizations and using the media to "sell" the importance of immunization.[51] Guinee and his staff would be responsible for coordinating home inspections, citywide education campaigns, and surveillance.[52] Mollified by the creation of the bureau, APHA president Paul Cornely visited McLaughlin in her office to apologize for his remarks; the association's public relations counsel issued a retraction and Cornely told the *Times* that his charges of racism had been based on "a wrong set of facts."[53]

The infusion of funds enabled the department to increase its screening more than fourteenfold, from about 7,000 children tested in 1968 to some 70,000 in 1970 to almost 100,000 in 1971, when close to 2,000 new cases of lead-poisoned children were found. Screening was done through the department's district health centers and child health stations, at Head Start programs, day care facilities, and health fairs, and—the most expensive and time-consuming method—by outreach workers going door to door. These efforts were complicated by the high level of mistrust that many residents felt toward government officials.

In an assessment of the department's efforts three years after the Bureau of Lead Poisoning Control was created, three health officers who served in the lead belt candidly acknowledged the program's limitations. Only about one-third of children were retested six months after the initial screening, as was recommended, and of those, more than half still had abnormally high blood lead levels. Evidence suggested that many of the children lost to follow-up were returning to toxic environments where they faced renewed exposure to lead. The Health Department received lackluster cooperation from the New York City Housing Authority, the city's largest landlord, which saw the extent of the problem as hopeless and dragged its feet on its emergency repair program. Checks by the department found that only about 60 percent of apartments where lead had been abated met the standards laid out in the health code.[54] Repairs were done not to the entire home but merely to the portion of the apartment where the positive paint sample was found. "Topical repairs to a systematically ill house," the health officers noted, "will not cure its continuing disintegration."[55] Screening, treatment, and abatement—no matter how vigorously applied—remained Band-aids on a vast problem that had been decades in the making.

In public health, there were sometimes small-bore solutions that could achieve remarkable results without altering deeply rooted social conditions. The difficulty of addressing lead paint poisoning contrasted sharply with a successful initiative around the same time to address another problem that disproportionately affected poor minority children in slum housing.

In the summer of 1967, employees in the department's Bureau of Health Statistics noticed a sharp uptick in the number of children dying as a result of falling from windows and fire escapes. The falls were especially common in the South Bronx and northern Manhattan. The typical victim was a preschool boy, African American or Puerto Rican, being raised by a single mother who worked outside the home. A disproportionate number of the falls occurred in five- or six-story walk-up tenement buildings. (Under the city's zoning laws, six stories was the maximum height allowed without requiring an elevator.) Many of the families had recently moved from rural parts of the U.S. South or from Puerto Rico and were unfamiliar with the potential dangers of leaving children unattended in high-rise buildings. Virtually all the falls occurred between May and September. From 1965 to 1969, some two hundred children died from falls in the city, accounting for about one-quarter of deaths of children under age five; children who fell also suffered a range of major injuries that left the victims with lifelong disabilities, including concussion, laceration, and internal injuries to kidneys, spleens, and bladders.[56]

The connection between injury and poor housing conditions was clear. Noting that one child who had fallen five stories survived because he landed in a pile of garbage, one analysis observed, "It is a sad commentary on our society that at the present time the illegal accumulation of refuse about these buildings appears to save more lives than any legal measures requiring appropriate window guards."[57] Unlike remediating a lead-painted environment, however, a narrowly targeted intervention was available.

The Health Department launched a two-year pilot program to distribute free window guards to residents of the Tremont neighborhood of the Bronx, which had the highest concentration of falls. The campaign, with the slogan "Children Can't Fly," included mass media ads and one-on-one education through outreach workers and community-based organizations. At the same time, the department stepped up its data gathering by partnering with police and hospital emergency room staff to report all window falls, and public health nurses made follow-up visits to households where a fall had occurred. In 1974, when declining numbers of falls indicated the success of the prevention program, it was expanded into all five boroughs. The "Children Can't Fly" theme was repeated through public-service announcements in English, Spanish, Chinese, and Haitian Creole. The department distributed more than 16,000 window guards free to some 4,200 families.[58] Between 1973 and 1975, the number of recorded falls was cut in half and the number of deaths from falls declined from 57 to 32.

The successful prevention of falls threw into stark relief the intractability of the lead paint problem. The technical difference between the two issues—windows could be barred far more easily than walls could be rebuilt and repainted—only partially explained the contrasting outcomes. A critical difference was that the window guards program imposed no financial burden on landlords. The Health Department bore the cost of the guards and the effort of getting them into homes. The importance of this fact would be highlighted during the city's fiscal crisis, when the department was forced to shift the cost of the window guards to landlords, who immediately (and unsuccessfully) mounted a court challenge to stop the move.

"Controversial Programs for Unpopular People"

In the summer of 1970, as the expanded lead poisoning campaign shifted into high gear, the Health Department launched an effort to enroll thousands of heroin addicts into new treatment clinics dispensing the synthetic opiate methadone. It was one of the most ambitious and aggressive rollouts of a health program in the city's history—and all the more remarkable because the department had done little since its founding to address the problem of narcotic use.

While various professions and interest groups—notably law enforcement and psychiatry—had sought to claim "ownership" over drug addiction and define its solution during the twentieth century, public health had historically remained on the sidelines. Few city or state health departments had programs to prevent heroin addiction. Congress had funded the establishment in 1929 of two hospitals under the aegis of the U.S. Public Health Service, in Fort Worth, Texas, and Lexington, Kentucky, dedicated to treating addicts who would otherwise be languishing in federal prisons. The facilities were hospitals in name only, however, since there were few effective therapeutic options at the time, and their connection to mainstream public health activities was tenuous.[59]

Defining the problem was complex. Was heroin addiction an illness or a crime? A physiological disorder or a mental one? Was it a moral weakness and character defect? A tragic but predictable consequence of social injustice and deprivation? A rational response to difficult life circumstances? As the prevalence of heroin use increased in the post–World War II era and concerns rose about its association with crime—especially by juveniles—the views of narcotic addiction as a crime and an illness coexisted uneasily. During the 1950s, new federal laws strengthened the penalties for possession of heroin, but some jurisprudence moved in the opposite direction: in the 1962 case *Robinson v. California*, the U.S. Supreme Court threw out a state law that made drug addiction a crime punishable by ninety days in jail. The court held this to be cruel and unusual punishment, akin to criminalizing mental illness or venereal disease.[60] In 1963 a presidential advisory commission on addiction called for dismantling the Federal Bureau of Narcotics and carving out a new role for the Department of Health, Education, and Welfare. Sometimes the therapeutic and punitive approaches overlapped: in 1966, New York governor Nelson Rockefeller approved an $81 million control program that prominently featured compulsory inpatient treatment, known as civil commitment, for addicts.[61]

Throughout the postwar years of growing public anxiety about the problem, the New York City Health Department's responses remained reactive and piecemeal and consisted largely of applying—with little apparent effect—the stalwart approaches that had long been used against infectious diseases: education, laboratory services, and surveillance. In 1961 the department created the position of narcotics coordinator, who gave talks to schools and community groups; one district health center in each of the five boroughs was designated to provide information, referral, and counseling on the subject.[62] The Bureau of Laboratories provided urine testing for community-based treatment programs to verify that the increasing number of addicts in treatment were staying clean.[63] When Nelson Rockefeller announced his civil commitment program for addicts, the Health Department considered amending the city health code to allow for a similar program locally, but determined that recent jurisprudence on due process made such an approach vulnerable to constitutional challenge.[64]

The most innovative attempt to adapt the infectious disease approach to addiction came in the area of surveillance. A 1963 amendment to the city health code created a narcotics registry and made it mandatory for anyone giving care to an addict to report that person.[65] The rationale was the same one that underpinned other types of disease notification: understanding the scope of the problem and the demographic patterns of those afflicted was essential to planning and providing services.[66] Reporting to the registry remained spotty, however, as was the case with surveillance more generally. The most complete reports came from the nonprofit organizations that the city funded to provide detoxification and rehabilitation services; the worst levels of compliance came, not surprisingly, from private physicians, whose cooperation with the city's disease surveillance laws had long been desultory.[67]

Partly owing to the absence of systematic and reliable surveillance, the prevalence of heroin addiction remained murky. In New York City, estimates of the number of addicts ranged from 30,000 to 100,000. What was clear, based on the evidence from the narcotics registry and reports from the hospital, criminal justice, and human services sectors, was that the city accounted for an outsized share of the nation's addicts; that they were disproportionately male, African American or Puerto Rican, and poor; and that their numbers in the city were growing steadily.

When John Lindsay took office in 1966, he had an interest in the problem of drug addiction but no coherent vision of how to approach it. The city's drug treatment world was a hodgepodge of halfway houses and therapeutic communities that often adhered to rigid principles of abstinence. The city's Community Mental Health Board funded voluntary organizations to provide counseling and supportive services to addicts, while other agencies were funded by private donors or state contracts.[68] A few months after Lindsay took office, several Health Department employees who felt that the agency should be doing more about the problem submitted a proposal for a dedicated Bureau of Drug Addiction.[69] Lindsay decided, however, that the problem was too important and complex to be housed within the Health Department. Not only did he turn down the proposal, but he transferred the department's drug education activities into a newly created mayoral Office of the Coordinator of Addiction Programs.[70] A year later, Lindsay further elevated the issue by creating a new mayoral agency, the Addiction Services Agency, which he housed not in the Health Services Administration superagency but in the Human Resources Administration, which ran the city's welfare programs—a move that reflected the belief that heroin use was a problem with societal rather than physiological roots.[71]

Health department employees who were concerned about addiction, especially those who worked in the district health centers in neighborhoods with the highest rates of drug use, were upset about the transfer of authority for the programs, limited though they were. Their dissatisfaction increased when it became apparent that Efren Ramirez, the psychiatrist Lindsay had recruited to run the Addiction Services Agency, was an incompetent administrator. Steven Jonas, the district health officer in the Bedford neighborhood of Brooklyn, sought to partner with community-based drug prevention organizations that could offer services in the center, but found that he could not get the approval he needed from Ramirez. "I feel that the time has come to blow the whistle on this man," Jonas wrote angrily to health commissioner Edward O'Rourke after months of trying unsuccessfully to set up a meeting with Ramirez. "He is not only doing nothing, but by sitting on monies already given to his agency he is effectively preventing the development of urgently needed programs for which financing is available."[72] The Addiction Services Agency achieved lackluster results in its first two years, and Ramirez would resign just ahead of calls by a City Council member for an investigation into the agency for fraud and waste.[73]

Meanwhile, public alarm about drug use was increasing, and the Lindsay administration felt increasing pressure to stanch the problem. Rising rates of theft, burglary, and mugging were blamed on addicts stealing to support their habits. Fear of racial and ethnic "others" on drug-fueled crime sprees was an old trope that had driven hard-line policies for decades.[74] Nelson Rockefeller's 1966 drug prevention initiative emphasizing civil commitment had in large measure been a response to the putative connection between drugs and crime.

Into these old concerns were now woven new fears. The hippie movement centered in the Haight-Ashbury neighborhood of San Francisco and the East Village in Manhattan seemed to middle-class observers to be fueled by marijuana and hallucinogens. The rise of the youth counter-culture presented the frightening prospect of affluent high school and college students lured into degeneracy and lawlessness as they progressed from glue-sniffing to a "hard drug" netherworld.[75] At the same time, America's involvement in the Vietnam War deepened, and reports of widespread heroin use by U.S. soldiers fighting in Southeast Asia raised the specter of thousands of veterans returning home as addicts.[76]

One approach that held out promise in a generally bleak therapeutic landscape was methadone maintenance therapy. Methadone had been developed in Germany before World War II as a synthetic substitute for morphine. It had been used experimentally at the U.S. Public Health Service hospitals in Lexington and Fort Worth as a short-term tool to ease withdrawal from heroin. In the early 1960s, two researchers at The Rockefeller University, Vincent Dole, an endocrinologist, and Marie Nyswander, a psychiatrist, began to study the use of methadone as a long-term substitute for heroin. The two hypothesized that the metabolism of some heroin addicts became so damaged that they could no longer function without receiving some form of opiate. Dole and Nyswander found that methadone fulfilled the physical craving but, unlike heroin, did not produce euphoria, psychomotor impairment, or sedation. Patients taking methadone could resume normal social and occupational functioning. Long-term, perhaps indefinite maintenance was necessary: methadone could "correct" but not "cure" the physiological damage that heroin had caused.[77]

Dole and Nyswander evaluated the treatment at different doses and in different settings and published their results in a series of seminal journal articles.[78] Impressed by the early results, outgoing mayor Robert Wagner in late 1965 had approved a $1.4 million grant from the city's Department of Hospitals to operate a methadone maintenance program out of the Beth Israel Medical Center.[79] Not everyone viewed the concept of opiate substitution as benign, however, and methadone maintenance quickly drew charges that it substituted one addiction for another. Much of this criticism came from partisans of abstinence-based drug programs.

A doctor who ran a treatment clinic in Harlem said that prescribing methadone was "like giving the alcoholic in the Bowery bourbon instead of whiskey in an attempt to get him off his alcoholism."[80] The director of the Synanon Foundation labeled Dole and Nyswander's research "dangerous" in a *New Republic* article titled "Stoned on Methadone."[81]

Partly because of such concerns, and partly because the issue of drug use was such a political hot potato, officials in the Lindsay administration repeatedly dodged questions from the press about whether, when, and how the city might expand methadone treatment beyond the Beth Israel program.[82] By the summer of 1968, however, the accumulation of scientific evidence on the efficacy of methadone had won over some previously skeptical political figures in the city, including, most crucially, African American and Puerto Rican community leaders such as congressional representatives Charles Rangel and Herman Badillo; Roy Innis of the Congress of Racial Equality; and Clarence Jones, the co-owner of the *Amsterdam News*.[83]

Backed by the more favorable climate of opinion, and under pressure to show results in the city's fight against addiction and crime, Lindsay's advisers began exploring ways to expand and decentralize methadone treatment. Top managers in the Addiction Services Agency were devoted to abstinence-based, addict-run therapeutic communities and ideologically hostile to methadone, so Lindsay's advisers turned to the Health Department to lead the expansion. Lindsay's special assistant for narcotics, Michael Dontzin, recommended "a modest program at the outset"—two or three new outpatient clinics that would operate out of district health centers.[84] Mary McLaughlin drafted a plan for methadone programs in the centers on the Lower East Side of Manhattan and in Mott Haven in the Bronx.[85]

After several weeks of meetings that had advanced well into the details of planning and budgeting, however, the plans fell through, and Lindsay and his team once again bypassed the Health Department as the home for addiction programs. Lindsay did not have a close relationship with then-commissioner Edward O'Rourke, and the health services administrator, Bernard Bucove, expressed skepticism about whether the department was the most appropriate home for the initiative. Lindsay did not trust either man to operate such a novel and politically sensitive program.[86]

Instead, Lindsay's team determined that the best course would be to house the program in a newly created nongovernmental agency, the Addiction Treatment and Resource Corporation, run by the Vera Institute of Justice, a think tank that had made a name for itself studying the impact of policy innovations in the realm of criminal justice such as alternative sentencing and bail reform. The mayor's office secured funding through a research grant from the National Institute of Mental Health (NIMH). In the spring of 1969, in the midst of his reelection campaign, Lindsay announced in a City Hall ceremony that the Addiction Treatment and Resource Corporation would open a program in Bedford-Stuyvesant. Tellingly, Lindsay described it not as a health initiative but as a "major new crime prevention effort."[87]

Almost immediately after Lindsay was reelected in 1969, two major shifts in policy occurred, neither of which could have been foreseen even a year earlier. First, the cautious approach to creating a decentralized methadone program was abandoned, and second, the Health Department moved to center stage in this expansion. The impetus behind both of these changes was Lindsay's hiring of Gordon Chase as the new health services administrator (figure 2.1).

Chase was a stunning departure from the previous two HSA chiefs. Unlike Howard Brown and Bernard Bucove, Chase was not a physician. Only thirty-seven years old, he had joined the Lindsay administration in 1968 to run the finances of the city's Human Resources Administration. He came with a stellar résumé, having done stints in Washington, D.C., on the staff of President Kennedy's national security adviser, McGeorge Bundy, and later at the Agency for International Development (AID) and the Equal Employment Commission (EEC). He had strong experience in budgeting and personnel. That he was not a doctor clearly signaled Lindsay's belief that the problems plaguing the city's health services were bureaucratic, not medical.[88]

While everyone agreed that an outstanding manager was needed to lead the Health Services Administration, the idea that someone with no scientific credentials could meet this challenge was an affront to the city's medical establishment, always fiercely protective of professional prerogatives and long resentful of nonphysicians controlling any aspect of health care. Doctors responded with outrage to the news of Chase's appointment. The president of the New York Academy of Medicine sent a hand-delivered letter to Lindsay calling Chase "professionally unqualified."[89] The four physician members of the Board of Health opposed the move; Louis Loeb, the only nonphysician on the board, praised the choice.

Gordon Chase shared Lindsay's view that heroin addiction was an urgent problem and that methadone was the most promising way to address it. The dramatic expansion of the therapy would be one of Chase's most important legacies as HSA administrator. The program run by the Addiction Treatment and Resource Corporation would continue, but now, in addition, methadone would be available in clinical outposts throughout the city. Chase moved swiftly to draft a proposal for the city's addiction strategy that gave top priority to methadone maintenance therapy and secured state funding to support the expansion.

Figure 2.1   Gordon Chase

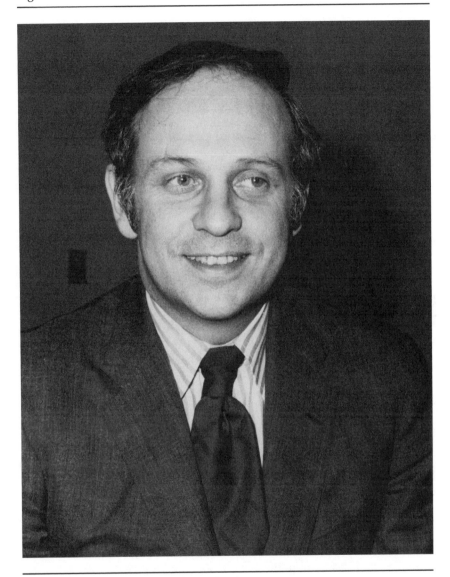

Source: Courtesy New York City Municipal Archives.
Note: Gordon Chase, whom Mayor Lindsay named to the post of health services administrator in 1969. Chase was widely admired within city government for his managerial
ability, but the city's doctors opposed his appointment because he did not hold a medical
degree.

Chase believed that methadone programs should be administered through the Health Department because the district health centers provided a natural infrastructure through which the clinics could operate.[90] Lindsay, for his part, was happy to turn the issue over to the Health Department now that Chase was in charge. He considered Chase a skilled and efficient manager who could achieve results, while he saw the Addiction Services Agency as a place where innovation was unlikely to thrive.[91] That a major new program to combat drug use would be housed outside of the mayoral agency dedicated to that issue had the potential to raise red flags for potential funders, however, so Chase and Lindsay finessed the issue by naming the Addiction Services Agency the official grantee for the state funding but channeling the money into the HSA through a subcontract.

Chase put even more distance between methadone maintenance and the city's drug treatment establishment by appointing an unknown, relatively junior Health Department employee to manage the new program. Chase's neighbor in his Upper West Side apartment building recommended Robert Newman, an idealistic young physician whose experience in city government consisted of one year of running the Health Department's nutrition survey. Newman's inexperience with drug prevention or treatment and his lack of connections to any of the key players in the addiction community might have made him an unlikely choice to head the program, but Chase saw these seeming limitations as strengths. Unburdened by any of the ideological biases or alliances that characterized the fractious and often dogmatic narcotic treatment community, Newman would be able to focus purely on measurable results: making methadone available to as many participants as possible. Setting and meeting quantitative goals was Chase's core strategy for managing the city's health services.[92] In the realm of drug addiction, the number of addicts enrolled in methadone programs became the key metric of success.

Although Newman was "in" the Health Department, he was not "of" it. His office was not at 125 Worth Street, and he carried out his work with little interaction with Commissioner Mary McLaughlin or anyone in the headquarters bureaucracy. Gordon Chase eschewed the usual protocol of communicating about the methadone program through McLaughlin, who was Newman's nominal boss; instead, Chase dealt with Newman directly, calling him multiple times a day to ask for updates on how many addicts had been enrolled and how the new sites were progressing.[93] Chase was determined that the program would reach the numerical targets that signaled success, and Newman, through a combination of youthful drive and unfamiliarity with the typical slow pace of city government, matched him step for step.

Because heroin addiction was so closely associated in the popular imagination with crime and social decay, one of Newman's most important—and difficult—tasks was gaining community buy-in for the methadone clinics. Over the next two years, Newman held three to four community meetings per week where he presented the program to neighbors. When residents got wind that a methadone clinic was to begin operating in their neighborhood, they wasted no time communicating their concerns to their City Council members and congressional representatives, who in turn put pressure on the mayor's office and the Board of Estimate, which held the purse strings to the city budget. Newman sought to defuse these concerns by laying out the benefits of methadone and convincing community members that the program would not lead, as they feared, to a worsening of the neighborhood.

In spite of his assurances, however, a proposed methadone maintenance clinic often became a lightning rod for all the dissatisfaction that city residents were feeling about the declining quality of city life and municipal services. At one meeting, after Newman had given a lengthy presentation about the benefits of methadone, an audience member demanded to know why her garbage had not been collected the previous week; when he tried to explain that a different city agency was responsible for that service, the attendees accused him of passing the buck. In virtually every case, Newman recalled, a planned clinic opened only "after a protracted, uphill struggle against neighborhood opposition."[94]

Given these difficulties, Newman's success was all the more impressive. Within a year of taking the helm, he had gotten seventeen clinics treating some 1,200 patients up and running; two years later, there were forty-four clinics serving between 100 and 600 patients each.[95] In addition to the district health centers, treatment units were opened at private and public hospitals and other outpatient facilities. Each unit had a small staff of a half-time physician, four counselors, a nurse, and a clerical worker.[96]

The dramatic growth of methadone maintenance therapy in New York paralleled similar expansion around the country. Richard Nixon's drug czar, Jerome Jaffe, a psychiatrist at the University of Chicago, was a major supporter of methadone, and federal funding for the treatment rose dramatically; within three years, some 80,000 people were receiving methadone maintenance therapy nationwide. In a remarkably short time, however, methadone became a victim of its success. It metamorphosed from panacea to pariah as commentators from across the political and ideological spectrum began to attack it. Liberals criticized methadone as a "quick fix" that attempted to paper over drug abuse patterns that were deeply rooted in economic and social injustice; conservatives charged that dispensing a synthetic opiate perpetuated drug abuse and its attendant problems rather than solving them.[97]

These criticisms were not new—they had surfaced as soon as Dole and Nyswander began to publish their results in 1965—but they had been more muted when the program was small and experimental. Attacks on methadone increased in proportion to the growth in its use and visibility. Members of the public who saw clients on their blocks conflated the attempted solution with the problem itself and reacted as if the city government were foisting drug abuse on the community rather than trying to address it. Rumors circulated of methadone patients selling the drug on the black market. Methadone's image problem would hit its nadir several years later when *New York* magazine published a lurid exposé, titled "Psst . . . Kid, Wanna Be a Junkie? Try Methadone!" in which a freelance reporter told of his success in scamming the drug from a private clinic in lower Manhattan and selling it on the street.[98]

New York City's expansion of its methadone maintenance program took place in an ambiguous legal context. Methadone had been approved by the Food and Drug Administration (FDA), but not for extended use, and drug officers in the Treasury Department questioned whether it fell within the realm of normal practice of medicine. In response to this uncertainty, a series of congressional acts constructed a complicated and restrictive regulatory framework for the drug. These rules governed patient eligibility and dosing and the types of facilities that could dispense the substance.[99] The guidelines were designed to prevent diversion that might lead to increased drug use in society. In addition to the federal regulations, state and local governments were allowed by law to impose additional guidelines that were more, but not less, restrictive.[100] This legal regime effectively quashed a plan that Mary McLaughlin proposed to Lindsay in the fall of 1970 to make methadone available for private physicians to prescribe.[101]

For the brief interval when Robert Newman was expanding the city's methadone programs, the Health Department seemed poised to assume a major new role in addiction. This involvement proved ephemeral, however. The department would soon cede responsibility for methadone maintenance therapy. The decentralized network of clinics that Newman built up would remain, but authority for them would be transferred to the state health department as part of the retrenchment resulting from the city's fiscal crisis.

Nor did methadone prove to be the magic bullet that some supporters had envisioned. Narcotics-related deaths in New York State rose by about one-third in 1972. Data such as these caused the pendulum to swing back toward the view of addiction as a crime rather than an illness and led Governor Nelson Rockefeller to propose a draconian set of anti-drug measures, including harsh penalties for possession and sale, mandatory minimum sentences, and limitations on plea bargaining.[102] Rockefeller was reportedly frustrated about the ongoing ineffectiveness of drug treatment in making a dent in the prevalence of narcotic use; cynics claimed that he was seeking to bolster his conservative bona fides for an anticipated presidential run. A broad range of medical and civil liberties groups condemned the new criminal justice measures when Rockefeller signed them into law in 1973. Gordon Chase, who by then was on his way out of city government and could speak bluntly, called them "simplistic and impractical." [103]

Rockefeller clearly had public opinion on his side, however. Many states copied elements of the drug laws that would immortalize his name. These laws, like the federal restrictions on methadone therapy, were of a piece with the broader societal backlash against what were perceived as the liberal excesses of the 1960s and the social policy experimentation that, according to critics, had brought higher rates of drug use and other cultural ills. Methadone maintenance clinics were destined to remain, according to an analysis in the 1990s, "controversial programs for unpopular people." [104]

A Woman's Right

In the spring of 1970, as Vincent Guinee was ramping up the outreach and testing for lead poisoning in the city's slum neighborhoods and Robert Newman was mapping out a strategy for methadone clinics, a veteran Health Department physician named Jean Pakter was working around the clock drafting new regulations on where and how abortion could be performed in New York City. Some of Pakter's colleagues, including the devout Roman Catholic who headed the Bureau of Nursing, had misgivings about the state's recent legalization of abortion. Pakter did not. She viewed the availability of abortion as "a sad medical necessity" given the life circumstances of many women, and she saw the guidelines she was developing as consistent with the work she had done for two decades to ensure the best possible outcomes related to maternity and family planning. [105]

Caring for the health of new and expectant mothers was a venerable part of the public health mission dating to the "maternalist" initiatives of the Progressive Era, when well-baby clinics and visiting nurse programs flourished. [106] That mission grew more complicated as scientific, social, and legal factors—including the development of the birth control pill, the rise of the feminist movement, and new jurisprudence on privacy—transformed the nature of reproductive health services.

A measure of these changes could be found in the stance of the city's health agencies toward family planning. Throughout the 1950s, there had been an unwritten rule in the Health Department that anyone asking about birth control was to be referred to Planned Parenthood. [107] The eighteen institutions run by the Department of Hospitals had a similar policy—unofficial but clearly understood—against offering information about family planning. In 1957, at a citywide conference on maternal mortality, the director of obstetrics at Kings County Hospital attacked this policy in front of one hundred of the city's medical elite, prompting Morris Jacobs, the hospitals commissioner, to retort, "I do not consider it the function or responsibility of the municipal hospitals of this city to disseminate birth control information." Alan Guttmacher, the president of Planned Parenthood, swiftly condemned Jacobs's remarks, setting off months of acrimonious public debate that ended with the ban on birth control information being dropped.[108]

The licensing of the birth control pill in 1960 accelerated the pace of change. So did the federal dollars flowing from the Kennedy and Johnson administrations. Congressional amendments to the Social Security Act in 1963 created a new funding stream for maternal and child health administered through the Children's Bureau, which the following year made a $1.4 million grant to the Health Department to reduce infant mortality by giving early prenatal care. In the first year of the grant, seven satellite clinics opened in district health centers in poor neighborhoods, including Bedford, Brownsville, East Harlem, Central Harlem, and Morrisania. The maternity and infant care clinics were operated in partnership with nearby hospitals, which furnished obstetricians and certified nurse-midwives.[109] The clinics provided family planning counseling along with condoms, diaphragms, and oral contraceptives.[110] By 1968 family planning services were being offered in twenty-one Health Department locations around the city, at either district health centers or child health stations.[111]

The city's rapidly expanding involvement in family planning during the 1960s provoked surprisingly little public debate, especially considering the brouhaha a decade earlier over birth control in public hospitals. The proposed legalization of abortion, however, was another matter entirely. New York's abortion law, dating from 1830, was one of the country's most restrictive, permitting the procedure only when necessary to save the life of the mother. The forces that had driven more liberal family planning services began to converage around the issue of abortion. Arrayed on one side was a coalition of feminist activists, liberal politicians, Protestant and Episcopalian churches, and medical, legal, and civil liberties groups. On the other stood the Catholic Church and legislators with the moral conviction that abortion was wrong. In the middle were large numbers of legislators who were either ambivalent about the procedure or reluctant to take on such a polarizing issue.

Organized efforts to ease restrictive state abortion laws had been under way since the late 1950s, when Planned Parenthood had asked the American Law Institute to draft a model act for reform.[112] The landmark 1965 Supreme Court case *Griswold v. Connecticut* had given activists new ammunition in their fight. *Griswold*, which overturned a state law banning the use of contraceptives by married couples, marked the first time the Supreme Court found a constitutionally protected right to privacy—William O. Douglas famously discovered the right in the "emanations" and "penumbras" of various clauses in the Bill of Rights—and the decision opened new legal frontiers within which proponents of abortion rights hoped to make their case.[113] In the wake of *Griswold*, activists in New York State redoubled their efforts at reform.

Initially they focused on broadening the circumstances under which a woman could terminate a pregnancy. Albert Blumenthal, the chair of the Assembly Committee on Health, introduced a bill in 1966 to expand the provisions to allow abortions to preserve the mother's health, if the pregnancy was the result of rape or incest, or if the mother was under fifteen years old or mentally ill. One of the key strategies of proponents was to frame abortion as an issue not of morality but of public health.[114] Blumenthal invited several prominent doctors from New York City to testify in Albany in support of the measure. Howard Brown, the health services administrator, told Assembly members that the number of deaths related to abortions was increasing at a time when maternal mortality overall was declining. Brown also noted the stark disparities in outcomes for poor women of color: the majority of deaths from illegal abortions occurred in northern Brooklyn, the South Bronx, and Harlem.[115] Louis Cooper, a professor of pediatrics at New York University Medical School, admitted to the committee that doctors in both private and city-run hospitals knowingly broke the law by performing abortions on women who were not legally eligible for them.

Efforts to reframe abortion as a health issue were only partly successful, however. The three days of hearings on Blumenthal's bill often devolved into emotionally charged arguments about morality, evil, and "the slaughter of the innocents"; one witness, the Albany district attorney, demanded to know whether the members of the Assembly health committee were atheists.[116] The bill never made it out of the codes committee onto the floor of the Assembly.

Bills introduced in each of the next two years met similar fates. During this time, however, the political ground was shifting in favor of reform. Most critically, the feminist movement gained strength, and women increasingly exerted influence through meetings with representatives, letter-writing campaigns, and leafleting. The National Organization for Women (NOW), founded in 1966, quickly became a prominent political voice, while militant groups such as the Redstockings, the October 17th Movement, Women's Liberation, and the New York Radical Women shook up staid legislative processes with raucous protests. A dozen members of the Redstockings crashed a state Assembly hearing at 125 Worth Street and called for repeal of the abortion law; the women demanded to know why the roster of fourteen expert witnesses scheduled to testify before the panel consisted of thirteen men and a nun. In a refrain increasingly heard from activists of all stripes, the women claimed that they, not the committee members or the witnesses, were the "real experts."[117]

Opinion polls indicated increasing public support for liberalized abortion, and the legislatures of several states, including Alaska, Hawaii, and Washington, passed abortion reform measures. New York governor Nelson Rockefeller announced his support for abortion reform, and pro-reform members joined the state legislature in 1968. In the spring of 1969, the National Association for the Repeal of Abortion Laws (NARAL) was formed in New York City. It was against this backdrop that Constance Cook, an upstate Republican who was one of three women in New York's 207-member legislature, agreed to carry a bill. A NOW member, Cook was an influential and savvy legislator who was able to mobilize support among colleagues with differing agendas and varying levels of comfort with reforming or repealing abortion restrictions.[118]

Cook introduced a bill in the spring 1969 legislative session with Franz Leichter, a Manhattan Democrat, as co-sponsor. The original version of the bill repealed all abortion restrictions, but Cook and Leichter, in a concession to gain support from more conservative colleagues, added provisions limiting abortion to the first twenty-four weeks and requiring parental consent for minors' abortions. It was clear to supporters that the vote would be close, and Cook kept the bill alive with last-minute parliamentary maneuvering even after it appeared to have been defeated. On April 10, upstate Democrat George Michaels, whose district was heavily Roman Catholic, reversed his vote at the last minute. "I realize, Mr. Speaker, that I am terminating my political career," Michaels said, choking back sobs as he cast his vote, "but I cannot in good conscience sit here and allow my vote to be the one that defeats this bill." (Michaels was defeated in the primary election a few months later.)[119] When Governor Rockefeller signed the bill two days later, New York went from having one of the most restrictive abortion laws in the country to one of the most liberal. As of July 1, all abortions would be allowed up to the twenty-fourth week of pregnancy, and after that to save a woman's life.

The law required that abortion be provided by a licensed physician, but it was silent on where and how the procedure could be done. The Board of Health, because of its role in clinical standard-setting, suddenly found itself at the center of fierce public debates. The state board would set guidelines as well, but, as was often the case, New York City's regulations would be far more consequential because it was expected to account for the vast majority of abortions performed in the state. It was the board's responsibility to promulgate rules for the city on where abortions could be carried out and the standards that would govern the conduct of the procedure, and it would ultimately fall to the Health Department to put the board's regulations into operation through its inspection and enforcement functions.

The board had the option of promulgating no regulations, a course preferred by some abortion rights activists who wanted no barriers to access. But many observers believed that regulation was essential to ensuring the fulfillment of the new law's promise. Deaths from botched abortions performed in ill-equipped facilities would generate bad press that might jeopardize the movement under way in other states to enact similar reforms. "The success or failure of the entire liberalized abortion program," predicted Shirley Mayer, the department's head of maternity services, "depends on whether or not the hospitals and clinics can provide safe and adequate treatment to thousands of additional patients."[120]

To craft the new regulations, the members of the Board of Health turned to Jean Pakter, one of the most experienced and respected figures in the department. A pediatrician who had trained under the eminent Viennese doctor Bela Schick in the 1930s, Pakter had joined the department after World War II and during more than two decades of service had been responsible for some of the city's most successful initiatives in maternal and child health. As the head of the Bureau of Maternity Services and Family Planning, she had been a passionate advocate for the health of expectant mothers and was devoted to remedying the disparities in birth outcomes for poor women of color. Pakter had gone to Albany during the hearings on the Cook-Leichter bill to present data on maternal mortality in the city resulting from illegal abortions. It was now her charge to craft rules that would determine how widely available abortion would be.

Pakter turned for advice to the Advisory Committee on Obstetrics and Gynecology, a nineteen-member group of local clinicians whom the Health Department had convened since 1968. Under the gun with less than three months until the new law took effect, they worked late into the night, often at Pakter's Upper East Side apartment, for weeks.[121] They grappled with questions about the types of facilities that should be allowed to perform abortions and the kinds of equipment and personnel that should be required. They sought to craft regulations that would make the procedure as widely available as possible and as safe as possible, knowing that each of these goals might undercut the other. Estimates of the number of abortions that might be performed annually varied from 50,000 to 250,000, and there was speculation that New York State would become a magnet for women from all over the country.[122] While demand was unknown, supply would largely be determined by where the procedure was allowed. Should it be limited to hospitals only? Should it be allowed in clinics not affiliated with a larger institution? Should private physicians be allowed to perform it in their offices?

Pakter and her colleagues were concerned that doctors' offices too often lacked the conditions, expertise, and equipment needed to perform abortions safely. Excluding a large number of potential practitioners, however, could limit women's options in what was likely to be an overburdened system, and the additional delays that women would face under such rules might mean deaths from later-term abortions, when complications were more frequent. Further, private physicians would be able to offer the procedure at lower cost, whereas allowing it in hospitals only was likely to keep the price between $400 and $1,000. Outlawing abortion in doctors' offices might have the effect of driving poor women into the back-alley procedures that the legislation was explicitly designed to end.

In May, Pakter's group submitted a first draft of the guidelines that suggested limiting abortions to hospitals. When the planned restriction was reported in the press, it was met with fierce criticism. Franz Leichter, who had co-sponsored the legalization bill, warned Commissioner Mary McLaughlin that it would be "unwise and unfortunate" for the Health Department to violate the spirit of the new law by placing restrictions on where the procedure could be performed.[123] The *Times* editorialized that such a limitation would amount to "aborting abortion reform."[124]

By the time the guidelines were published for public comment, the hospitals-only stance had been softened somewhat. Physicians would still be prohibited from performing abortions in their offices; violators would face a $1,000 fine and up to a year in prison. Clinics would be allowed to offer abortions, but they would have to meet an extensive list of technical requirements, including a blood bank, clinical and X-ray labs, a fully equipped operating room, and a staff of obstetricians, anesthesiologists, and nurses. Any clinic offering the procedure would also have to be located less than ten minutes away from a hospital for quick access in case of complications.

The regulations were published for public comment on July 1, 1970, the day the new law took effect. The same day, NARAL sponsored a teach-in at New York University Medical Center where physicians—in open defiance of the proposed regulation—offered guidelines to private practitioners on performing office-based abortions.[125]

Two weeks later, a public hearing on the regulations was held at 125 Worth Street. Outside, two lines of picketers faced off: one demanding full access to abortion, the other chanting against all abortion (see figure 2.2).[126] Inside, at a five-hour hearing, Pakter explained the rationale for the regulations and some fifty witnesses testified. The president of the Greater New York Hospital Association supported the restrictions on grounds of safety, but most of those who spoke urged that few or no limitations be placed on availability. One physician testified that the long waiting time that most hospitals were forecasting—four to five weeks—"converts a simple early abortion into a relatively dangerous late operation." A twenty-one-year-old woman who had had an abortion in a private doctor's office said that she was testifying in order to "dispel all the horror stories you've heard and try to convince you that this can be done safely, cheaply, comfortingly and even happily without going to a hospital."[127]

After the public comment period, the board reviewed additional data about the number of abortions requested and performed during the initial weeks of the new law and the number and kinds of complications. When members reconvened on September 17, they voted unanimously to adopt the guidelines as Pakter and the advisory committee had proposed them. The guidelines were consistent with recommendations put forth by the state medical society and the city's five borough medical societies. But a NARAL official denounced the board's action in a *New York Times* op-ed, saying that the action "mutilated" the state's law and created a two-tier system that unfairly restricted the options of poor women.[128]

The Bureau of Maternity Services and Family Planning prepared an extensive publicity campaign to educate women about the availability of the new service, including television and radio announcements, subway cards and other posters, and half a million copies of a brochure entitled "If You Want an Abortion. . . ."[129] The bureau also contracted with Planned Parenthood to operate a telephone hotline that made appointments for any woman seeking an abortion and directed them away from institutions that were overbooked toward hospitals with greater availability (see figure 2.3).[130]

Monitoring the new guidelines would be daunting, with close to one hundred hospitals gearing up to offer a procedure that was new for many of them and required specialized training and equipment. All of the ninety-six hospitals that would be performing abortions would have to be visited at least once during the first six months after the law went into effect and twice a year thereafter; hospitals that did not offer maternity services and those that had previously received poor reports from the Health Department would have to be visited more frequently. Any maternal death during an abortion would have to be investigated to determine whether it was the result of unavoidable circumstances, failure to observe the new code requirements, or problems with the code itself. Finally, statistics on the total number of abortions performed and demographic information on patients would have to be collected. Most hospitals cooperated by filing the required form for each procedure performed and a weekly statistics report.[131]

In the first year of the new law, an estimated 168,000 abortions were performed at about one hundred facilities. The majority of patients traveled to New York City from elsewhere; only 37 percent were city residents. Women came from all of the fifty states. Four out of five abortions

Figure 2.2   Protesting Abortion Regulation

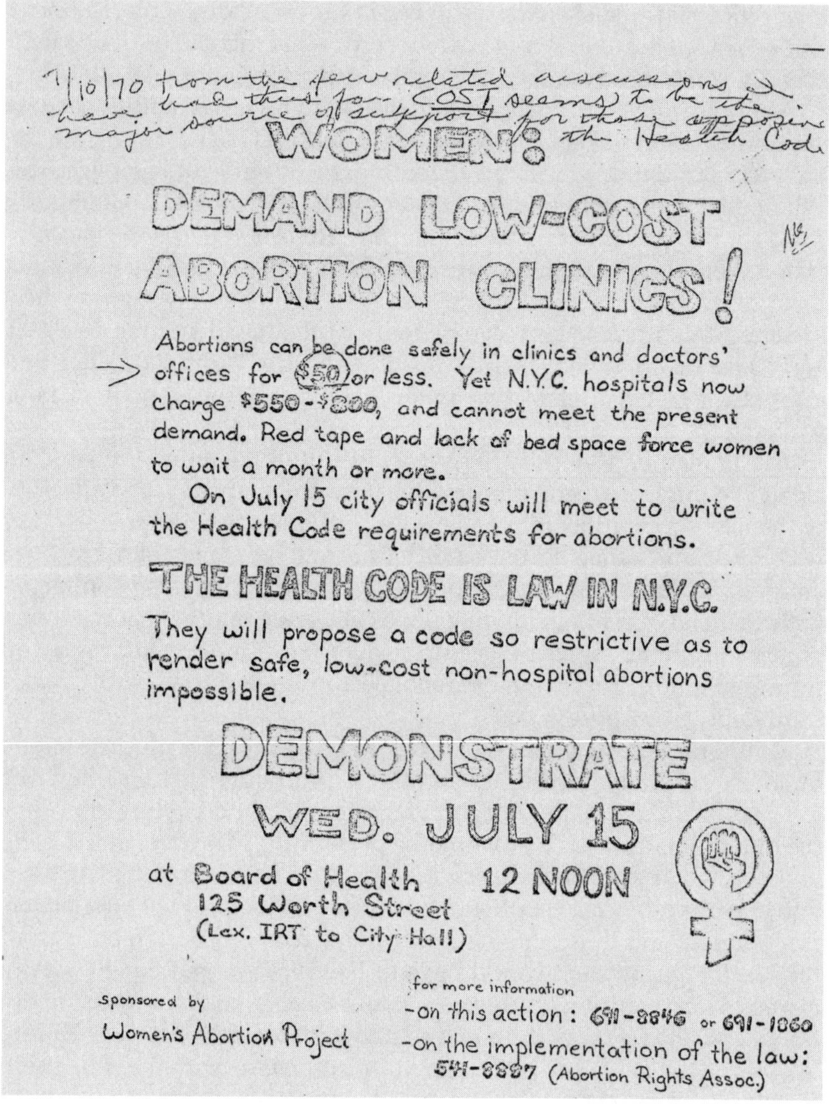

Source: Courtesy New York City Municipal Archives.
Note: A flyer announcing a July 1970 rally protesting the Board of Health's proposed restrictions on where abortions could be performed. Some abortion-rights activists claimed that restricting the procedure to hospitals would make it inaccessible to poor women. At the top of the flyer, an unidentified Health Department employee has written: "7/10/70 From the few related discussions I have had the COST seems to be the major source of support for those opposing the Health Code."

Figure 2.3   Abortion Hotline

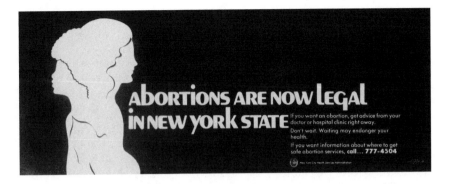

Source: Courtesy New York City Municipal Archives.
Note: After abortion became legal in the New York State in 1970, the New York City Health Department contracted with Planned Parenthood to operate an information hotline, which it publicized with a series of posters.

were done in hospitals. About 43 percent of women receiving abortions were nonwhite, and about 10 percent were Puerto Rican.

In 1971 New York City recorded its lowest maternal mortality rate on record, fulfilling the hopes of those who had predicted that the change in the law would lead to fewer deaths from women having the procedure done in illicit and unsafe conditions.[132] Free-standing clinics devoted to abortion proliferated. By 1972 there were twenty-one such facilities operating in the city; they performed about half of all abortions and disproportionately served women who came from outside the city. Costs of the procedure varied significantly, with the voluntary hospitals being the most expensive (and performing the smallest percentage among the types of facilities).[133]

New York was one of several jurisdictions that the U.S. Supreme Court cited when it ruled, two and a half years after Pakter and the obstetrics advisory committee completed their work, that the Constitution protected a woman's right to abortion. "Mortality rates for women undergoing early abortions, where the procedure is legal, appear to be as low as or lower than the rates for normal childbirth," the Court stated in *Roe v. Wade.* "Consequently, any interest of the State in protecting the woman from an inherently hazardous procedure, except when it would be equally dangerous for her to forgo it, has largely disappeared."[134] The battles sparked by *Roe* would be a central front in the "culture wars" waged in the last decades of the twentieth century. That these clashes often took place at the level of state and federal government policy makes it easy to forget the pivotal role played by the New York City

Health Department and Board of Health in ensuring that abortion was not just legal but safe.

Public Health and the People

The initiatives on lead paint, methadone, and abortion revealed, in different ways, how the social turmoil of the 1960s complicated the mission of the Health Department. Changing popular attitudes about the plight of the urban poor, the causes and consequences of drug use, and the reproductive rights of women catalyzed new public health programs and changed the direction of existing ones. The three issues, though diverse in their particulars, all raised the question of whether and how public health professionals should respond in the context of societal inequity and exclusion.

One driver of change during these years was an increasingly activist federal government that supported new programs. The 1960s were flush years for health and social welfare spending nationwide, and much of it benefited local public health. The flow of money into New York City through an assortment of categorical programs was incoherent, however. The vagaries of funding streams expanded some programs, like family planning and methadone maintenance, dramatically, while others, like lead paint abatement, went begging. For example, Lindsay's budget office tried to convince the federal Department of Housing and Urban Development (HUD) to fund the city's lead testing and abatement through the Model Cities Program, an ambitious effort to renew blighted inner city areas, but the agency refused.[135]

In the cases of lead paint abatement and abortion regulation, public health involvement was also driven by the demands of radicalized community members, who used new forms of direct action that had become common in the civil rights movement. Protests, demonstrations, and sit-ins all played a role at pivotal moments in the debates over both issues; activists also had to gain the support of politicians and legislators to achieve their goals. In the case of lead paint, advocates won their key demand of expanded testing for lead poisoning and stronger health code rules to force abatement. In the case of abortion regulations, in contrast, the Health Department largely retained professional control, rebuffing the demands of activists who wanted the procedure to be available with no restrictions.

The case of methadone maintenance was somewhat different. The question of how to respond to rising numbers of heroin users was largely an interprofessional struggle. Law enforcement and addiction treatment experts were equally committed to their own view of the nature of drug use and resisted the reframing of the problem as a physiological condition that should be managed in a manner analogous to treatment for diabetes or other chronic medical conditions. To the extent that a "community" viewpoint was present at all, it was the opposition of neighborhood residents where methadone clinics were proposed. These residents generally rejected the move to treat addiction as a health problem when it seemed that such a course of action might bring the problem closer to their front door; they preferred instead to have the government deal with drug users through traditional law enforcement means. Yet in the widespread expansion of methadone clinics, public health professionals were able, to a surprising extent, to circumvent the opposition of those who favored drug policies emphasizing interdiction and criminalization.

Finally, the debates over all three of these issues were strongly overlaid with moral judgments: about the obligations of society to the poor, about the meaning of addiction, and about the rights of women and their fetuses. The language of values pervaded the discussions as the Health Department sought to craft policies and programs. Lead paint poisoning was not just a health problem but a moral outrage (claimed proponents of more aggressive outreach and abatement); narcotic use should be treated like other illnesses, not like a weakness of character (argued methadone supporters); abortion was a medical procedure, not a sin (said feminists and most public health professionals). These struggles gave lie to the notion that public health was, or could be, a purely technical and value-neutral enterprise.

Chapter 3

Dropping Dead

IN THE early 1970s, the Health Department's staff continued to grapple with whether and how to address issues beyond their traditional purview—as they had done with lead paint, heroin addiction, and abortion—and what role they should play in providing clinical care. These debates reflected a broader soul-searching in American public health about the field's mission and purpose. Should it be a force for social justice and political change? Should it return to its nineteenth-century roots and attempt to reassert its authority over areas such as housing and environmental sanitation? In New York City, however, such questions would soon become moot. Powerful economic forces were taking shape that would create an unprecedented fiscal crisis for the city and the Health Department. In 1974 the city would enter a period of chaos—economic, social, political—and the imperative to slash budgets and personnel would overtake all other priorities. To the extent that there was an overarching mission of public health in the city after 1974, it was survival in the face of adversity.

Innovation and Its Limits

The sense that the public health profession "had run out of things to do"—as one member of the New York City Board of Health put it—grew steadily in the postwar years.[1] Many of the problems related to infectious diseases that had preoccupied earlier generations of public health workers seemed to have been solved. Heart disease, cancer, and stroke had become the country's leading causes of death in the 1920s, but there was no clear course of action—no analog to vaccines or antibiotics—against diseases with complex and poorly understood etiologies. As a result, few state and local health departments addressed chronic illnesses thought to be related to diet, smoking, and other "lifestyle" factors. In the 1960s, the nascent environmental movement brought renewed attention to the toxic hazards lurking in the air and water, but responsibility for these issues was typically vested in specialized agencies of environmental protection whose staff had a professional identity distinct from public health and felt little connection to health departments.[2]

Just as the profession had failed to innovate in preventing diseases of consumption or the environment, so had it been unable to carve out a role for itself in remaking the health care system. Surgeon General Luther Terry's 1963 exhortation that the profession "belonged in the field of medical care" had gone largely unanswered by the rank and file. A few key public health leaders—notably New York's health commissioner, George James, and hospitals commissioner, Alonzo Yerby—gave input to decisionmakers in Washington during the creation of the era's signature achievements, Medicaid and Medicare, but the profession generally remained marginal to the implementation of the programs. Both conceptually and administratively, Medicaid remained within a welfare paradigm, housed in state and local welfare departments.[3]

Among his profession's sharpest critics was the president of the American Public Health Association, Paul Cornely. In his keynote address at the group's 1970 annual meeting in Houston, he chided his colleagues for neglecting the "hidden enemies of health" lurking in modern consumer society and for failing to put forth any concrete proposal for a national health plan during the preceding decade, when the possibility of so much change had been on the table. Cornely charged that the association had been "a mere bystander" on urgent social issues such as occupational health and environmental protection. Public health professionals, he claimed, remained "outside the power structure."[4]

At the same time that public health was confronting the limits of its traditional role, the medical profession was undergoing its own identity crisis. Politicians and prominent media commentators, joined by critics within the profession, decried a health care system that was costly, wasteful, and too focused on high-technology curative interventions at the expense of routine prevention.[5] Radical groups such as Health/PAC had launched this line of attack in the 1960s; picking up where activists had left off, academics of various disciplines produced a spate of books in the 1970s describing the modern medical enterprise as, at best, misguided and, at worst, malignant. Among the most widely read of these polemics were *Who Shall Live?* by the economist Victor Fuchs; *Medical Nemesis* by the philosopher Ivan Illich; *Effectiveness and Efficiency* by the physician Archibald Cochrane; *The Role of Medicine* by the historical demographer Thomas McKeown; and *Doing Better and Feeling Worse*, a collection of essays by some of the country's leading academics and policymakers, edited by John Knowles, a physician and the president of the Rockefeller Foundation.[6]

All of these works challenged the hegemonic notion that medicine was an unalloyed force for good in society. Attacks on the medical profession dovetailed with a newly prominent discourse of "personal responsibility." According to this line of reasoning, blame for society's ills rested on the lifestyle habits of individuals; the remedy for problems such as smoking, substance use, and sexually transmitted disease was not the ministrations of health professionals but better behavior from the citizenry.[7]

Criticism of what was often called the "medical industrial complex" might have redounded to the benefit of public health had anyone in the profession been able to make the case that preventive programs were a more just, effective, and efficient alternative. Yet skepticism about the power and goals of curative medicine was not accompanied by a corollary improvement in the standing or influence of public health. Through failures of imagination and will, public health leaders were slow to innovate within a new epidemiological context and unsuccessful at navigating a changing political environment.

The sense of purposelessness was reflected in a gloomy 1973 article by Assistant Surgeon General John Hanlon titled "Is There a Future for Local Health Departments?" Surveying the prospects for a vigorous course of action, Hanlon found little reason for optimism. "Something unhealthy," he lamented, "seems to have happened of late to public health. We seem caught in the doldrums or in some kind of professional Sargasso Sea."[8] He noted that the Department of Health, Education, and Welfare had recently stopped maintaining its registry of local health departments, clearly signaling how marginal the federal government considered these units to be.[9] The most urgent health issues of the day, from the environment to universal insurance coverage, seemed to transcend the parochial concerns of individual cities. Traditional public health as it was practiced at the local level was in danger of becoming little more than a residual category, a hodgepodge of data collection and petty regulation.

New York City's Health Department had mixed results navigating this unsettled environment. The ultimately fruitless efforts to increase the department's involvement in ambulatory care illustrated the difficulty of asserting new roles. In contrast, the department's initiatives against lead poisoning and heroin addiction showed that ventures outside the traditional public health bailiwick could be successful. The latter efforts had been spearheaded by Gordon Chase, the health services administrator, and they carried his hallmarks: a hard-charging managerial style, a talent for circumventing bureaucratic obstacles, a penchant for quantification and goal setting, and an eye for politically appealing programs responsive to problems that were widely perceived as urgent. During John Lindsay's second term, from 1970 through 1973, these characteristics defined the city's public health decisionmaking. Chase's leadership won praise from many of the skeptics in the medical community

who had initially opposed his appointment, but it also created dissatisfaction and dissent within the Health Department.

Much of the conflict grew out of the bifurcated structure of the Health
Department and the Health Services Administration superagency. For
the first several years after Lindsay created the superagency, it had had
little impact on the city's public health activities, beyond imposing an
additional layer of bureaucracy that sometimes made the implementation of programs slower and more cumbersome. The first two health services administrators, Howard Brown and Bernard Bucove, had been
preoccupied with the city's perpetually troubled municipal hospital system, and neither had stayed in the job long enough to affect the direction
of public health.

Things changed with Lindsay's hiring of Gordon Chase. As an out-
sider, Chase was not beholden to the city's many entrenched health care
interests, nor was he burdened by preconceived notions of how responsibility for health problems should be divided. He also enjoyed a much
better working relationship with Lindsay than either of his predecessors
had. Chase was a devotee of program, planning, and budgeting systems
(PPBS), a project management technique in which problems were broken down into "inputs" and "outputs" that were to be manipulated into
optimal results, regardless of the content of the problem. PPBS was popular in Lyndon Johnson's administration, where Chase had worked before coming to New York; it was also favored by Mayor Lindsay's "good
government" advisers, especially in his Bureau of the Budget.[10] Chase
had used PPBS in his efforts to improve management at the city's Human Resources Administration, where he had won Lindsay's admira-
tion and convinced the mayor that similar results could be achieved in
the health arena.

One of Chase's first moves clearly signaled his belief in the importance of management techniques: he hired the consulting firm McKinsey
& Company to survey the Health Department.[11] He then went about setting up what was essentially a shadow department at 125 Worth Street.
Whereas the health services administrator had previously operated with
almost no staff of his own, Chase recruited into the HSA a cadre of two
dozen aides—typically giving them the generic title of "program ana-
lyst"—who had management expertise but no public health background.[12] None was older than the thirty-seven-year-old Chase. They
developed their own priorities, initiatives, and procedures and explicitly
excluded the Health Department's professional staff who were nomi-
nally responsible for the issues.

One of Chase's most ambitious undertakings was to convert selected
child health stations, which provided screening and preventive services
but no treatment, into full-service clinics. Located in the city's poorest

neighborhoods, often in public housing projects, the centers had once represented the cutting edge in progressive well-child care. By the 1960s, however, their shortcomings were increasingly difficult to ignore. After years of deferred maintenance, most of the stations badly needed renovations.[13] The services, generally performed by part-time hourly physicians, had failed to keep up with the state of the art in pediatric medicine. And children found to have a problem requiring treatment were unlikely to receive appropriate follow-up care because of their parents' difficult life circumstances and lack of a regular doctor.[14] The department had piloted a full-service pediatric clinic in the Bedford District Health Center, but plans for upgrading and expanding more of the centers had repeatedly foundered through a combination of bureaucratic inertia, lack of funds, and opposition from unions concerned about possible layoffs should the conversion involve a partnership with a nearby hospital. Chase was determined to move the plans forward.

He placed the task in the hands of his program analysts, to whom he gave management authority over budgeting, staffing, and construction. The conversions began in late 1972 and continued through early 1974. In all, nineteen of the seventy-six child health stations were converted to "pediatric treatment centers" offering a full range of both diagnostic and curative services.[15] A subsequent evaluation found high acceptance of the facilities and generally improved utilization, especially in areas where there were few alternative providers nearby.[16] Even skeptics applauded the achievement. Its success depended, critically, on Chase's ability to get around many of the bureaucratic hurdles related to hiring and capital costs that had stymied Mary McLaughlin in her efforts to create the family care centers.

Not all of Chase's initiatives won acclaim, however. Health problems were not widgets, critics argued, and numbers alone could give an incomplete or misleading picture of success. A program of blood pressure screening in community settings throughout the city in 1971 and 1972 illustrated the potential pitfalls of Chase's approach. It was "successful" in the sense that it enabled the city to report that it had screened large numbers of individuals and uncovered many with high blood pressure. People with expertise in health services, however, pointed out what Chase's analysts could not or would not recognize: screening conducted in community settings was of questionable reliability and validity; it failed to reach those most at risk of hypertension; and without procedures in place to ensure follow-up care, the vast majority of those found to have high blood pressure would not end up receiving treatment for it.[17] Health Department veterans charged that efforts such as these were poorly thought out and undertaken more for the short-term political gain that they held for Lindsay than their overall significance for public health or their relative merit compared with other pressing needs.[18]

Chase's staff brushed aside such criticisms and insisted that substantive experience in health was irrelevant, or at least secondary, in designing programs. "When presented with a choice between [hiring] less capable persons with health backgrounds and more analytic persons without health experience or training," two of his deputies later wrote, "we often chose the latter. Generalized health knowledge was often superfluous when dealing with highly particularized problems in a rapidly changing context like that presented by the City of New York."[19] The dismissive attitude reflected in this comment illustrated that the tensions between the HSA and the Health Department were related not just to substance but to style. Chase's program analysts barely concealed their disdain for the department old-timers who had risen through the public health ranks.

One casualty of the conflicts between the department and the superagency was health commissioner Mary McLaughlin, whose years of frontline experience exemplified the type of background that fell out of favor under Chase. She repeatedly clashed with Chase in her efforts to protect the autonomy of Health Department operations and keep the HSA program analysts from doing end-runs around the department's professional staff. Her refusal to get out of Chase's way led Lindsay to replace her at the end of 1971 with Joseph Cimino, a mild-mannered environmental scientist who had run the department's poison control program. Cimino, though more accommodating of Chase than McLaughlin had been, was no figurehead: he was a thoughtful and dedicated public servant who brought great scientific rigor to the post. He oversaw a major reorganization in the reporting relationship between the central office and the health officers working in the five boroughs.[20] But during Cimino's two-year tenure as health commissioner, it was Gordon Chase and the HSA staff who were the dominant forces in public health policymaking.

The end of the Lindsay mayoralty brought a close to the Chase regime and the Health Services Administration superagency. Lindsay's political fortunes, which had seemed boundless when he was first elected in 1965, plummeted during his second term, and after a disastrous decision to switch parties and an aborted run for the presidency, he announced in March 1973 that he would not seek reelection. Chase resigned a few months later, earning Lindsay's praise as a "truly brilliant" administrator.[21]

That fall, Abraham Beame, who had served as comptroller under Wagner and Lindsay, was elected mayor with the backing of most of the city's Democratic establishment and labor unions. Beame was a colorless bureaucrat whose chief claim to the office was—ironically, it would turn out—managerial and accounting competence. (His campaign slogan was "He knows the buck.")[22] Beame called the superagency concept an "administrative disaster," and as a candidate he pledged to eliminate the Health Services Administration along with two other superagencies that Lindsay had created, Human Resources and Housing and Development.[23] Dismantling superagencies was complicated legally, so the HSA continued to exist on paper, but it effectively ceased functioning once Beame took office. The health commissioner was given the (now-ceremonial) joint title of health services administrator and once again reported directly to the mayor; Chase's staff of program analysts swiftly followed their former boss out the door.[24] The City Council would ultimately approve legislation in 1977, formally abolishing all nine of the superagencies that Lindsay had created.[25]

To lead the once-again independent Health Department, Beame chose Lowell Bellin, who had won wide respect for his efforts to end Medicaid fraud and waste in the late 1960s (see figure 3.1). Bellin had left the department in 1972 to join the faculty of the Columbia School of Public Health, but with the HSA out of the way he wanted the job of commissioner and lobbied aggressively for it with Beame's advisers.[26] Once back at 125 Worth Street, he wasted no time in repudiating Chase's legacy of "project management." Bellin passionately believed in public health as a rigorous, science-based discipline, and he found Chase's approach anathema. As a colleague of both men later recalled, Bellin considered Chase to be "a *wunderkind* without the *wunder*."[27]

It is revealing that the subject of Bellin's first speech as commissioner, to the Public Health Association of New York City, was not a new programmatic initiative but his efforts to reverse what he saw as the department's institutional decline over the previous four years under Gordon Chase and the baleful influence of the Health Services Administration. Bellin never mentioned Chase's name, but it was clear to everyone whom he was criticizing. Bellin told his audience that under the leadership of his predecessor, "committed amateurism and chutzpah had supplanted relevant education and experience in health affairs." While Chase had considered his staff of program analysts to be skilled problem-solvers who approached public health issues with fresh eyes and much-needed innovation, Bellin saw them as "Sorcerer's Apprentices gone wild." Bellin's speech described his efforts to "re-professionalize" the department by recruiting staff with substantive expertise in traditional public health disciplines such as epidemiology, environmental science, and medicine.[28]

The task of recruitment was not an easy one. The department had had increasing difficulty attracting skilled public health workers over the prior decade, both because the center of gravity had shifted to the superagency, where such a background was not valued, and because of stagnating salaries in the field. In his favor, Bellin was able to draw upon an

Figure 3.1   Bellin Takes Charge

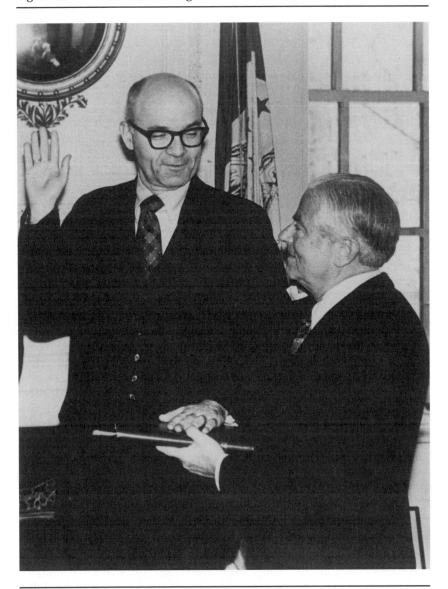

Source: Courtesy New York City Municipal Archives.
Note: Lowell Bellin (left) is sworn in as health commissioner by Mayor Abraham Beame in January 1974. Before the end of the year, New York City would begin its slide into insolvency.

extensive network of professional connections, especially among his former students at the School of Public Health at Columbia, and he was a charismatic leader (a quality he shared with both Lindsay and Chase). In convincing young professionals to come work at the Health Department, which offered a lower salary than they would draw in the private sector, he presented the opportunity not as a sinecure civil service position but as a chance to gain valuable experience in the exciting urban "laboratory" of New York City before moving on to other jobs.[29]

Even as he set about rebuilding the department, Bellin confronted a constrained fiscal environment. Federal funding for public health programs, which had steadily (if unevenly) expanded during the 1960s, began to shrink, and the idea that the government should be responsible for generous social welfare provisions went into retreat. The Democrat-controlled Congress of Richard Nixon's first term had prevented the elimination of most Great Society programs and indeed oversaw a dramatic expansion in Social Security benefits. The first budget of Nixon's second term, however, made deep cuts to the HEW and signaled a new period of retrenchment. Nixon dismembered the Office of Economic Opportunity, the intellectual and financial nerve center of the War on Poverty, and farmed out its constituent parts to the Departments of Labor, Commerce, and HEW. The Model Cities Program, which had once been a source of support for public health initiatives, was phased out in 1974.[30]

Nixon's administration, under attack in the Watergate investigation, eventually restored some funding that had been slated for elimination, but the writing on the wall was clear: the Great Society was at an end.[31] In New York City, the grim budget numbers prompted the Health Department's maternity and infant care program, heavily dependent on federal grants for its family planning, prenatal, and well-baby services, to lay off several dozen employees.[32] As the national economy contracted into a recession in late 1973, the outlook grew worse.

Economic woes at the national level were—not coincidentally—soon joined by budget problems closer to home. In late 1974, near the end of his first year as commissioner, Bellin received an urgent directive from the city's Office of Management and Budget (OMB). He would have twenty-four hours to identify some $1.5 million, or about 3 percent, to cut from the amount of city funding in the department budget. Bellin turned for assistance to his closest adviser, Pascal "Pat" Imperato, an infectious disease doctor he had recruited to run the Bureau of Preventable Diseases. The two hastily cobbled together a recommendation to eliminate almost seventy positions from the Bureaus of Social Work, Nutrition, and Health Education.

Bellin and Imperato knew that other city agencies were being asked to make similar cuts and that the unusual urgency of the OMB request was an ominous sign of the city's financial condition. They did not know that their deliberations marked the beginning of what would become the largest reduction of the department's budget and personnel in its history.

"Welcome to Fear City"

Under Mayors Wagner, Lindsay, and Beame, New York City spent more money than it took in and borrowed to cover the difference. This untenable strategy came to an end when lenders determined that the city was no longer a good credit risk.[33] The imbalance between what the city took in and what it paid out had complex causes, some specific to local policies and politics and others rooted in far-reaching demographic and economic trends that were affecting many of the nation's big cities. The retrenchment that came in the wake of the insolvency colored every aspect of city life and determined the fate of public health activities both directly and indirectly for at least two decades, its influence being felt long after the city had returned to fiscal stability.

On one side of the ledger were rapidly increasing municipal expenditures, both in areas that were traditionally part of city budgets, such as police, fire, and sanitation, and for services, such as public assistance and higher education, that most cities did not provide (these expenses typically being borne by the states). Indeed, the largest increases in the city's budget were expenditures on welfare and education. Between 1961 and 1976, city spending in each of these areas increased tenfold. The growth in these areas can be attributed partly to a commitment on the part of the city's leaders to social democratic ideals of equal opportunity and generous safety net provisions. It was also a response to the threat of civil unrest by newly radicalized poor communities.

In the area of welfare policy, the city's public assistance rolls expanded dramatically during the 1960s. The change was driven in part by a grassroots movement led by the National Welfare Rights Organization (NWRO), a coalition of groups around the country with headquarters in Washington, D.C. Activists working with federal antipoverty agencies sought to end the practices that had long been used, either covertly or explicitly, to limit welfare rolls, such as citing technicalities to throw people off for eligibility violations. New York City was at the vanguard of the welfare rights movement; among its chief theorists and proponents were Richard Cloward, a Columbia University social work professor, and Mitchell Ginsberg, the city's welfare commissioner. Welfare recipients staged demonstrations organized by the NWRO at the offices of the Department of Social Services and flooded offices with applications in a bid to get the city to increase payments.[34] Under Ginsberg's direction, the Welfare Department made it easier for potential clients to sign up and retain benefits, changes that prompted the conservative *Daily News* to give the commissioner the contemptuous nickname "Come-and-Get-It

Ginsberg." The city's Aid to Families with Dependent Children (AFDC) caseload roughly quintupled in the 1960s and early 1970s, from around 50,000 clients to 250,000.[35]

In the realm of education policy, the spending increases were triggered by the adoption in 1970 at the sixteen-campus City University of New York (CUNY) system, which had been tuition-free since its founding in 1847, of an "open admission" policy: any high school graduate would be allowed to attend. As with the growth in welfare spending, the CUNY decision was partly a result of direct action by activists. African American and Puerto Rican students had staged demonstrations that shut down CUNY's flagship City College campus in 1969. The protests, during a time of heightened racial tensions and a hard-fought mayoral race, hastened the adoption of the new policy, but plans for open enrollment had in fact been in the works for several years. Moreover, the policy was not specifically designed to assist ethnic minorities, nor were these groups the primary beneficiaries: working-class white students had been those most likely to receive a score just below qualification for admittance to CUNY.[36] Whatever its intent, the new policy almost doubled the size of the incoming freshman class; total enrollment in 1970 was around 200,000, double what it had been a decade earlier. To handle the influx of new students, many of whom required remedial instruction, the size of the full-time staff grew from some 15,000 to more than 20,000.

In part to deal with the greatly increased CUNY class size and the rapidly rising welfare rolls, city government grew by about 50 percent, from 200,000 employees to almost 300,000. Between 1970 and 1974 alone, the municipal workforce expanded by 33,000 while the city shed almost 120,000 private-sector jobs.[37] The cost per employee also rose dramatically. City workers unionized at a rapid clip throughout the 1960s, and civil service unions negotiated generous wage and benefits packages for their members.[38] Lindsay, having been badly bruised in the labor skirmishes of his first term, gave expensive concessions to unions during his 1969 reelection campaign. By 1974, the city's labor costs had quadrupled from a decade earlier.

Meanwhile, broad national trends in employment and housing were adversely affecting the city's financial position. Federal policies in areas such as highway construction and tax incentives for home ownership encouraged an exodus of the middle class to new developments outside of the city, draining the city's taxpayer base.[39] Working-class blacks and Puerto Ricans seeking better employment opportunities were drawn to the city in large numbers as the middle class fled to the suburbs. Between 1960 and 1970, the city lost about one million middle-class white residents and gained about the same number of poor or working-class black and Puerto Rican residents. Even as this transformation was occurring, the light manufacturing sector and the garment and construction industries, which had traditionally provided blue-collar work for city residents, were shrinking as once-reliable jobs moved to other regions of the country or overseas. White-collar employment, including jobs in the financial, insurance, and real estate sectors, also declined sharply after 1969. In the terminology of the political scientists Wallace Sayre and Herbert Kaufman, in their influential analysis *Governing New York City*, the city's "service demanders" grew more numerous and their needs more urgent while the "money providers" became fewer and lost much of their fiscal strength.[40]

Mayors Wagner, Lindsay, and Beame all used a variety of questionable fiscal gimmicks to cover the gap between what the city took in and what it gave out—for example, relying on unrealistically optimistic budget projections and advancing the collection date to June 30 for taxes that were due July 1 in order to count the revenues for the current fiscal year. Lindsay balanced the budget during his first term, but each year after his reelection he ran large deficits financed through short-term notes and long-term bonds. By 1975, the city's deficit had ballooned to $3 billion.

The major financial institutions had long turned a blind eye to the city's questionable practices, partly because they earned substantial fees and commissions from servicing the city's debt. In 1973, however, the national economy entered a steep recession triggered by the Arab oil embargo and the costs of the Vietnam War. The bankers, hard-hit by their many loans to multinational corporations and developing countries, became increasingly skittish about continuing to roll over the city's debt. In the fall of 1974, the banks began to dump the notes and bonds they held, which worsened the market for the city's securities. In March 1975, they announced that they would no longer continue to underwrite the city's debt obligations. New York City was without creditors.

Beame's efforts to deal with the unfolding crisis were, in the eyes of most observers, feeble and inadequate.[41] In May, New York governor Hugh Carey stepped in and created the Municipal Assistance Corporation, an independent public agency that could sell bonds to meet the city's credit needs. The corporation initially seemed to promise a way out of the crisis, but by the end of the summer it had been unable to find buyers for the city's debt. In September, Carey made an even more drastic move, creating the Emergency Financial Control Board (EFCB), which placed fiscal control of the city into the hands of a seven-member body: the governor, the state comptroller, the mayor, the city comptroller, and three gubernatorial appointees who were corporate executives. The EFCB was given plenary authority over all aspects of the city budget, including expenditures, borrowing, and contracts with municipal unions.

Under the terms of the legislation that created the EFCB, the city would be required to balance its budget within three years.

When the creation of the EFCB proved insufficient to entice buyers for the city's securities, Carey asked the federal government to serve as a lender of last resort, but President Gerald Ford demurred. In a speech at the National Press Club at the end of October, Ford declared that he would veto any bill to federally guarantee the city's bonds, and the president added insult to injury by blaming the city's predicament on its own poor management. The day after the speech, the *Daily News*, with the flair for melodrama for which it was renowned, ran on its front page what would become an iconic image of the crisis: the boldface headline "Ford to City: Drop Dead." That the headline was inaccurate—Ford in fact wanted the city to escape insolvency, since its default would cause turmoil in the nation's financial markets—was beside the point. It captured a larger truth about the city's self-image. To many New Yorkers, it did seem that their city was on the verge of dropping dead. (Ford eventually reversed his position and supported a bill extending $2.3 billion in federal loans to the city.)

Throughout the chaotic months of 1975, the specter of imminent collapse—of a government unable to pay its employees or conduct its business, respond to fires, educate children, or collect garbage—hovered over the city. Public spectacles mounted by city workers and advocacy groups heightened the sense of crisis. Having been largely excluded by the powerful banking and financial interests from the formal decision-making about the city's future, they took to the streets for demonstrations and guerrilla actions. Garbage piled up as sanitation workers staged wildcat strikes and work stoppages. Ten thousand members of municipal unions demonstrated at the headquarters of First National City Bank (later Citibank), one of the institutions that had dumped city securities and then refused to continue lending. The United Federation of Teachers organized a "day of mourning" at which some 15,000 teachers, parents, and students wearing black armbands marched on City Hall to protest education cutbacks. At transportation hubs such as Grand Central Station and the Port Authority Bus Terminal, members of police and fire unions handed out leaflets illustrated with a hooded death's-head under the headline "Welcome to Fear City," warning that New York would become too dangerous to visit should proposed cuts to public safety services be made. Several hundred police officers who had received pink slips marched onto the Brooklyn Bridge, where they blocked traffic, rocked cars back and forth, and flattened the tires of the trapped motorists.[42]

"London life in the Hitler Blitz of 1940 must have been something like life in New York these days," *Times* columnist Russell Baker wrote in the fall. "New York goes to bed every night wondering if it will still be there by dawn."[43]

Life-Preserving, Life-Enhancing

As the crisis unfolded over the spring and summer of 1975, it became clear that the initial round of cuts that Lowell Bellin had been ordered to make to the Health Department budget would be only the beginning. He assembled a team of five close advisers who would help him decide how to make the further reductions that were certain to be necessary. Bellin chose the group partly based on the key positions they held in the department, but he considered their backgrounds and temperaments as well. He valued colleagues who were plainspoken and willing to disagree and defend their positions; he also wanted input from people with training in medicine and academic public health. His desire for these qualities influenced the composition of his inner circle during the crisis.

Pat Imperato, the first deputy commissioner (the official second-in-command at the department), was Bellin's primary adviser. Imperato had trained in infectious diseases during an era when that specialty had fallen out of fashion; he was skeptical toward the conventional wisdom that contagions would soon vanish as a threat to health. As a member of the CDC's Epidemic Intelligence Service (EIS), he had worked on the global smallpox eradication program in West Africa. His in-the-trenches background impressed Bellin, and since joining the department his creative efforts to reorganize key aspects of the epidemiology program had earned his boss's respect. Peter Levin, the associate commissioner for program planning and analysis, was a health services researcher trained at Yale and Johns Hopkins whom Bellin had tapped in his efforts to "re-professionalize" the department. Levin functioned as a kind of jack-of-all-trades in the department. Jean Cropper was one of Bellin's former students at Columbia whom he had brought in to lead environmental health services; Cropper's diverse responsibilities included restaurant inspections, monitoring the quality of water on city beaches, control of rats, and the window guard program. Haynes Rice was an African American physician with a master's degree in business administration who had been a top administrator at Harlem Hospital Center. Bellin had recruited Rice to serve as the department's liaison with the city's public hospital system. Finally, Louis Neugeborn, a thirty-year department veteran and the chief administrative officer, was an expert in all matters related to budgets, personnel, and city government.[44]

The team first came together in early 1975, after the OMB had requested the initial round of cuts. The department's annual budget was approximately $90 million. About $50 million of that came from city tax levy; the remainder consisted of grants from the state and federal governments for specific programs such as venereal disease control and immunization, which were both largely funded by the Center for Disease Control.[45] It was city tax levy from which the cuts would have to come. Anticipating demands for steep reductions, the team held a series of painstaking meetings in which they pored over computer printouts listing dozens of programs and thousands of employees.[46]

Three core principles guided the group's decisions about what to cut. First, each department function was categorized as either "life-preserving" or "life-enhancing," with the former having priority. Life-preserving services included infectious disease control activities such as immunization programs, while life-enhancing programs included dental clinics, health education, and nutrition counseling. "Nobody ever died of bad teeth and bad gums," Bellin said. "I had to weigh that against diphtheria inoculations. I didn't have money for both."[47] Second, the group sought to sustain even downsized programs with a small nucleus of core staff so that no department service would completely or permanently disappear. Finally, programs targeted for cutting would be those for which alternative providers existed in the city. This principle pointed toward the elimination of what were known as "personal health services"—the individual screening and preventive education that the district health centers and child health stations offered—since these were, at least in theory, also available through private practitioners and the outpatient departments and neighborhood clinics run by the city's hospitals.[48]

With these guidelines in place, Bellin's team convened weekly meetings with affected deputy and assistant commissioners and program managers throughout the agency to get their feedback on the merits, drawbacks, and potential consequences of the cuts that were being planned. Especially key was input from the district health officers, who oversaw the personal health services in each of the city's thirty health districts and who provided utilization data for each health center or child health station.[49] In laying the groundwork for potential elimination of some of the department's clinical facilities, Haynes Rice also worked in close consultation with the Health and Hospitals Corporation (HHC), the semipublic agency that ran the public hospitals, to ensure that, should cuts in personal health services be necessary, they would be made in locations where HHC would be able to step in as provider.

The major cuts in the Health Department budget came in three rounds over fourteen months. In May 1975, after Beame released what he called a "crisis budget," the OMB sent another round of cuts to the Health Department totaling $18 million. Beame soon came out with a less draconian "austerity budget," and the demand for cuts was reduced to a (still painful) $5 million. In spite of having no expertise in public health, the mayor's accountants had identified 255 specific positions they wanted to eliminate; many of the cuts, not surprisingly, were ill advised. For example, the OMB recommended closing the tropical medicine clinic in northern Manhattan, evidently believing that New York's nontropical latitude made the facility superfluous, without realizing that it was the only facility in the city able to provide treatment for many rare but deadly conditions, including ongoing care for about seventy patients with Hansen's disease, or leprosy. The accountants swiftly backpedaled when Pat Imperato conjured up the specter of dozens of untreated lepers spreading their disease on the city subways (a frightening though misleading scenario, since leprosy is rarely transmitted through casual contact).[50]

Because of the work of the previous four months, Bellin and his team were able to counter with a list based on their own prioritizations, which the OMB accepted. They eliminated the Health Research Council, which Leona Baumgartner had established in the 1950s to fund extramural studies of emerging health problems and intervention approaches.[51] In addition, a neighborhood maternity center in the Bronx was closed, and about $1 million was cut from the methadone maintenance program.

Deeper cuts soon followed. In the fall, the OMB demanded an additional $3 million in reductions. Bellin chose to discontinue city funding for the "ghetto medicine" program, one of the department's signature initiatives of the 1960s, which had enabled it to oversee the ambulatory care services offered in public hospitals' outpatient departments. (The state continued to fund a portion of the program, allowing it to continue in a much-debilitated form.) Finally, in July 1976, City Hall ordered that additional savings worth $4.4 million would have to be found. This time, the ax fell on personal health services, which had largely been spared thus far. Seven of the city's twenty district health centers were closed, along with twenty of the seventy-six child health stations and five of fourteen chest clinics, which were responsible for diagnosing and treating tuberculosis.

The department was also on the receiving end of orphaned city programs. In 1977 the department absorbed the Addiction Services Agency —or what was left of it. The city had cut off all funding, and the state had reduced funds as well, resulting in layoffs of about half the staff and the elimination of all direct services. All that remained were the contractual arrangements with community-based treatment services, about half the number as had been funded before the crisis.[52]

Some $10 million, or roughly 20 percent of the money the department received from the city, was lost in the three rounds of cuts. The largest cuts were made to the district health services, both in terms of personnel and expenditure; 1,500 of the positions cut, and $3.3 million of the budget, derived from closing district health centers, child health stations, and chest clinics. Some of the reductions represented housecleaning that might have been carried out even without the city's fiscal emergency. Imperato admitted to an audience at the New York Academy of Medicine that three of the seven district health centers that had been closed were underutilized and that their closure would have minimal impact on the city's health.[53] Yet there was no question that many valuable programs that enhanced the health and well-being of city residents all but vanished in 1975 and 1976.

The elimination of programs represents only part of the story of the crisis. Staff were laid off throughout the department, reducing capacity in every corner. When the first request for cuts had come down in November 1974, the department employed some 6,000 people, 4,400 full-time and 1,600 part-time. Over the following two years, the workforce shrank by 1,700, or 28 percent. The majority of this shrinkage was done through attrition resulting from retirements and resignations; only about 400 people were laid off. Although Bellin's team had been creative and determined enough to retain at least minimal continuity in some scaled-back programs, the remaining staff struggled to continue their work. When the staff of nutritionists, who provided counseling and education at district health centers and community organizations around the city, was cut from twenty-three to five in the first round of layoffs in November 1974, the program was effectively killed.[54] "As far as I'm concerned," said Catherine Cowell, the director of the nutrition bureau, "they've wiped out our entire service."[55]

When staffing shortages endangered two of the department's largest direct service programs, Bellin spared them through administrative legerdemain. The maternity and infant care clinics provided prenatal and family planning services with funding from the federal Children's Bureau, and the Women, Infants, and Children (WIC) program was supported by the Department of Agriculture to provide food and nutritional support for low-income women and their infants and children. The two programs should have been safe because most of their budget came from grants, but their ability to continue operation was jeopardized by a city-wide hiring freeze instituted at the start of the crisis, which applied even to externally funded positions. In response, Bellin chose to subcontract both programs to the Medical and Health Research Association (MHRA), a private nonprofit organization with close ties to the department. As an independent agency, the MHRA was not subject to the city's hiring freeze and could operate free from the city's civil service requirements.[56]

Bellin also used creative cost-shifting to keep alive one of the department's most successful initiatives, the window guard program to prevent deaths from childhood falls. Faced with having to curtail free distribution of the window guards, Bellin determined that the best approach would be to amend the health code to require that landlords provide them instead. In the spring of 1976, the board unanimously approved a new regulation put forth by Bellin mandating that landlords install window guards in all apartments where children age ten or younger lived. The new law, the first of its kind in the country, drew a swift condemnation from the city's real estate interests, and a property management company filed suit alleging that the department had overstepped its bounds and placed an unacceptable financial burden on landlords (a claim curtly dismissed by the state supreme court a few months later).[57]

Nor did opposition to the window guard regulation come only from the private sector. The city's largest landlord was the Housing Authority, which estimated the cost of implementing the new rule in city-managed buildings at between $8 million and $10 million.[58] Deputy Mayor John Zuccoti, who had formerly chaired the city's Planning Commission and had close ties to the real estate industry, convinced Bellin to phase the requirement in over three years, with only the highest-risk areas being forced to comply in the first year.[59] When Pat Imperato replaced Bellin as commissioner in 1977, Zuccoti took the opportunity of the leadership change to press his case again, threatening to have Imperato fired if he did not repeal the window guard legislation. Imperato held his ground, and Zuccoti backed down.[60]

One way the Beame administration sought to minimize layoffs and plug staffing holes in city agencies was to redirect money from the federal Comprehensive Employment Training Act (CETA), which Congress had passed in 1973 to reduce the sting of recession and rising joblessness. Although the intent of the act was to create public-service jobs for the unemployed, big-city mayors soon found it to be an all-purpose way to keep their municipalities staffed (often with patronage jobs). Early in the fiscal crisis, Beame received permission from the U.S. Department of Labor to use CETA monies to ease the amount of retrenchment. By 1978, almost one in six Health Department employees was being paid through CETA funds.[61] But CETA was only a stopgap: it funded a position for a maximum of eighteen months, so that while programs may have been saved from immediate elimination, their long-term stability remained tenuous.[62]

The Health Department had the highest rate of attrition of any city agency, with approximately sixty people leaving per month. The majority of these were younger middle managers and professional staff of the sort the department had had difficulty attracting.[63] The department's reduced circumstances foreclosed the possibility of undertaking the type of creative initiatives it had historically pioneered; New York City no longer seemed a place where public health professionals could carve out a career for themselves. "You could not have stayed there and thought, 'I'm going to make a career at the New York City Health Department,'" recalled Peter Levin, one of Bellin's inner circle. "Absolutely not."[64] At the same time, however, adversity also fostered a spirit of camaraderie.

"We were New York City in 'Ford to City: Drop Dead,'" one epidemiologist recalled. "And I think we were giving the finger to Ford. We were going to do it despite him."[65]

The Hospital Wars

The reduction and elimination of Health Department programs drew scant protest either from activists who typically mobilized around public health issues or from the mainstream or alternative press. The radical *Health/PAC Bulletin* ran a scathing assessment of the cuts—titled "The Fall and Fall of the New York City Department of Health"—alleging that the department's leaders were not doing enough to protect their interests, but the article was exceptional (and its readership limited). At a time when the entire infrastructure of the city seemed to teeter on the edge of implosion, it was not surprising that the most vigorous political agitation would surround cuts to the municipal services that most directly affected the public's sense of order and well-being, such as police, fire, education, and garbage collection.

The relative silence over the cuts to the Health Department was in stark contrast to the outcry that met proposed reductions in the city's public hospital system, whose supporters were numerous, powerful, and well organized. Much of their outrage came to be directed at Lowell Bellin because, in addition to being health commissioner, he served as chair of the board of the Health and Hospitals Corporation, the quasi-public entity that ran the city's nineteen municipal institutions.

The state legislature had created the HHC in 1969, capping a decade of study, debate, and controversy over what should be done about the nineteen hospitals that the city operated. The HHC was a public benefit corporation, a unit of city government that controlled its own budget; it was able to issue bonds, hire contractors, and make purchasing arrangements independent of city rules. It was not directly under mayoral control, although the mayor appointed all sixteen members of the board of directors, who in turn chose the president. The corporation's semi-independent status was conceived as a way to remedy the hospitals' chronic managerial and budgetary woes. The system's fiscal status remained wobbly after the creation of the HHC, however, and there was little evidence that the new bureaucratic arrangement had remedied the poor management that plagued the institutions under the old Department of Hospitals.[66]

In December 1974, as the Beame administration began to recognize the magnitude of the crisis and sent out its initial demands for cuts in agency budgets, the mayor's office asked that the HHC eliminate more than five hundred jobs. The board voted unanimously to refuse, and Beame was powerless to force the cuts because of the HHC's independent status. Bellin joined the unanimous vote against the cuts because he believed that Beame's request was hasty and poorly thought out, not because he believed that reductions were unwarranted. On the contrary, Bellin saw the HHC as rife with waste and inefficiency, and he asked the board to investigate the possibility of closing some institutions. In February 1975, the board called for the closing of eight of the city's least-used public hospitals.[67]

The city's insolvency lent urgency to the issue of hospital closings, but behind this proximal impetus lay a deep and long-standing ideological divide over whether the city should operate such an extensive safety net of health care for the poor. For most of the 1970s, it was widely believed that some form of national health insurance would soon be enacted. Congress and policy think tanks put forth a welter of competing policy and legislative proposals. In 1969, Massachusetts senator Edward Kennedy, the leading congressional proponent of reform, introduced a sweeping "health security" plan that would have eliminated the market for private insurance and replaced it with a national single-payer system. The Nixon administration, ideologically opposed to an expanded role for the federal government, countered with a proposal for a new private-sector initiative, the health maintenance organization (HMO). The dual calamities of the Watergate scandal and the economic recession overwhelmed all other events on the national political scene in 1974, and the window of opportunity for reform closed.[68] At the time of New York's fiscal woes, however, there remained a widespread expectation that some form of universal coverage was imminent.

This belief lay at the root of Bellin's doubts about the need for New York City to operate nineteen public hospitals. He believed that the city's experience after the enactment of Medicaid foreshadowed changes to come. The use of the municipal hospitals had dropped off as patients voted with their feet and chose to receive their care at the private institutions from which financial barriers had long excluded them. Bellin was convinced that as the two-tier system fell away, so would the need for the city to serve as the provider of last resort.[69] For their part, defenders of the public hospital system emphasized the vital role that oversight and accountability played in municipal ownership. They were less sanguine about both the prospects for universal health coverage and the ability of the private sector to meet the needs of poor patients.[70]

From the start, the disagreement was strongly inflected with racial politics. The hospitals slated for elimination primarily served the city's black and Latino residents, and news of the proposed closings fed into the widespread and not inaccurate perception in poor communities that they were bearing the brunt of the city's economizing. More significant, over half of the HHC's 40,000 employees were black.[71] While the hospitals had symbolic importance for the residents of the neighborhoods they served, it was their more concrete value as sources of jobs that made the prospect of their closure so incendiary. The fact that many of these hospitals were underused and badly managed was lost amid charges of racism and genocide. Delafield Hospital in Washington Heights, for example, which was the first casualty of the budgetary ax in 1975, had an occupancy rate of below 50 percent and had been cited for many violations of the state hospital code.[72]

Bellin's chief antagonist over the closings was John Holloman, the president of the HHC. Holloman was the first African American to lead the city's hospital system, and he enjoyed broad support among the city's black political leaders.[73] Holloman was a fierce defender of public hospitals and resisted calls to close any of them. Bellin and Holloman shared the ideal that poor individuals who had long been subject to substandard medical care should enjoy the same access and quality as the well-off, but they had diametrically opposing visions of how that should be achieved, with their disagreement centering on the role of government as a provider. That Holloman was black and Bellin was white added to the tense atmosphere surrounding the debates. Their differing positions on the closings set off a fierce power struggle between the two men, complete with accusations of budget numbers being distorted or concealed and memos being leaked to the press. Their disagreements escalated into a war of words, and by the end of the summer the atmosphere had become so poisoned that the board ordered the two men to stop putting out "unauthorized and often conflicting statements on corporation matters."[74]

As news of the impending hospital closings were reported in the press and outrage spread in affected communities, 125 Worth Street became a figurative and often literal battleground. Bellin came under attack from activists, union leaders, and local politicians; protesters became a constant presence at HHC board meetings on the fifth floor (see figure 3.2). In May 1975, some one thousand demonstrators massed on the building steps, attempting to enter a closed session of the HHC board.[75] On several occasions, protesters broke through the police guards and flooded into the room as board members—their papers, pens, and eyeglasses flying—dove under the table to avoid being manhandled by the crowd.[76] A protective cordon of sawhorses went up around the building, and for several months a busload of tactical police were stationed nearby on Foley Square to maintain order. Bellin was twice hanged in effigy from the lamppost at the corner of Worth and Lafayette Streets. Bulletproof glass was installed in the door leading to his outer office.[77]

The primary force behind the protests was an alliance of community groups and labor activists. Bellin had long had a prickly relationship with the advisory boards of hospitals, and their enmity increased as the

Figure 3.2   Protesting Bellin

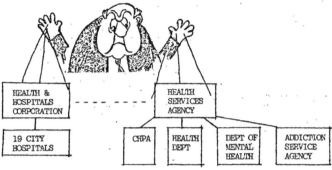

Tonight the Commissioner of Health is speaking on
"MAJOR URBAN HEALTH PROBLEMS," we say

DR. BELLIN IS A MAJOR

HEALTH PROBLEM

Who is Dr. Bellin? Mayor Beame appointed him Commissioner
of Health, head of the Health Department, BUT he is also...

* Chairman of the Health and Hospitals Corporation
  Board of Directors
* Chairman of the Comprehensive Health Planning Agency
* Acting administrator of the Health Service Agency

Source: Courtesy New York City Municipal Archives.
Note: A flyer for a protest of a talk by Health Commissioner Lowell Bellin, who came under attack during the fiscal crisis for his efforts to close public hospitals. The flyer emphasizes the multiple roles that Bellin played in the city's health care system.

possibility of closing some institutions grew stronger. The chair of the community board of Metropolitan Hospital Center angrily demanded that Mayor Beame fire Bellin. The board members wrote to Bellin, "Your constant and flagrant disregard for the poor people of this city will no longer be tolerated."[78] Two dozen black ministers marched into City Hall and occupied Mayor Beame's office, where they chanted, clapped, and conducted prayer services to demand Bellin's ouster. "His uncaring attitude and utter insensitivity," said Rev. William Jones, pastor of the Bethany Baptist Church in Brooklyn, "disqualify him for any position that has to do with the lives of ordinary people."[79] District Council 37, which represented health care workers, organized many protests. Victor Gotbaum, the head of District Council 37 and one of the city's most powerful political figures, also called for Bellin's resignation.[80] That someone openly skeptical about the need for a public hospital system should chair the HHC board was "a paradox that would be farcical if it weren't so serious," according to a DC 37 press release.[81]

Such attacks left Bellin unfazed. He was a skilled bureaucratic infighter (at HHC board meetings he took notes in Hebrew so that no one would know what he was writing), and he considered it a point of pride to defend an unpopular position that he believed was correct. But in the fall of 1976, his three-year leave of absence from Columbia, and with it the term as health commissioner he had promised Beame, came to an end. Extending his leave could place his tenure in jeopardy, he said, and with two children starting college, he needed to increase his salary above what he could earn in city government.[82]

As Bellin's replacement, Beame chose Pat Imperato, who had been Bellin's closest confidant and adviser throughout the fiscal crisis. During his brief tenure as health commissioner through the remainder of Beame's mayoralty, Imperato, as chair of the HHC board, found himself enmeshed in the same political struggles that had preoccupied Bellin. Almost immediately after he took the helm in January 1977, long-simmering tensions over Holloman's leadership of the HHC came to a head. The HHC board, after months of divisive debates, voted nine-to-seven to remove Holloman as president of the corporation. Protesters disrupted the meeting at which the vote took place, jeering, shouting, and threatening the board members; one protester broke through the police line and struck a board member who had voted for removal.[83]

The closure of hospitals—even ones that were demonstrably superfluous, underperforming, and cost-ineffective—sparked public outrage that was never seen in response to the elimination of the Health Department's preventive programs. That hospitals were the source of far more —and higher-paying—union jobs than were Health Department programs only partially explains the disproportionate attention. The involvement of so many constituencies and the persistence and intensity of their protests speak to the resonance of the hospital as a symbol of health. In the eyes of community members, politicians, and the media, curative medicine, not prevention, was the key to a community's wellbeing.

The battles over hospital closings that marked the tenures of Mayor Beame and Commissioners Bellin and Imperato raged on under their successors. In the 1977 mayoral election, Beame was doomed by his obvious impotence at preventing the city's slide into insolvency and his complicity in the years of financial gimmickry as comptroller under Mayors Wagner and Lindsay. From a crowded field of candidates, voters chose as his replacement Ed Koch, a colorful, garrulous congressional representative who was backed by most of the city's Democratic machine. Koch won the election with just under 50 percent of the vote.

As the new health commissioner, Koch's search committee selected Reinaldo Ferrer. A surgeon from Puerto Rico, Ferrer was an executive with the Beth Israel Medical Center who had been a protégé of Ray Trussel, the former hospitals commissioner and one of the city's most influential physicians. Ferrer had served as deputy secretary of health for Puerto Rico in the 1950s, but his primary expertise was in hospital management, not public health. Although Koch's administration denied that ethnicity played a role in his selection, the mayor had been under fire for failing to include any Hispanic commissioners in his first round of cabinet picks.

Koch in fact had little interest in the Health Department. The choice of health commissioner was significant to him almost entirely because the position represented a slot on the HHC board, over which he wanted to assert more control through his power to appoint members. In its eight years of existence, the HHC had proven a persistent cause of budgetary and political headaches. The lack of mayoral control was a source of frustration that Koch, a canny if not always adept politician, wanted to remedy.

In 1979 the Koch administration announced a plan to close four underused city hospitals, including two, Sydenham and Metropolitan, in Harlem. The plan came in the wake of a highly critical report by a state task force on the oversupply of hospital beds in the state and pressure from Governor Hugh Carey's administration on Koch to close institutions whose high costs were not justified by the need in their community.[84] Whatever the economic soundness of the rationale, the move proved to be politically disastrous for Koch. Sydenham Hospital was a historic institution in the heart of Harlem on 124th Street that had been the first in the city to allow black physicians to admit patients. African American community leaders bitterly denounced the proposal. The move was particularly offensive to Congressman Charles Rangel, who represented Harlem and had backed Koch in the past.

The proposed closings reignited the battles at 125 Worth Street. For over a year, protesters jammed HHC board meetings and public hearings. Ferrer was a target of particular vilification because he was part of the five-member task force of the HHC board that recommended closing the institutions, and his action was seen as a betrayal of his ethnicity. "You are killing blacks and Hispanics," a Puerto Rican City Council member from the Bronx shouted at Ferrer at one HHC board meeting, "and you will be tried publicly in our community for your crime."[85] Metropolitan was ultimately spared; Sydenham, the smallest and most expensive of the municipal hospitals, was shuttered at the end of 1980, a few months after police had carried out protesters who staged a ten-day sit-in. The episode permanently damaged Koch's relationship with black and Puerto Rican voters and political leaders and reinforced a deep suspicion of the city's health establishment.[86]

In the Wake of the Crisis

The battles over the Health and Hospitals Corporation kept the spotlight on 125 Worth Street during and after the fiscal crisis. The Health Department limped along in relative obscurity, however, its deficiencies drawing little attention. Services continued at minimal levels with little innovation or expansion. The problems facing the agency were exemplified by the condition of the school health program, through which physicians and nurses provided screening for thousands of youth.

School health had been hard-hit in spite of being one of the few public health programs with a well-connected and influential lobby behind it; advocates for children were among the city's most vocal, but even their support had been insufficient to protect the school health staff from cutbacks. Lowell Bellin had reduced the budget for the program by about one-third.[87] During and after the fiscal crisis, the number of physicians working in city schools shrank from 27 to 5; the number of school nurses dropped from 207 to 124. Nurses worked just one half-day per month in most elementary and junior high schools and had been eliminated from high schools altogether. Some schools had responded to the reductions by bringing in parents or hiring paraprofessionals to conduct health screenings such as hearing and vision tests.[88] The department stopped giving the new entrance examination in eighth grade in preparation for a student's progression to high school; as a result, a student might receive a routine physical only once in twelve years of school.[89] By the fall of 1980, an internal analysis had concluded that school health

> can no longer be considered a viable program. At current budget and staffing levels, program goals are not and cannot be realized. The strain of attempting to perform functions developed in the 1960s with resources available in the 1980s has resulted in demoralization and the loss (or potential loss) of clinicians and nurses as a result of little or no job satisfaction.[90]

Although insufficient money was the primary source of the problems, the report also noted a failure to streamline administration and use resources more efficiently. In a thinly veiled criticism of Commissioner Reinaldo Ferrer, the report condemned "the seeming reluctance by the Department to seek implementation of recommendations that could improve the delivery of services within programmatic, personnel and fiscal constraints."[91] For example, several experts both inside and outside of the department had recommended a major overhaul of the way the routine examination for newly admitted students was given. Providing the examinations in the district health centers rather than on-site at each school would eliminate time-consuming travel between schools by physicians. Such a plan would also ensure consistent availability of bilingual staff and better quality control; perhaps most advantageous, it would allow the department to receive Medicaid reimbursement for the exams.

Given the enfeebled state of the school health program, it was all the more remarkable that it was able to respond when local politicians and officials at the Center for Disease Control sought to mount an ambitious effort to improve the immunization status of the city's schoolchildren. Outbreaks of vaccine-preventable diseases, especially measles, were a recurring problem in many American cities in the 1970s, a consequence in part of the failure of states and the federal government to sustain funding for immunization programs. In 1977 the CDC launched a national push to get school districts to implement laws requiring youth to be vaccinated before they could attend school. Although these mandates were on the books in almost all states, they tended to languish unenforced because authority was typically vested with local boards of education, which were burdened with many other administrative requirements and did not consider disease control a priority.[92] There was strong evidence that New York City was among the localities where lax enforcement had resulted in preventable outbreaks of measles.

New York City Council president Carol Bellamy, a frequent critic of Koch who was especially interested in child health, championed the issue of school immunization and pressured the Health Department and the Board of Education to work together to implement the CDC's drive, dubbed "No Shots, No School." Verifying the immunization status of the more than one million students in the school system and giving shots to those who needed them would have been an undertaking of mind-boggling complexity even under the best of circumstances. Not only was the school health program reeling from the staff losses of the previous several years, but the Board of Education was dealing with its own cutbacks that had resulted in diminished capacity to keep records of all types. The mobility of the student population, especially those from poor families, further complicated matters. Some students moved three or four times during a school year; in some schools, as much as 40 percent of the student population turned over during the year.[93]

Beginning in 1978 and continuing over four years, the department waged a multipronged campaign to overcome these barriers. The effort not only required coordination among numerous bureaus within the department, including legal, school health, and immunization, but also necessitated delicate negotiations with officials at the Board of Education headquarters and with principals and personnel throughout the school system.[94] Teams from the Health Department conducted massive audits of student records in schools throughout the city. They found widespread failure to keep adequate records, and in 1978 the education official responsible for the records was fired.[95] Each fall, the department set up special immunization clinics around the city, where parents could bring children to get their shots before it was time to start classes, and conducted emergency clinics on-site at selected schools. At the same time an aggressive advertising campaign, including billboards, flyers, and mailings, was launched to educate parents about the "No Shots, No School" policy. Youth who lacked the vaccinations required under state law were forbidden to attend school until they had been brought up to date, although it was not until the fall of 1981 that the policy was strictly and consistently enforced.

The protection of thousands of schoolchildren from preventable diseases came at a cost. By the end of the 1980 to 1981 school year, the Health Department had fined eleven school principals for not cooperating with the effort.[96] School officials and teachers alike resented the disruption of their work. Parents often became hostile when their children were sent home. And some youth advocates questioned the ethics of using school exclusion to control disease, given that many poor children were already at risk of truancy and dropping out. Even former commissioner Pat Imperato questioned the effort in a letter to the *Times*. While being careful to praise the department's school health and immunization staff, he argued that mandatory vaccination was a "latter-day version of an outdated public health police action" and "unworkable in a highly heterogeneous urban society."[97] Although the wisdom of the school mandate policy may have been debatable, there was no question that the department's "No Shots, No School" campaign was a logistical triumph and a testament to the dedication and skill of dozens of department employees at a time of unprecedented challenges. It was also successful: the city recorded eight hundred cases of measles in 1978; in the first five months of 1982, it had eleven.[98]

In its ambition and ultimate success, "No Shots, No School" was anomalous. There were few high-profile initiatives in the years following the fiscal crisis, and the department's performance remained lackluster in many areas. Indeed, even as local politicians praised the success of the immunization drive, they noted that the overall school health program remained substandard; a study by the State Board of Regents found that students were not receiving adequate checkups and that, among other problems, schools were experiencing outbreaks of head lice.[99]

Numerous other areas were problematic. Because of staff losses, inspections of restaurants for sanitary violations and apartment units where lead paint exposure was suspected were running far below optimal levels.[100] The office that collected Medicaid reimbursements for medical and dental services was understaffed, resulting in the loss of badly needed department revenue. The Bureau of Vital Records was unable to meet the demand for birth and death certificates. Citizen complaints about delays in answering phones and rude customer service from areas of the department that dealt with the public were skyrocketing.[101] The department had to severely curtail its case-finding and prevention activities for gonorrhea and syphilis because of staff cutbacks.[102]

Some in the public health community blamed the department's performance on inadequate leadership at the commissioner level. No one disputed that the aftermath of the fiscal crisis was one of the most challenging periods in the department's history. Reinaldo Ferrer was under constant pressure from Koch's office to increase department revenue (by instituting fees for licenses, laboratory services, or birth certificates, for example) even as it cut expenditures.[103] Nevertheless, prominent members of the city's public health establishment alleged—some in oblique terms, others more explicitly—that Ferrer was an ineffective advocate for the department's interests who had failed to stand up to the mayor's demands, much less press for an increase in resources.[104]

One oft-repeated charge was that Ferrer had too readily acquiesced to the transfer of department programs to the state. Since the mid-1960s, the state health department had repeatedly tried to assert authority over the city as part of the Rockefeller administration's efforts to rein in home rule and accrue power in the capital. The state had sought to wrest control of the city's vital statistics reporting, for example, a move that the previous commissioners, Bellin and Imperato, had both vehemently resisted.[105] Under pressure during the fiscal crisis, Imperato had reluctantly surrendered the department's Medicaid auditing program, which Bellin had pioneered, to a new Office of Health Systems Management that Governor Hugh Carey created to control the state's hospital expenses.[106]

Unlike his predecessors, Ferrer embraced such transfers as a way to meet budget reduction targets.[107] He ceded to the state's Department of Substance Abuse Services operation of the methadone maintenance clinics that Robert Newman had established—a move that saved the city some $4 million annually, but which critics claimed would result in longer waits and poorer service. Independence from the state was a point of pride in the city's public health community, but the dismay over the loss of programs was more than just a matter of professional honor. Critics charged that the state health department was insufficiently staffed, too willing to cave in to political pressure, and lacking in understanding of the complex social milieu of New York City.[108]

Ferrer was also caught up in an embarrassing scandal surrounding the Office of the Chief Medical Examiner, which was responsible for performing autopsies and issuing death certificates. The office had been part of the Health Department since Beame had abolished the Health Services Administration superagency, and it was plagued by administrative and financial problems.[109] In 1979 Ferrer attempted to remove the chief medical examiner, Michael Baden, a highly regarded forensic pathologist. Ferrer claimed that Baden ran the office poorly and had committed numerous breaches of medical and administrative standards. The most damaging of Ferrer's allegations was that Baden, in a speech at a hospital grand rounds, had revealed that New York governor Nelson Rockefeller, whose autopsy Baden had performed, died during sexual intercourse. (Baden denied disclosing any details of the governor's death.) After being demoted to a lower-level civil service position, Baden sued; the case would drag on for several years before being resolved largely in favor of the city.[110] The affair became a lurid sideshow that drew Ferrer's time and energy away from the city's public health needs.

Insiders in the Koch administration claimed that the mayor was less than pleased with Ferrer's performance. Koch valued loyalty, however, and Ferrer stood by the mayor throughout the hospitals uproar, even as prominent African American and Latino members of the administration resigned in protest. Ferrer was also Koch's only Puerto Rican commissioner at a time when allegations of racism against the administration had become commonplace.[111]

Ferrer's reputation hit its nadir in April 1980 when the *Village Voice* splashed a photo of him on its cover under the boldface headline "A Sick Joke."[112] The article was a blistering attack on Ferrer's stewardship of the Health Department and his performance on the board of the Health and Hospitals Corporation. The article's ad hominem vitriol was extreme even by the standards of the *Voice*, where bare-knuckled political attacks sometimes veered into character assassination. Reporter Anna Mayo ridiculed Ferrer's thick Puerto Rican accent and unidiomatic grammar, calling him a "buffoon" who looked like "a Shriner up from a small town in Florida." (Mayo also took the occasion to mock what she saw as the effeminacy of Marvin Bogner, the department's public relations officer, whom she described as "prancing" and "chirping.") The article included on-the-record denunciations of Ferrer from numerous health professionals, community leaders, and politicians.

When Ferrer resigned in April 1981, citing a desire to spend more time with his ailing wife, few members of the medical or public health establishment, much less the labor and community groups that had fought so bitterly with the Koch administration over the hospital closings, mourned his departure.

Decline and Fall

Laments about New York's decline—about how dirt, crime, and vice had grown worse than ever—were as old as the metropolis.[113] By the end of the 1970s, however, the city seemed to have crossed a grim threshold. The failure of elected officials to keep the government solvent, the reduction of so many public services, and the resulting deterioration in the quality of life seemed to many observers qualitatively different from past crises.

One of the city's most infamous calamities encapsulated the zeitgeist. Around 8:30 on the night of July 13, 1977, a series of lightning strikes at Consolidated Edison power stations north of New York City set off a chain reaction through the system that fed energy to the electrical grid. An hour later, the power failed and the city went dark. During the sweltering, humid night that followed, large swaths of the city combusted into a Hobbesian inferno of violence and lawlessness. Mobs of looters threw trash cans through store windows, ripped away metal storefront shutters, and made off with anything they could carry. Governor Hugh Carey sent in state troopers to assist local police in keeping order. At daybreak, some of the most economically depressed areas of the South Bronx, Harlem, Bedford-Stuyvesant, and Bushwick resembled war zones. By the time power was restored, eighteen hours after it went out, more than 1,600 stores had been ransacked and some 1,000 fires set. Close to 4,000 people had been arrested.[114]

Riots had ripped through the city's poor neighborhoods before, yet there had been in those earlier conflicts the sense that something significant—the struggle for racial equality and social justice—was at stake. The actions of the looters during the blackout of 1977, though clearly rooted in racism and economic oppression, had an aura of nihilism and crazed futility that seemed new and disturbing. The events were even more troubling when contrasted with a power failure that had struck New York City in 1965, when residents had responded not with violence and crime but with cooperation, civility, and good Samaritanism.

The blackout of 1977 came to symbolize New York City's decline and fall. In dozens of ways both large and small, the city seemed an increasingly dangerous and unpleasant place by decade's end. Municipal services across the board had been slashed. Parks were filthy and decaying. The Parks Department had lost about one-quarter of its budget and half of its workforce; the Sanitation Department lost more than one in five of its employees, the Police Department one in six.[115] In the subway system, which had been the city's lifeline and public sphere since the turn of the century, service was erratic and cars were vandalized and covered with graffiti, while the fare was almost double what it had been a decade earlier. The number of felonies committed on the subway tripled during the 1970s.[116] Times Square, in the heart of Manhattan, had become a cesspool of peep shows and massage parlors.[117] In 1979 the city recorded a record number of homicides, and a higher percentage of them were "murder by stranger," which criminologists considered a key metric of violence in a community.[118] Unemployment in the city hovered around 9 percent, compared with 6 percent nationally. The city had lost some 800,000 residents during the 1970s, more than 10 percent of its population. One in five residents lived below the poverty level.[119]

In the midst of so much adversity, the decimation of the Health Department barely registered, either among political leaders or with members of the public who would have been the beneficiaries of preventive services. It is rare for the elimination of public health programs to be felt immediately. Prevention by its nature generally produces effects that become apparent, if at all, incrementally and over the long term. That the city would suffer consequences from cutbacks in so many areas—health education, substance use treatment, tuberculosis control, and many others—seemed certain. Exactly how those reductions would be felt remained to be revealed.

Chapter 4

A Plague of Politics

R EPORTS OF prolonged, unexplained lymphadenopathy in the homosexual population in New York City recently prompted a record review of cases reported by several clinical investigators." So
began a research protocol written by Health Department epidemiologists
in May 1982. In collaboration with officials at the Centers for Disease
Control, they were preparing to undertake a systematic review of pathology records at hospitals around the city to better understand the mysterious cases of swollen lymph nodes and other ailments that physicians had
begun seeing. "Because increased consciousness of disease patterns in
the homosexual subculture in the past several months could partially account for the recent 'appearance' of this apparently new syndrome, we
plan to assess unbiased data sources for secular trend information."[1]

The dispassionate technical language of the research protocol contrasted sharply with the emotional debates that were beginning to swirl
around the new disease that had appeared in the city. More than one
hundred men had become ill, and about forty had died. There was no
effective treatment. No one was sure what was causing the condition or
how it was spread. It did not yet have a name, although it would soon be
labeled acquired immune deficiency syndrome (AIDS). The people most
affected by the disease, the sick and dying and their friends and loved
ones, were beginning to demand action, but no one agreed about what
exactly should be done. The moral opprobrium surrounding the behaviors—sexual contact between men, illicit drug use—that were suspected
of spreading the disease cast a shadow over efforts by public health professionals to intervene.

The Health Department's initial encounters with AIDS were a throwback to an earlier epoch when frightening new illnesses appeared seemingly from nowhere and defied all efforts to stop them. But this was also
a distinctly modern plague, striking in a post–civil rights era when communities challenged expert judgments and demanded a role in public
health decisionmaking; measures to control the spread of disease sparked

acrimonious debates about privacy, discrimination, and stigma. In the first years of the epidemic, the department would be caught in a crossfire of competing and often irreconcilable demands from affected individuals and groups, politicians, government officials, and medical professionals. The tools in the public health armamentarium that had been successful in the past—outbreak investigation, surveillance, education, screening, regulation of hazardous environments—would be scrutinized and, often, condemned. Critics would charge the department with elevating political considerations over the needs of public health. The lesson to emerge from these years, however, was that the two realms were inseparable.

Rumors of Disease

In the late 1970s, physicians in New York and Los Angeles began to see patients with baffling, tenacious, and often grisly constellations of illnesses. Some of the conditions were rare, such as Kaposi's sarcoma (KS), a skin cancer seen almost exclusively in elderly Jewish men of Mediterranean descent. Others were complications from common microbes that healthy immune systems were able to control, such as the lung infection *Pneumocystis carinii* pneumonia (PCP). The diseases were accompanied by a set of generalized symptoms, including swollen lymph glands, diarrhea, fatigue, weight loss, and drenching sweat during the night. Most of the patients were men in their twenties, thirties, and forties. Some of them reported use of injection drugs, which was known to suppress the immune system. For many others, however, there was no explanation for their inability to fight off disease; the only thing they seemed to have in common was their sexual orientation. The physicians treating them were confused and dismayed: men this young did not simply sicken and die for no reason.[2] A growing sense of unease spread in the close-knit communities of gay men in New York, Los Angeles, and San Francisco.[3]

The initial cases were pieces of a still-incomplete epidemiological puzzle, too fragmentary even to appear as instances of the same phenomenon. As more men began to be seen with similar symptoms, alert physicians and officials at the CDC in Atlanta took note, and pieces of the puzzle began to click into place. Infectious disease doctors in New York City who came together for a regular case conference reported on the strange clustering of similar cases in 1980 and 1981.[4] In the summer of 1981, two reports appeared in the *Morbidity and Mortality Weekly Report*. The first, on June 5, described a cluster of patients with *pneumocystis carinii* pneumonia in Los Angeles; the second, on July 3, reported on cases of KS and PCP among twenty-six men in Los Angeles and New York. With the first report, the CDC ran an editorial note speculating that "some aspect of a homosexual life-style" might be responsible for the condition.[5]

Polly Thomas, who had recently completed a pediatric residency at Yale, was preparing that summer to start work with the Health Department's Bureau of Preventable Diseases. She had joined the Centers for Disease Control's Epidemic Intelligence Service (EIS), a two-year program through which young physicians received training in epidemiology and outbreak investigation—"medical detective" work—while stationed in a city or state health department. New York City was not a sought-after posting for an EIS officer in the summer of 1981. The once-renowned Health Department had fallen on hard times, and the gritty urban environment promised few compensatory attractions. But Thomas asked to be stationed there because her husband had gotten a job in the city. During a monthlong training and orientation in Atlanta in June, she read a short item in the *New York Times* about the apparent outbreak of immune suppression in homosexual men and thought it might prove to be an interesting project to work on.[6]

Thomas was presented with three tasks upon arriving at 125 Worth Street in July. The first was to begin surveillance. Thomas phoned local hospitals, clinics, and private physicians, asking them to submit reports about any patients they might see with symptoms that looked like unexplained immune suppression. Second, Thomas and Stephen Friedman, the assistant commissioner of preventable diseases, began to review all death certificates from KS and PCP that had been filed in the city in the previous several years. Third, Thomas began interviewing patients as a way to generate hypotheses about what might be the cause of the illness.[7] As more cases were reported during the fall, Friedman pulled staff from the venereal disease control program, who were highly skilled at taking sexual histories, to assist with the interviews.[8]

As the inquiry widened, Thomas and Friedman, joined by new staff and additional CDC officers seconded to New York City, became part of a nationwide network of investigators studying the new disease. They began crisscrossing the city, drawing blood and pulling medical charts, asking questions of frightened patients and baffled doctors, listening carefully through hours of interviews, sifting through reams of notes looking for patterns—conducting the kind of shoe-leather epidemiology that had been the public health stock-in-trade for decades. These descriptive and analytic studies were the means through which the biological, clinical, and epidemiological features of the disease came to be understood (see figure 4.1).

The first coordinated investigation began in October 1981. Friedman and Thomas worked with their counterparts in San Francisco, Los Angeles, and Atlanta on a case-control study in which men with the illness were compared with a selected group of healthy men, matched as closely as possible for age and race. In hourlong interviews, subjects were questioned on an exhaustive range of topics: their income, education, occupa-

Figure 4.1   A Mysterious New Epidemic

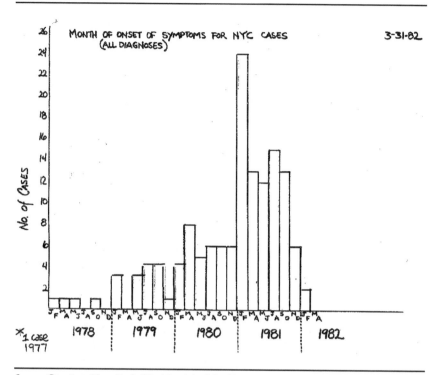

Source: Courtesy New York City Municipal Archives.
Note: A hand-drawn graph by Health Department epidemiologists from March 1982 shows the temporal distribution of diagnosed cases of the immune suppression in the city. The first cases of the mysterious syndrome, which did not yet have a name, had begun to appear in 1978, but the connections between the cases were not recognized until three years later.

tion, and family ancestry; their history of travel and exposure to toxic substances; their medical history, including previous sexually transmitted diseases and prescription medications taken; and "lifestyle" habits, such as recreational drug use. Each subject was asked an extensive and specific list of questions about his sexual history, including age of first sexual activity, estimated number of partners per year, proportion of partners encountered in sex clubs and bathhouses, and frequency with which penis, tongue, and hands had been inserted into mouths and rectums. All patients were also asked to donate blood for laboratory testing.[9]

The most prominent differences to emerge between the cases and controls were the number of sexual partners, the proportion of partners met in bathhouses, and exposure to inhaled stimulants. (When it was later determined that the illness included an asymptomatic phase, the researchers on this study realized that many of the people they had interviewed as controls were almost certainly cases who had not yet developed symptoms.) These findings suggested at least three plausible hypotheses. One was that the infections represented a common exposure to some toxic substance that might be found in public sex venues. A likely cause was thought to be "poppers," small vials of amyl nitrate that were used to enhance sexual pleasure. A second theory was that repeated infections with multiple sexually transmitted pathogens had broken down the men's immune systems. A third possibility was that a new and unidentified virus was circulating.[10]

Several other investigations were undertaken in 1982 as the case-control study was going on. Since many of the patients described in the first articles in the *Morbidity and Mortality Weekly Report* (*MMWR*) had had persistent swelling of the lymph nodes, investigators reviewed the pathology reports on all lymph node biopsies that had been performed at seven New York City hospitals and conducted chart reviews of men who had been seen for lymphadenopathy.[11] Thomas and Friedman interviewed the known and suspected sexual contacts of the man known as "Patient Zero," who had been one of the initial cases diagnosed with KS at New York University Medical Center and reported in the second *MMWR* article (see figure 4.2).[12] The Canadian flight attendant later immortalized in journalist Randy Shilts's account of the epidemic, *And the Band Played On*, was thought to have infected dozens of men.

As the epidemiologists continued to search for clues, the circle of infection seemed steadily to widen. In late 1981 and early 1982, cases were reported to the CDC of what appeared to be the same condition in women and in men who reported no instances of sexual contact with other men, challenging the initial speculation that "some aspect of the homosexual lifestyle" was responsible for the immune deterioration. In the summer of 1982, cases of KS or opportunistic infections in Haitians were reported in five states and cases of PCP in three hemophiliacs, who regularly received the blood product Factor VIII. These new cases threw into question the hypotheses of infection via poppers or immune system breakdown after repeated infections with sexually transmitted diseases and instead suggested a contagious agent such as a virus that was spread through blood or blood products.[13] In late 1982, a case-control study of patients who identified as heterosexual found that a history of injection drug use was common to almost all of them, reinforcing the idea that a blood-borne pathogen was responsible.[14]

When physicians in the Bronx and in Newark, New Jersey, reported the first cases of infants with opportunistic infections and unexplained

Figure 4.2   Investigating Patient Zero

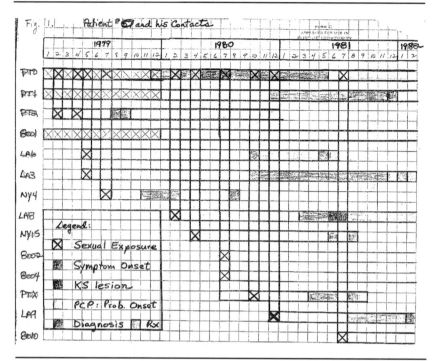

Source: Courtesy New York City Municipal Archives.
Note: A hand-drawn graph showing the sexual contacts of "Patient Zero," the Canadian flight attendant who was the focus of one of the early epidemiological investigations conducted by the Centers for Disease Control in collaboration with the Health Department. The cells show each contact's date of sexual exposure, symptom onset, and diagnosis with an opportunistic infection.

immune suppression in November 1982, Thomas and Friedman worked with colleagues in New Jersey and the CDC to determine if this was the same condition that was being seen in adults. To seek out possible additional cases, they reviewed all requests that pediatricians had made over the previous several years for pentamidine, a rarely used drug for treating PCP. (An unusually high number of requests for the drug had been one of the ways in which CDC officials had picked up on the initial outbreak of immune suppression among gay men.) They also examined death certificates from 1978 through 1982 of all children under age five who had died of pneumonia, and when possible, they interviewed the parents.[15] In more than half the cases, one or both parents was an injection drug user or was born in Haiti; among children for whom no parental risk could be identified, many had received blood transfusions. It became increasingly clear to Thomas, Friedman, and their fellow investigators that the most likely cause of the disease was a viral infection with an epidemiology similar to that of hepatitis B.

For a year the condition did not have a formal name, though it was often referred to colloquially as gay-related immune deficiency, or GRID, even after numerous cases were identified in people who were not gay. In July 1982, the CDC formally labeled the new condition acquired immune deficiency syndrome, or AIDS. The *MMWR* of September 24, 1982, officially defined AIDS as "a disease, at least moderately predictive of a defect in cell-mediated immunity, occurring in a person with no known cause for diminished resistance to that disease. Such diseases include KS, PCP, and serious OOI [other opportunistic infection]." At the same time, however, the CDC conceded the imprecision of its definition: patients might manifest a variety of other conditions not currently included in monitoring (notably, tuberculosis); conversely, some of the people currently considered cases might be suffering from a different ailment.[16]

Over the two years that all of these investigations were being carried out, the Health Department staff working on the new problem grew steadily. By mid-1983, about twenty people were involved in the AIDS investigations; most positions were supported by city funds, although several were funded by a cooperative agreement with the CDC.[17] As the number of cases continued to rise, the Bureau of Preventable Diseases became concerned about the completeness of their information, and in January 1983, the department shifted from passive to active surveillance. Staff members were assigned to visit all city hospitals, each of which now had a dedicated staff member responsible for collecting the data.[18]

Although the Health Department staff generally had a good working relationship with their CDC-based colleagues, tensions did arise over some of the decisions made in Atlanta. One of the major concerns of Health Department staff was protection of patient confidentiality. Jim Monroe, an investigator who was brought in from the Bureau of Venereal Disease to assist with the interviews of AIDS patients, objected to the CDC's request that case reports be sent to the agency with patient names to ensure an unduplicated listing. Sensitive to gay men's concerns about their names being sent to federal bureaucrats, Monroe fought successfully for a policy under which case reports were forwarded to Atlanta in anonymized form, using a numerical code called Soundex.[19] The concerns about the dangers posed by privacy breaches foreshadowed the greater conflicts that would arise once the causal agent of the new condition was identified and a blood test became available in 1985.

Others in the Health Department worried that the CDC was insufficiently attentive to the social and political implications of the epidemiological conclusions they were drawing. Rebecca Reiss, an interviewer who assisted Polly Thomas and Stephen Friedman on the "Patient Zero" cluster investigation, strongly objected to what she saw as the CDC's indiscriminate use of the concept of "risk group." In an *MMWR* report, the CDC had identified the populations in whom the disease had primarily been found (homosexuals, Haitians, hemophiliacs, and heroin addicts) even as it conceded that these groups, which became known colloquially as the "4-H groups"—the term a modern-day scarlet letter—included individuals who were not infected. Reiss would ultimately resign her position because of qualms about the ways in which the CDC's studies had, in her view, "often been hastily translated into harmful generalizations regarding all people in 'at risk' groups."[20]

As Health Department and CDC investigators began sifting through interview data, medical charts, and blood samples to try to map the epidemiology of the mysterious illnesses, a parallel process of anxious discovery and conjecture was taking place among gay men as they sought to understand what might be making their friends and loved ones sick. A month before the *MMWR* report of June 5, 1981, appeared, the *New York Native*, a biweekly newspaper for the city's gay community, ran a three-paragraph item buried amid several short articles on page 7. The author was Lawrence Mass, a gay physician who wrote the paper's medical column. Headlined "Disease Rumors Largely Unfounded," the article reported on eleven cases of PCP that had recently been seen at Bellevue Hospital.[21] The occurrence of the rare disease in people not obviously immune-compromised was strange and potentially worrisome, but, Mass reassured readers, only some of the cases were among gay men.

After the second *MMWR* article, a new urgency took hold. The *Native* elevated the story to its front page in an article headlined "Cancer in the Gay Community." Mass speculated on the cause of the apparent outbreak. "Perhaps certain homosexuals in certain urban centers," he wrote, "have been breathing, eating, drinking, or wearing unusual things, behaving in unusual ways, or frequenting unusual locations."[22] Several months later, the first newsletter of Gay Men's Health Crisis (GMHC), a community organization that had been founded to deal with the epidemic, included a column titled "AID and What to Do About It" that reflected the ongoing uncertainty (and inconsistent nomenclature). "There continues to be no incontrovertible evidence to suggest that AID is overtly contagious," the column stated. "Informed speculation, however, suggests that an infectious agent—perhaps a virus such as cytomegalovirus or Epstein-Barr virus—is at least a critical factor in the outbreak."[23]

One of the most outspoken community members was the physician Joseph Sonnabend. An avuncular South African who had done immunological research before setting up a private practice primarily serving gay men in Greenwich Village, Sonnabend had seen many patients with the new condition. He vehemently rejected the "new virus" theory as epidemiologically implausible and politically dangerous. He explained his concerns in a letter to the city's new health commissioner, David Sencer, in mid-1982. "It is indeed a very serious matter," he wrote, "to suggest that members of any minority group may be carriers of what in effect is a cancer virus."[24] Instead, Sonnabend advanced the theory that the biological culprit was cytomegalovirus (CMV), a type of herpes virus endemic in adults. Infection with CMV was generally asymptomatic, but, Sonnabend believed, the virus ran wild in the bodies of gay men because their immune systems had been weakened by repeated attacks from sexually transmitted diseases and consequent treatment with anti-biotics.[25] In August 1982, Sonnabend put forth his theory in a column in the *Native* titled "Promiscuity Is Bad for Your Health."

Sonnabend's theory was given a wide audience by two activists who were his patients, Michael Callen, a composer and musician well known in the downtown arts scene, and Richard Berkowitz, a self-described hustler who had been a gay rights organizer in college. Believing their illnesses had been caused by the high levels of sexual activity commonly practiced by newly liberated gay men living in large cities, they wrote a manifesto that ran in the November 8–21, 1982 issue of the *Native* under the headline, "We Know Who We Are: Two Gay Men Declare War on Promiscuity." The two men blamed "the accumulation of risk through leading a promiscuous gay urban lifestyle" for the immunological break-downs that were being seen.[26]

Many gay men, however, found the theory that too much sex was causing the new disease not just spurious but offensive. To these critics, the very notion of "promiscuity"—an ill-defined term freighted with moral and political baggage—had no place in public health discussions; the views of Callen, Berkowitz, and Sonnabend represented little more than internalized homophobia and self-hatred.[27] Lawrence Mass, in an article titled "The Case Against Medical Panic," compared Callen and Berkowitz to Jerry Falwell, founder of the Moral Majority. The question of whether it was necessary or wise to publicly call attention to the new disease—or even whether the disease was cause for alarm—revealed deep divides among gay men. After Callen and Berkowitz's call to arms ran in the *Native*, the influential gay magazine *Body Politic* ran a rebuttal titled "The Real Gay Epidemic: Panic and Paranoia." Rather than urging gay men to speak out, the author warned of the potential dangers that such actions could trigger: "Lesbians and sexually active gay men are going to have their rights denied and infringed upon—all because 400 cases of a disease have appeared among 20 million of us."[28]

Two years after the first reports in the *MMWR*, more than 1,600 cases of AIDS had been identified in the United States—almost half of them in New York City. Four out of ten people with the disease had died. As new cases doubled every six months, pressure built on health officials at all levels of government to respond. But with the causal agent yet to be identified and questions remaining about how the disease might be transmitted, it was not clear what could be done to stanch the flow of sickness and death.

Skeleton and Muscle

One of the people who took an interest in Reinaldo Ferrer's resignation from the post of health commissioner was David Sencer, who read a newspaper article about the departure in April 1981 and then wrote a letter to Ed Koch asking to be considered for the job. Sencer was working at Becton, Dickinson & Company, a medical technology firm in New Jersey, but until recently he had held one of the most influential public health jobs in the country: director of the Center for Disease Control. He had joined the CDC in 1960, when it was still the Communicable Disease Center, after a decade with the U.S. Public Health Service working on tuberculosis control in rural Idaho and Georgia. He had risen through the ranks to become the CDC's director in 1966.

Sencer's eleven years at the helm of the CDC were a time of growth for the agency and some high-profile successes, notably its leadership of the global smallpox eradication campaign. The years had also been marked by controversy. Sencer had convened an advisory panel that recommended not to discontinue the Tuskegee syphilis study before it was scandalously exposed by a whistle-blower and a journalist in 1972. In 1976, Sencer had shepherded an ambitious and controversial plan to vaccinate all Americans against a feared epidemic of swine flu. The epidemic failed to occur, and the vaccine was suspected of causing dangerous side effects. The episode quickly entered the annals of public health disasters, and he lost his job because of it.[29] The commissioner's post in New York City offered Sencer the chance to return to the world of public health. The challenge of reversing what was widely seen as a long period of decline for the department appealed to him. "When things are the worst," he told the *Times*, "that's the best time to build."[30]

As he set about rebuilding, Sencer was guided by a clear vision of what the Health Department should be. During the flush years of the 1950s, Leona Baumgartner had enhanced the Health Department's mission and prestige by the ad hoc creation of programs to meet a wide range of health needs. Although a great admirer of Baumgartner's skills and dedication, Sencer believed that the department had become spread too thin over the years, taking on too many functions that had only a tenuous connection to public health or were more appropriately carried out by other city agencies—licensing day care facilities, providing dental care for schoolchildren, and regulating the safety of the horses that pulled carriages in Central Park, to name just a few. He believed that municipal health departments should limit themselves to programs that were truly preventive in nature and could not be fulfilled by other segments of the health care system.

Sencer's was a minimalist view of public health that hewed closely to concepts of primary prevention and population-level interventions. The clinical care services that the department had sought to expand during the 1960s were better handled by hospitals and other institutions, he believed, and the social welfare functions that at various times had fallen into the public health ambit were, in his view, the responsibility of other professions. The department in Sencer's vision should function as coordinator and convener, facilitating the work of other organizations. It would be the "skeleton" for the "muscle" provided by other individuals and institutions.[31]

With a poker face and thick glasses, David Sencer had a low-key, diffident manner that disguised an acute grasp of the political and bureaucratic dimensions of public health work. He had gained a reputation at the CDC as an expert administrator with an encyclopedic memory. At 125 Worth Street, he would become a hands-on manager who roamed the offices, directly approaching employees at all levels of the organization and asking them about particular problems related to their work. He pored over the department's surveillance reports, looking for trends in the data that he believed warranted further attention. Sencer made it a priority to rebuild the department's science base, in terms of both personnel and technology. He leveraged his contacts at the CDC and networked extensively among members of the city's health care community in search of talented staff he might recruit.

When Sencer assumed his position on the first day of 1982, the new disease striking gay men was just one of many pressing issues that demanded attention. There were several urgent health problems, including a troubling rise in the incidence of tuberculosis and an outbreak of penicillin-resistant gonorrhea. There were also numerous administrative, bureaucratic, and budgetary challenges to confront.

First, Sencer had to take stock of an agency weakened by years of attrition following the city's fiscal crisis and the relentless demands for economizing from the Emergency Financial Control Board and the Koch administration. The department's annual budget was $102 million, compared with $90 million at the start of the fiscal crisis; adjusted for inflation, its budget had shrunk by almost half in eight years. There were some 3,700 employees, almost 40 percent fewer than in the early 1970s.[32] The department was a technological backwater. The biostatistics unit was using computer punch cards to tabulate the city's births and deaths, a decades-old technology that failed to permit the kinds of sophisticated analysis that could identify emerging problems in sub-populations.[33] Attracting talented staff, which had always been a challenge because of relatively low public-sector salaries, became even more difficult as the department lost its reputation as a place where cutting-edge public health work could be done. There was little depth in epidemiology; family planning and maternity services barely existed. The district health centers were grim, dingy, and crumbling from years of deferred maintenance.[34]

Local budgetary constraints were compounded by the new ethos of limited government that reigned in Washington, D.C. In the summer of 1981, Congress passed a budget bill that cut or eliminated about two hundred domestic spending programs. Health and human services programs were especially hard-hit by the cutbacks. Hundreds of thousands of poor women and children were thrown off public assistance rolls as billions of dollars were cut from Aid to Families with Dependent Children, Medicaid, food stamps, and child nutrition.[35] As part of the "new federalism" philosophy designed to return budgetary control to the states, categorical federal funding for public health programs such as maternal and child health and alcohol and drug abuse were transformed into block grants.[36] Proponents argued that block grants allowed states and cities flexibility to determine their own priorities closer to home and eliminated redundant administration.[37] But the amount of the block grants was less—often far less—than the sum of what the categorical programs had been.[38] Areas that continued to be funded categorically, such as immunization and venereal disease, were reduced by as much as one-fifth. Overall, federal aid to state and local governments declined about 20 percent in the first two years of the Reagan administration.[39] Funding was ended for the Comprehensive Employee Training Act, the Nixon-era program that had enabled the Health Department to maintain staffing in several bureaus.

The local budgetary situation was only a little brighter. City agencies still lived under the tyranny of the Office of Management and Budget's "program to eliminate the gap," or PEG, through which commissioners and their staffs were asked to produce scenarios for meeting various budget reduction targets. One of Sencer's first memos to his deputies asked for ideas for program initiatives but warned that "new funds are going to be difficult if not impossible to come by."[40] At the same time, however, the city's fiscal situation had stabilized since the depths of the fiscal crisis to the extent that commissioners could also ask the mayor's office for money to meet new and emerging needs.[41] A month after taking office, for example, Sencer requested a $2.8 million special needs package that included funding for enhanced venereal disease surveillance to help deal with the gonorrhea outbreak.[42] Staffing in the program remained tenuous, however, with key positions often going unfilled for months at a time.[43]

Sencer also stepped into a turf war over one of the department's largest programs, school health, through which dozens of nurses and part-time physicians provided screening and medical referral in hundreds of city schools. The program had become the focus of long-standing frictions between the Health Department and the Board of Education. The "No Shots, No School" campaign from 1978 through 1981 had brought many of these tensions to the fore, as health officials and school administrators battled over the division of labor and resources in the Herculean task of vaccinating thousands of students. Tensions increased when eleven school principals were brought before the Health Department's administrative tribunal and fined for their failure to exclude unvaccinated pupils.[44]

In early 1981, schools chancellor Frank Macchiarola launched an effort to wrest control of all school medical and nursing services from the Health Department and place them under the aegis of the Board of Education. Numerous advocacy groups, including the Citizens Committee for Children, the United Parents Association, and the New York Pediatric Society, opposed the plan, arguing that the Board of Education was ill prepared to operate such a large and complex health program. The plan was shelved when Macchiarola left his job, but deep discontent remained among the city's many child advocates over the quality and quantity of school-provided health services, which had deteriorated markedly during the 1970s. Reorganizing and revitalizing the system was a top priority.

Sencer also had to confront the long-standing question of the department's involvement in ambulatory care. He resisted the idea of the Health Department as a safety net provider for the poor; he believed that the department should "divorce itself from all curative programs except those that are themselves a means of primary prevention (such as ambulatory treatment of tuberculosis)."[45] The district health centers and child health stations, in his view, would be better operated by the Health and Hospitals Corporation and integrated into the functioning of the public hospitals. After the bruising battles over the hospital closings, however, scaling back any clinical facility remained a political third rail. Although Sencer floated the idea of consolidating some district health centers and child health stations with nearby HHC facilities, he quickly backtracked after hostile reactions from community groups and politicians representing the affected areas.[46] When Sencer announced that he was withdrawing his plan, the chair of the City Council's health committee called the decision "a victory for the poor, the underprivileged and the City Council of New York."[47]

How to Have Public Health in an Epidemic

Sencer's initial responses to AIDS exemplified his "skeleton and muscle" philosophy that the department should stick to the core functions of public health while supporting other parts of the health system. The Bureau of Laboratories acquired a T-cell sorter to run tests on the blood of people diagnosed with the new condition. Sencer won permission from the Food and Drug Administration for the department to serve as a distributor in the city for an investigational drug against one of the AIDS-related infections, *mycobacterium avium intracellulare*, and make it available to physicians for use with their patients. He also tried unsuccessfully to interest the National Institutes of Health in setting up a network of clinical research on the new disease in New York City, with the Health Department serving as a clearinghouse for funds and information.[48] He began convening meetings for health care personnel dealing with the new condition to discuss what they were seeing and to share findings.[49] Thirty-five invitations were sent out for the first gathering, in March 1982; an overflow crowd of ninety people, mostly physicians, packed into the third-floor conference room at 125 Worth Street. Polly Thomas and the other staff working on the various studies in progress—the case-control studies, the cluster investigations, the biopsy studies—reported on what they were learning about the new condition, showing their handwritten data on overhead projectors.[50] Clinical issues predominated, but by the second meeting concerns about patient privacy were already surfacing.[51]

In January 1983, Sencer began convening the Interagency Task Force on AIDS, made up of representatives of the Health and Hospitals Corporation, the Human Resources Administration, and the Department of Mental Health, Mental Retardation, and Alcoholism Services.[52] That month, he also notified Mayor Koch's office that he intended to create an office of gay and lesbian health concerns, primarily to coordinate the work going on in the community around AIDS.[53] To head the office he recruited Roger Enlow, a young rheumatologist and immunologist who had collaborated with the department on the study of lymph node enlargement and who was a member of the New York AIDS Network, an advocacy organization.

The role of coordinator and convener was adequate in the first days of the epidemic, when little was known and little could be done. As AIDS continued to spread, however, and the need for health and social services increased, the limits of this model became apparent. The city's enormous health and human services sector was resistant to centralized coordination or direction. (This was the same problem that had bedeviled the city's first health services administrator, Howard Brown, as he sought to rationalize the system under Mayor Lindsay.) Sencer had little leverage to influence the quality or quantity of AIDS care in public hospitals, the availability of substance use treatment, or the provision of emergency housing, social work, and counseling.[54] Critical gaps remained in all of these areas.

Some of these gaps were filled by a new organization, Gay Men's Health Crisis, founded at the beginning of 1982. Sustained by an indefatigable corps of volunteers working out of makeshift offices, GMHC quickly emerged as a primary source of information and services around the new disease, organizing practical and emotional support programs, a hotline, and community forums where physicians treating large numbers of AIDS patients reported on what they were seeing.[55]

Other gaps—especially in funding—were filled by the state health department. In the summer of 1983, Governor Mario Cuomo signed legislation creating the New York State AIDS Institute, reporting to David Axelrod, Cuomo's health commissioner. The institute was the culmination of lobbying by gay activists, who were able to convince liberal members of the state legislature that the epidemic outstripped the fiscal and administrative capacity of New York City. The institute devoted more than $5 million of state funding to research and education, which supported contracts with community-based organizations and hospitals to provide clinical and social services. Axelrod had asserted a stronger role for Albany than his predecessors, and in the eyes of many activists, the state became a more effective and consequential player in the fight against the disease than New York City.[56]

A particular source of discontent among activists was the Health Department's scant public education about the new disease. The department's Bureau of Preventable Diseases produced a threefold brochure in May 1983 in question-and-answer format with basic information about the epidemiology, clinical signs, and transmission of the condition.[57] The brochure was distributed to health care providers, however, not to the general public or groups thought to be at heightened risk, and its plain, text-heavy format was hardly the stuff of effective public education campaigns.

Part of the minimal response can be attributed to gaps in the scientific understanding of the new condition. Throughout 1982 and into 1983, even as expert opinion coalesced around the theory of a blood-borne virus similar to hepatitis B, uncertainty remained about the disease's etiology and modes of transmission. In May 1983, the *Journal of the American Medical Association* ran a report by James Oleske, who had been among the first to identify cases of pediatric AIDS and whose report raised the possibility that some children had become infected through routine household contact. The article cautioned that the epidemiology of AIDS "may now have taken an ominous new turn."[58] Amid such uncertainty, Sencer did not believe that the science base existed for prevention guidelines. "To make recommendations before there is sufficient evidence to support them," Sencer said in early 1983, "is at least as bad as not making any recommendations."[59]

The Health Department's most outspoken critic was Larry Kramer, a prominent gay playwright and author who had cofounded GMHC. With his abrasive and dogmatic manner, Kramer was a relentless critic of official inaction. In March 1983, Kramer wrote an article for the *Native* titled "1,112 and Counting" (the number of AIDS cases that had been diagnosed in the United States), which demanded greater attention to the new disease and attacked virtually everyone involved in the city's response: Mayor Ed Koch and other political leaders, the city's medical and public health establishment, and gay men themselves, whom Kramer accused of a complacent unwillingness to abandon sexual profligacy. David Sencer came in for harsh criticism in the article, as did Stanley Brezenoff, head of the Health and Hospitals Corporation. The two men, Kramer charged, had done "an appalling job of educating our citizens, our hospital workers, and even, in some instances, our doctors. Almost everything this city knows about AIDS has come to it, in one way or another, through Gay Men's Health Crisis."[60]

This accusation was exaggerated. While the Health Department had done little in the way of educating the lay public, it had been central to informing the city's health care workers about the new condition. Many department staff members, including Polly Thomas and her fellow investigators in the Bureau of Preventable Diseases and Roger Enlow and his colleagues in the Office of Gay and Lesbian Health Concerns, had met with professional groups and employers and had trained hundreds of health care providers.[61] Nevertheless, the failure to produce mass educational messages for the lay public remained a serious weakness in the department's response to the new disease.

Gay activists angry over what they saw as the city's sluggish response alleged that Ed Koch was a closeted homosexual (a charge the mayor vehemently denied) and did not want to risk appearing overly sympathetic to the problems of the gay community. Critics also charged that Sencer, having mistakenly sounded an alarm over swine flu in 1976, was now erring in the opposite direction, refraining from taking any action as long as doubt remained about its scientific soundness or potential consequences. While there was a kernel of truth in this, Sencer had other reasons for maintaining a low public profile around the disease. For prevention purposes, he considered individual and small group presentations to be more effective than mass media. "Education efforts are best done on face to face bases rather than with heavy dependence upon brochures and pamphlets," he wrote. He also believed that messages put forth by community groups such as the Gay Men's Health Crisis were more credible and persuasive than those coming from the Health Department, since these organizations had "a degree of trust from the affected community that officialdom does not always have."[62] In May 1983, the department gave its first funding, a $100,000 contract, to GMHC to support the organization's education and prevention programs, and it would continue to provide grants for GMHC's work.[63]

The most significant educational effort in the epidemic's early years was a community-produced initiative. In the spring of 1983, activists Michael Callen and Richard Berkowitz, who had warned in the pages of the *Native* about the dangers of sexual promiscuity, undertook their own homegrown public health campaign. They wrote a forty-page pamphlet titled "How to Have Sex in an Epidemic: One Approach," based on their recommendations in their *Native* article from the previous fall, and used their own funds to print five thousand copies. Their advice was specific and blunt: Don't get semen or fecal matter in your mouth. Don't get semen in your rectum. Alcohol and poppers impair judgment; use them carefully, if at all. Shower before and after sex.[64] The two men carried copies of their pamphlet to bookstores in Greenwich Village, where it sold for $3.75.

That community members were paying out of pocket to distribute the kind of prevention messages that were ostensibly within the purview of the Health Department was a point of embarrassment and even anger for some department staff members. When the head of the Bureau of Venereal Disease resigned in 1982, a major reason was his frustration over what he perceived as the department's sluggish response to AIDS; he believed that there should have been far more aggressive outreach and education efforts, especially programs for high school students.[65] Pat Maher, who worked with Roger Enlow in the Office of Gay and Lesbian Health Concerns, also quit in frustration over the department's failure to more aggressively educate the public. "We were making the case for a subway poster campaign," she later said, "and I'll never forget being told, 'We don't need that. Anybody who needs to know about AIDS already knows about it.'"[66] In the spring of 1985, assistant commissioner Peggy Clarke, who was in charge of health education, and Ellen Rautenberg, assistant commissioner for policy and planning, attended a performance of Larry Kramer's polemical play *The Normal Heart*, which dramatized the societal neglect of the epidemic. Although mortified when one of the play's protagonists complained about the failure of the Health Department to produce educational materials, they had to concede that Kramer had a point.[67]

An Epidemic of Fear

The department's lack of public education was all the more pronounced in contrast with increasingly prominent—and alarmist—coverage in the popular media. In 1981 and 1982, most of the country had remained oblivious to the new disease, even as the death toll climbed into the hundreds—a silence plainly due to journalists' indifference to or discomfort with homosexuality and drug use. Lawrence Altman, the medical reporter at the *New York Times*, told David Sencer, "The *Times* is a family newspaper—we don't talk about that."[68] (A notable exception was an inflammatory story in *New York* magazine in the summer of 1982 titled "The Gay Plague."[69])

In 1983, however, reporters discovered the epidemic and began to churn out a steady stream of stories, usually sensationalistic and often warning about the ominous spread of the disease to "innocent victims." Such coverage was fed partly by the views of some scientific experts who remained unconvinced that the disease spread only through intimate contact. In a *JAMA* editorial accompanying James Oleske's report on suspected household transmission, Anthony Fauci of the National Institute of Allergy and Infectious Diseases had warned that "the scope of the syndrome may be enormous."[70] The overriding question raised by the resulting news coverage was whether the disease would remain reassuringly contained within distinct groups of "others" or whether it would gain entry into the "general population."[71]

In the spring of 1983, members of the city's Interagency Task Force on AIDS lamented "the tidal wave of publicity on contagion" and debated how best to "reduce the reported levels of panic being generated by the media."[72] The members suggested a "massive distribution" of the Health Department's Q&A fact sheet to counter the trend. It seemed plausible that the fact sheet, though it carefully avoided categorical assertions about the illness, might help to tamp down public fears. "Although a cause for the syndrome has not been found," the brochure stated, "it appears that *intimate, direct* contact, such as sexual contact or injection into the blood, is required. There is no evidence that AIDS is spread through the air or by other forms of casual contact that commonly occur in the workplace or school."[73] The Oleske report had thrown this last assertion into question, however.

The department did not follow the recommendation of the Interagency Task Force on AIDS to distribute the brochure widely. Whether such an action would have significantly reduced the public anxiety surrounding the disease is unclear, and whether it would have moderated the negative views of AIDS patients is doubtful. Throughout history, societies have reacted to new contagions with fear, disgust, and the urge to blame and scapegoat. AIDS provoked all of these responses, and in an especially pronounced fashion because it struck groups whom many people already viewed with distaste. In May 1983, the *Post* ran a syndicated column by the conservative political commentator Patrick Buchanan in which he declared that homosexuals had "declared war on

Nature—and now Nature is exacting an awful retribution." Jerry Falwell, leader of the Moral Majority, jumped on the bandwagon in July by claiming that God was "spanking" homosexuals for their sins.[74] A corollary of this view was that, since people with AIDS had brought the illness on themselves, they had no right to object to whatever punitive measures might be visited upon them in the name of disease control.

Reports circulated widely of people with AIDS being fired from their jobs and evicted from their apartments, even denied burials by funeral homes.[75] Some health care providers refused to care for AIDS patients, citing both disapproval of the way the sick had contracted the illness and fear that the disease might be transmitted from patient to caregiver. The Health Department received calls from medical students asking which hospitals had reported the most AIDS cases so they could be sure not to request a residency there.[76] Lawmakers also sought to control the disease through coercive measures such as isolation and quarantine. Legislation was often driven by sensational cases, as when the Connecticut legislature considered a bill to expand the state's quarantine provisions to include AIDS after a prostitute was alleged to have knowingly spread the disease.[77] That such measures would have been virtually impossible to enforce on a wide scale and unlikely to affect the course of the epidemic was generally lost in these debates.

In this climate, the question of how to prevent the spread of disease was inextricably linked to the issue of protecting the privacy rights of those infected and at risk. In May 1983, Sencer established a committee on confidentiality to review the procedures on the reporting of AIDS cases to the department and craft guidelines that would ensure the protection of patient identities. He also shepherded an amendment to the health code to extend to reports of AIDS cases the same confidentiality protections that applied to other sexually transmitted diseases.[78]

The combination of public fear and scientific uncertainty placed Sencer on the defensive, however. When a sanitation worker who had no known risk—a twenty-six-year-old married man with three children, who denied having engaged in homosexual contact or injection drug use—fell ill with what appeared to be AIDS, the case alarmed municipal workers and unions and seemed to confirm the worst scenarios that had been raised by the Oleske reports on potential routes of transmission. Sencer, along with Mayor Koch and William Foege, head of the CDC, sought to reassure the public at a hastily called news conference. The following week, two New York City Council members, Joe Lisa of Queens and Michael Long of Brooklyn, introduced a measure that would allow the quarantine of people diagnosed with AIDS; the bill would also bar them from working in restaurants and require mandatory reporting of sexual contacts by all people with the disease.[79] Testifying before the City Council health committee when the measure was discussed, Sencer declared, "I can see no scientific reason to incarcerate an individual because he has a disease." Lisa countered, "You're not going to stop people from having sexual contacts just by telling them not to. What great violation of civil rights is it to try to protect the public from a fatal disease that is doubling every six months?"[80]

Neither Lisa nor Long had consulted with the Health Department before introducing the bill, and it was clear that neither had thought through the legal, ethical, or logistical implications of attempting to enforce the measures they were proposing. The effort was emblematic of the reactionary policy responses in the epidemic's early years, as proposals were put forth by politicians who had scant understanding of public health and who were indifferent or hostile to the groups most likely to be affected.

Concern about civil rights and the potential for discrimination grew more acute in April 1984, when researchers working simultaneously in the United States and France announced that they had identified a new retrovirus that was the causal agent of AIDS. Originally called HTLV-III, the virus was ultimately dubbed HIV, or human immunodeficiency virus. Officials at the U.S. Department of Health and Human Services promised that a blood test to detect HIV would soon be available. There were many questions about the test's medical significance. What proportion of people who carried the virus would go on to develop the illness? Might some people—perhaps even a majority—never become sick? Even more troubling than the clinical uncertainties were the social ramifications of the test. Would testing become mandatory for some populations? Who would have access to the results? Would people identified as positive be marked with "carrier" status that could impair their ability to keep their job, maintain their housing, or obtain insurance? Would they be subject to draconian measures such as quarantine?

Anticipating the availability of the test, Sencer convened a meeting in the summer of 1984 to elicit the opinions of gay activists, physicians, and civil rights groups. A clear consensus emerged from the gathering: there was far more peril than promise in the new test. "High-risk groups should be told precisely what dangers they face" from taking the test, GMHC's executive director Rodger McFarlane told Sencer. "Further, they should be advised of the limitations of scientific knowledge and use of any information gained through such testing, especially as it bears on their future health and employment security and insurability."[81] McFarlane was especially concerned about the possibility, broached by the CDC, of using the test results to create a national registry of people who should be barred from donating blood. Such a list could, in the twenty states with sodomy laws, be tantamount to a roster of criminals.

Over the next several months, as licensure of the test grew imminent, many segments of the community voiced similar concerns. In October 1984, the *Native* editorialized strongly: "No gay or bisexual man should allow his blood to be tested." Stephen Caiazza, the president of New York Physicians for Human Rights, a gay doctors' organization, called the test "pernicious." In the spring of 1985, shortly after the test had come onto the market, GMHC took out an advertisement in the *Native* discouraging readers from learning whether they carried the virus.[82] City Council president Carol Bellamy asked Sencer to establish strict confidentiality procedures to prevent accidental or deliberate disclosure of test results by physicians. After reviewing a draft of the consent form the department was preparing for use with the test, Bellamy asked that it be amended to emphasize even more strongly the risks of housing and employment discrimination that HIV-positive people might face.[83]

Sencer saw the test as a tool for protecting the blood supply, but he believed that too much remained unknown for it to be freely available without safeguards. After considering the positions of community leaders and consulting with department staff members, Sencer settled on a policy designed to minimize the social harms that might result from being identified as HIV-positive. New Yorkers would be able to have their blood tested only in carefully circumscribed situations. Aside from use by blood banks for screening donors, the test would be available only as part of a study conducted by the Health Department to assess its sensitivity, specificity, and clinical significance. The Bureau of Laboratories would process each blood sample it received using each of the three commercially available tests and would run T-cell counts, a marker of immune system function, on all blood samples. Commercial laboratories were prohibited from using any of the test kits except as part of a protocol of the department or a department-approved researcher. Physicians could test their patients' blood only if they agreed to participate in the department's study and provide the department's consent form, which strongly emphasized the risks that a positive result posed to the patient's emotional well-being and employment and insurance status.[84] At a time when other cities and states were moving to make the test widely available, the policy guaranteed that few people would learn their status.

In a mass mailing to the city's 27,000 physicians at the beginning of April, Sencer explained the department's policy. "Many people who feel they are at risk of AIDS because of their life style will want to be immediately tested. They should be strongly urged not to seek the test at this time," the letter advised. "If the test is truly positive, we do not know the prognostic significance. If it is falsely positive, it will cause worries that need not exist. And a negative test does not always mean a person is free of infection."[85]

Soon after the test was licensed, however, fissures appeared in the wall of community opposition. Many people began to question whether the potential for stigma, discrimination, and psychological distress should outweigh all other concerns. There was a clear public demand for the test. In March, the Department had set up a hotline to answer questions about testing, staffed by eighteen counselors, which within a few months was receiving around four thousand calls per month (see figure 4.3).[86] Those in favor of greater access to testing saw the city's position as both unacceptably paternalistic and detrimental to the public health. The former executive director of the National Gay Task Force argued that learning one's HIV status was an essential step toward protecting oneself and others. Stephen Caiazza of New York Physicians for Human Rights, who had initially opposed testing, reversed his position after learning that more than a dozen patients in his practice had donated blood so that they could find out their status.[87] By the end of 1985, the president of the American Association of Physicians for Human Rights had changed his position as well.[88]

As community reactions shifted, so did the official positions of public health organizations. The Association of State and Territorial Health Officials issued a strongly pro-testing position paper in the summer of 1985, and the CDC recommended the following March that all Americans be voluntarily tested.[89] The Health Department's continued caution surrounding use of the test drew criticism from some public health experts. King Holmes, a professor of medicine at the University of Washington and a nationally recognized authority on sexually transmitted diseases, wrote to Sencer urging him to reconsider the policy; Holmes considered it "repugnant" that the department would refuse to allow laboratories to perform any test that both the patient and physician wanted.[90]

Positions within the department varied. Wendy Chavkin, a young physician with the Bureau of Maternity Services and Family Planning who was a strong advocate for the rights of poor women, chaired an internal working group that recommended against pregnant women being tested. The key issue for the group was the lack of any clear benefit: clinical medicine had nothing to offer the women who might test positive, while there was a risk of stigma, discrimination, and the threat of violence from intimate partners. The group's recommendation contained a proviso that it was subject to revision should therapeutic prospects for the disease improve. "We all agreed," Chavkin later recalled, "that if there were to be treatment, it would change everything."[91] Rand Stoneburner, who directed the AIDS Surveillance Unit, grappled with the issue but ultimately felt that the test's value was limited. "We think that if a person is in a high-risk group, the message for them about behavior changes is the same whether they're antibody-positive or -negative."[92] But Mary Ann Chiasson, an epidemiologist who worked with Stoneburner, felt that the failure to make testing widely available amounted to an abdication of public health responsibilities to the gay community.[93]

Figure 4.3   AIDS Hotline

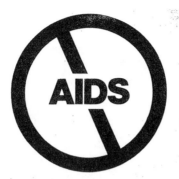

IF YOU WANT TO STOP AIDS, YOU HAVE TO KNOW THE FACTS:

- **AIDS** IS NOT SPREAD BY CASUAL CONTACT;

- **THERE** IS NO BLOOD TEST WHICH CAN TELL YOU IF YOU HAVE AIDS, OR IF YOU'RE GOING TO GET IT;

- **BLOOD** BANKS ARE NOW SCREENING ALL DONATED BLOOD FOR A VIRUS CONNECTED TO AIDS, THE "HTLV–III" VIRUS, TO KEEP THE BLOOD SUPPLY SAFE.

FOR QUESTIONS ABOUT HTLV–III, ABOUT AIDS, **AND** ABOUT BEING AT RISK, CALL

(1–718–HTLV–III)
(1–718–485–8III)

NEW YORK CITY DEPARTMENT OF HEALTH.
ALL SERVICES CONFIDENTIAL.

Source: Courtesy New York City Municipal Archives.
Note: When a blood test for the AIDS virus became available in April 1985, the Health Department set up a hotline to answer questions about the disease and the test. The virus would eventually be named human immunodeficiency virus (HIV), but at the time it was known as HTLV-III.

Irwin Davison, the department's legal counsel, also saw the policy as a misguided. "AIDS is the biggest thing to come along," he said, "and [if] we aren't going to test, what are we about?"[94]

By the end of the year, the department had bowed to public pressure and relaxed the restrictive policy, allowing hospitals to perform the test. They were required to use the department's consent form, however, which strongly emphasized the risks over the benefits of the test.

Battlegrounds: Bathhouses and Schoolyards

Two of the most contentious debates in the AIDS epidemic's early years involved the Health Department's policies regarding environments where the disease might spread. One debate involved bathhouses, sex clubs, and other settings where multiple public and semipublic sex acts occurred; the other involved schools, where parents feared that their children might be infected by the heedless actions of HIV-positive classmates. In both cases, community members asserted the right to control their own risks and to challenge the Health Department's judgment and interpretation of evidence.

One of Roger Enlow's first acts as the director of the department's Office of Gay and Lesbian Health Concerns was to convene a meeting of all the city's bathhouse owners. In July 1983, he and Dennis Passer, the president of New York Physicians for Human Rights, hosted two working sessions to discuss with the owners how they could educate their patrons about the risks of sexually transmitted diseases in general and AIDS in particular.[95] The Health Department could have used its regulatory powers to order bathhouses closed on the grounds that they posed a danger to public health, just as it could shutter restaurants serving tainted food. That it should refrain from doing so struck many observers as absurd. The department's own epidemiologists, after all, had determined that having a high number of partners in bathhouses was one of the strongest predictors of infection.

But both Sencer and Enlow—along with virtually the entire staff of the Bureau of Preventable Diseases—believed that sites of infection could also serve as venues for prevention. Bathhouse patrons were not going to stop having sex, they reasoned; the bathhouses provided a setting for the efficient distribution of educational and persuasive messages about reducing risk. Enlow told Neil Schram, the president of the American Association of Physicians for Human Rights, that closing the bathhouses "would simply result in a displacement of behavior already deeply ingrained in many gay men and, perhaps more importantly, another clientele which frequents the baths, and only the baths, which might not be reached any other way."[96]

Some experts believed, moreover, that the risk posed by bathhouses might have been high in the late 1970s, when people now showing symptoms were most likely to have been infected, but that it had greatly diminished since then. Alan Kristal, an epidemiologist with the Bureau of Preventable Diseases who had been active in the New York AIDS Network, an advocacy group, before David Sencer recruited him to join the department, had done an analysis based on interview data collected in San Francisco about the number of partners reported by gay men and the percentage of those partners encountered in bathhouses. After estimating the number of gay men still attending the baths, he calculated that closure would have a negligible effect on transmission patterns; at most, it would reduce the number of AIDS cases by one-quarter of 1 percent. "No public health official would institute a public health intervention based upon such a tiny expected benefit," Kristal said.[97] A later study by other researchers would confirm that sexual encounters in all public venues dropped off dramatically after the advent of AIDS, with attendance at bathhouses declining the most.[98]

While some opponents of closure based their objections on empirical questions about risk, others raised philosophical and political concerns. Civil libertarians argued that activities in bathhouses took place between consenting adults and should therefore remain outside the purview of state regulation. Gay rights activists warned that any measures to limit sexual freedom would be the first step in an antigay campaign, with disease control providing a pretense for moralistic prohibitions. Thomas Stoddard, a gay lawyer with the New York Civil Liberties Union, saw closing the bathhouses as the entering wedge toward the suppression of other businesses catering to gays and lesbians, such as bars and movie theaters—culminating, in the grimmest scenario, in the reenactment of antisodomy laws in places where they had been repealed.[99]

Even as Enlow was negotiating with bathhouse owners, political forces seemed on the verge of forcing the government's regulatory hand. Governor Mario Cuomo was under pressure from some of his conservative constituents, including members of the clergy who viewed the gay liberation movement with suspicion, to clamp down on public sex venues. He directed state health commissioner David Axelrod to investigate whether such establishments contributed to the spread of AIDS.[100] Axelrod could have bypassed the city and invoked the state health code to shut these businesses. He concluded, however, that such a move would violate civil rights and have no clear benefit for public health. For now, the bathhouses would remain open.

After the meeting that Enlow convened, New York Physicians for Human Rights prepared a set of guidelines for reducing the risk of infection and requested that bathhouse owners prominently post them. The guidelines closely followed the safe sex recommendations developed by

Michael Callen and Richard Berkowitz—shower before and after sex, use condoms, avoid ingesting semen and fecal matter—and concluded with an exhortation to "take better care of yourself and your partners."[101] Gay Men's Health Crisis created an educational campaign with the slogan "Great sex is healthy sex," and the message was distributed via posters and pamphlets in bathhouses, backroom bars, movie theaters, and bookstores.[102]

Such efforts were premised on the belief that bathhouse owners would cooperate in the distribution of prevention messages. This assumption proved unwarranted, however. By early 1985, several gay activists who had become convinced that bathhouse patrons were not being provided with educational materials and condoms formed a group called the Coalition for Sexual Responsibility. The group saw the safe sex recommendations for customers as insufficient; explicit rules for the owners were also necessary. The group's members drew up a list of guidelines for lighting, condom distribution, and presence of posters and pamphlets designed to reduce risky sexual acts; they stopped short of recommending more far-reaching structural changes such as removal of doors from private areas.[103] When group members conducted a follow-up investigation several months later, however, they found that only two of the city's ten bathhouses were complying with the recommendations. The perception grew that community self-policing was inadequate.

Michael Callen, a cofounder of the Coalition for Sexual Responsibility, initially rejected the idea of government intervention, believing that the matter had to be handled within the gay community. Yet in a guest column for the *Village Voice* in March 1985, Callen conceded the need for outside regulation. "Who will take responsibility," he asked, "for altering the business-as-usual operation of commercial sex establishments during this health crisis? The gay 'community'? The state? The answer, I believe, should be both."[104] In Callen's view, the intervention of the Health Department was needed because gay men were "pathetically weak and disorganized" and lacked both the political will and the legal authority to police the establishments that served them. Callen's call for the assistance of the department was ironic given that health professionals and government officials had historically been forces for the oppression of gay sexuality. That he would now ask the department to intervene was a remarkable indication of the sense of crisis brought on by the continuing toll of sickness and death.

By the fall of 1985, a laissez-faire stance toward public sex establishments had grown untenable. The incidence of AIDS continued to climb; cases had roughly doubled over the previous year, and in June the city had reported its highest one-month incidence of the disease. Faced with the relentless spread, health officials in San Francisco, the other metropolitan area hardest hit by the disease, had opted to close the bathhouses.[105] Finally, there was increasing concern about the spread of the disease beyond the initially recognized "risk groups" into the "general population." In early October, Mario Cuomo announced in a press conference that he had asked state health commissioner David Axelrod to reconsider his earlier opposition to closure of the bathhouses. Axelrod subsequently explained that the governor's request was motivated by concern for "the spouses of bisexual males who did not know of their husband's proclivities and what impact that would have on the ultimate birth of children"—a revealing example of how the potential spread of the disease to "innocent victims" was driving the policy agenda.[106]

Cuomo's renewed push for closure coincided with the New York City mayoral election. Diane McGrath, the Republican candidate, called for the bathhouses to be closed. Ed Koch, now under pressure from both his mayoral opponent and the governor's office, asked Sencer to revisit the issue. Koch made clear his desire to avoid an embarrassing conflict between state and city policy.[107] Sencer continued to believe, however, that "closure of the bathhouses will contribute little if anything to the control of AIDS and has the potential to be counterproductive." Sencer was concerned about the ramifications of such an action on future work with affected communities. "Control of this disease, as in most diseases, is predicated on voluntary cooperation with public policy," he explained to Koch. "If we resort to individual coercion, will this lead the public to shun cooperation on other important issues?"[108]

The tide was clearly turning against the bathhouses, however. At the end of October, state health commissioner David Axelrod reversed his earlier position and now declared that the bathhouses were "a serious menace to the public health." He denied that Cuomo had pressured him to change his stance. Bypassing Sencer, he introduced a resolution that would amend the state health code to declare the bathhouses subject to closure as "public nuisances." Sixty days later, the resolution overwhelmingly passed the Public Health Council, the state's equivalent of the city's Board of Health.[109]

The amendment to the health code compelled the city to inspect the bathhouses to determine which should be closed. The city's lawyers believed that the Health Department, in light of its past opposition to closure, would be uncooperative in the effort, so they decided to dispatch inspectors from the Department of Consumer Affairs—normally concerned with matters such as the proper issuance of sales receipts and the price labeling of grocery items—to assess exactly what was going on in public sex environments. Over the course of two weeks, the inspectors observed "49 acts of high risk sexual activity (consisting of 41 acts of fellatio involving 70 persons and 8 acts of anal intercourse involving 16 persons)."[110] The first club to be shuttered under the new rule was the Mine Shaft, which some gay activists had long decried as the establishment where safe sex guidelines were most flagrantly disregarded; within a year, six of the city's ten bathhouses had been closed for violations. Along with the gay establishments, Plato's Retreat, a popular heterosexual club, was shut by the city—not for high-risk sex but for prostitution.[111]

The St. Mark's Baths, one of the clubs that had been considered cooperative in safe sex education efforts, brought suit against the state, arguing that the amendment to the health code violated its rights of privacy and freedom of association. The State Supreme Court dismissed the claim. "The privacy protection of sexual activity conducted in a private home," the court stated, "does not extend to commercial establishments simply because they provide an opportunity for intimate behavior or sexual release."[112]

After the first cases of AIDS were diagnosed in children in the fall of 1982, it was only a matter of time before the issue of transmission in schools would arise. The department's early educational efforts had included outreach to teachers and school principals; the department suggested that schools follow the guidelines that had been developed a few years earlier for preventing transmission of hepatitis B. Concerns among many educators persisted, however, especially after James Oleske's *JAMA* study suggested that the virus might spread among members of a household. In the summer of 1983, the director of a school for the deaf had written to the Health Department for guidance about dealing with children who might be infected; the staff were "not reassured by the lack of evidence that it may not be spread by casual contact."[113] Such fears hinged on the belief that schoolchildren—especially very young ones, the disabled, and those with special needs—were not in control of their bodily fluids and that schools presented a uniquely hazardous environment where the risk of contagion was heightened.

By early 1985, the CDC had concluded that there was no scientific reason to exclude children with AIDS from schools and was drafting official guidelines on the issue. Around that time, David Sencer began negotiating with the city's Board of Education on a new policy, anticipating that it would reflect the CDC's recommendations once they were released to the public. Two episodes that summer—one local and the other seven hundred miles away in the heart of the Midwest—powerfully influenced the events that would unfold in the fall.

In Kokomo, Indiana, residents mobilized to keep thirteen-year-old Ryan White, a hemophiliac who had contracted AIDS from contaminated blood products, from attending middle school. The superintendent issued an order barring White, who was forced to listen to his classes via speaker phone when the school year began in August. White's family sued, and the case would drag on throughout the school year, attracting national attention. That even one of the epidemic's "innocent victims" could be denied his rights and ostracized by his neighbors dramatically illustrated the fear that surrounded the illness.[114] At the same time that Kokomo residents were organizing to keep Ryan White out of school, a grassroots movement against "AIDS victims" was emerging in New York City in a distant corner of the borough of Queens. In July, the Health and Hospitals Corporation announced plans to transfer ten patients with AIDS from Bellevue Hospital to a wing of a partially vacant nursing home in Neponsit, an affluent beachfront neighborhood on a sliver of land at the southern edge of the borough. Residents there rose up in protest, and their City Council representatives forced the HHC to back away from its plan. A comment by a Neponsit resident during the controversy captured both the extremity of discomfort with the illness and the distorted ideas about its routes of transmission: "It's ridiculous to put AIDS cases a block away from residential facilities."[115] The mobilization by residents of Kokomo and Neponsit formed the backdrop to the decision by two community school boards in Queens to oppose the admission of children with AIDS to schools.

Since 1970, the New York City school district had been subdivided into thirty-two semi-autonomous community school boards, which had control over local matters, such as the physical plants of schools (and which often clashed with the central Board of Education, headquartered in downtown Brooklyn). On August 22, 1985, the community school board for District 27 passed a resolution declaring that children with AIDS had a "communicable disease" and should be subject to "appropriate isolation"—that is, barred from attending school.[116] The president of the school board sent a letter to all parents in the district notifying them of the board's action. A few days later, the school board in the adjacent District 29 passed a similar resolution. District 27, which included Neponsit, was mostly white, with a median income higher than the city overall; District 29 was majority black and included both middle-class and poor residents, though the median income in the district was also higher than the city median.[117] What the two districts shared was a more conservative political outlook than the city overall; a history of having disagreed with the central education bureaucracy over policy matters; a conviction that their interests were not well served by the decisions of government bureaucrats and scientific elites; and a belief that AIDS was, and should remain, outside of their neighborhoods.[118]

On August 27, the New York City Board of Education announced the policy it had developed in collaboration with the Health Department (see figure 4.4). Children with AIDS would be admitted to school on a case-by-case basis; ad hoc panels would make decisions after considering the child's age, health status, and other relevant behavioral factors. At

Figure 4.4   Press Conference on Children with AIDS

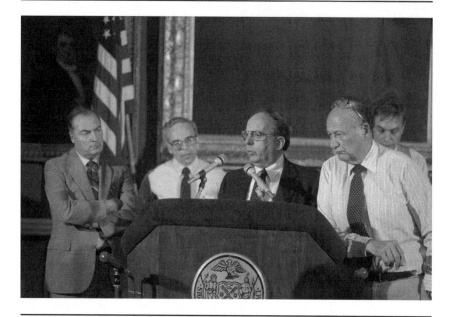

Source: William Sauro/The New York Times/Redux, with permission.
Note: Health Commissioner David Sencer (at lectern) and Mayor Ed Koch (right) answer questions at a press conference about the city's policy of deciding on a case-by-case basis whether children with AIDS would be allowed to attend school. At left are Board of Education president James Regan and Schools Chancellor Nathan Quinones.

the time there were about seventy-eight children under age twelve known to have contracted AIDS in New York City. Fifty-two were deceased; of the remaining twenty-six, four wanted to attend school.[119] In keeping with the new policy, Sencer appointed a panel, made up of two employees from the Health Department, employees from the Board of Education, and the president of the United Parents Association, to review the four cases. Not waiting for the panel's decision, officials from Districts 27 and 29 held a press conference on September 4 in which they called for a moratorium on enrolling children with AIDS in school. For the event, officials flew in Daniel Carter, the president of the Kokomo school board that had voted to keep Ryan White from attending school.

Three days later, on September 7, the panel reviewing the children's cases announced its decision. Of the four children with AIDS known to the city, one was determined to be well enough to continue attending school. The child was a second-grader who had been going to classes the previous three years. The school the child would attend was not named, nor was the child's gender revealed to the public. The day of the announcement, Samuel Granirer, the president of the District 27 school board, declared his intention to sue the city. Granirer was a well-to-do businessman with political aspirations who had been prominent in the battle to keep AIDS patients out of the Neponsit nursing home. Speaking to an overflowing crowd of more than five hundred Queens residents gathered in a school auditorium, Granirer defiantly rejected the policy put forth by the city. With a flair for dramatic gestures that he would display throughout the controversy, Granirer brought his nine- and eleven-year-old children to the stage and hugged them, declaring, "These are my two children. I worked very hard to get them to this age. And I don't want any bureaucrat in downtown Brooklyn telling me I have no right to protect these kids."[120]

With just two days before classes were to start, leaders of the two school boards sought to convince parents to keep their children out of classes. They blanketed their neighborhoods with flyers and drove through the streets with a bullhorn to reinforce the message. On September 9, the first day of classes, hundreds of parents protested outside of eight public schools in the two districts carrying signs such as SAVE OUR KIDS, KEEP AIDS OUT, OUR CHILDREN WANT GRADES, NOT AIDS, and TEACHER'S AIDES, YES; STUDENT AIDS, No. About 11,000 students from the two districts were kept home by their parents.

In absolute numbers, the boycott was unimpressive. The children kept home represented just 1 percent of the city's one million pupils; none of the other thirty community school boards mounted a similar challenge. But the protest carried symbolic significance far in excess of its numerical strength. Like the Ryan White case, it revealed the depths of the fears about people with AIDS and the lengths to which galvanized communities would go to keep the disease from entering their lives. Playing out in parallel with the controversy in Kokomo, and in the midst of the local battles over bathhouse closings and fears of the disease's spread into the "general population," the fight in Queens was tailor-made for the local press, which blanketed their pages with coverage. When Granirer's suit came to trial in late September, far more was at stake than the issue of children attending school. At a time of widespread fear, often verging on hysteria, about the potential spread of AIDS, a decision to bar infected children from school would give a judicial imprimatur to what most scientists considered a distorted view of the risks of casual transmission.[121]

Besides David Sencer, the most important witness from the Health Department was epidemiologist Polly Thomas, who had been a member of the ad hoc panel that reviewed the child's case. Neither Sencer nor

Thomas had ever testified in court, and with their cautious, carefully spoken demeanors, both approached the role of witness with trepidation. But the city's chief lawyer, F. A. O. Schwartz, who was arguing the case, prepped them both extensively about the kinds of questions they would face and the most effective way to answer. Robert Sullivan, representing the Queens parents, hammered at Sencer for his handling of the swine flu episode. In cross-examining Thomas—who was herself a mother of two toddlers—Sullivan demanded to know whether she would want her child to be tested for the virus if the child were bitten by a person with AIDS. Thomas's unhesitant reply of "I would not" drew gasps from the spectators. "I know of all the things that can happen to my kids," she later told the *Times*. "I have all these irrational fears. I know what it's like to be a mother. But I'm also a pediatrician and epidemiologist with the Health Department."[122] Several mothers in the two school districts later said that Thomas's answer made them reconsider their opposition to the city's policy.[123]

In addition to Sencer and Thomas, the city drew on a high-powered lineup of witnesses that included some of the city's most respected and well-known medical figures. Sullivan's array of witnesses was smaller and less distinguished, partly because most medical experts believed that the city's policy was correct, and partly because even those who remained doubtful about the possibility of transmission in schools saw little to gain from stepping publicly into the midst of such an emotionally and politically charged controversy. Sullivan's witness with the most impressive credentials was Ayre Rubinstein, a pediatrician and immunologist at Albert Einstein Medical College who was a nationally recognized expert on children with AIDS. Rubinstein at first refused to testify, but Sullivan subpoenaed him.[124] On the stand, Rubinstein said, "There's more to know" about transmission of the AIDS virus—a statement no scientist would ever dispute, but which Sullivan presented as a vindication of the Queens parents' position.

Throughout the five-week trial, the opposing sides in the case were operating without a shared understanding of the concept of risk and were thus, at a basic level, talking past each other. Scientists used such cautious qualifiers as "extremely unlikely" and "infinitesimally small" to describe the risks of transmission.[125] For the parents, however, the catastrophic nature of the outcome—a child contracting AIDS from a classmate—was far more salient than the remoteness of that possibility. In their eyes, no amount of risk was acceptable. The school board's lawyers hammered home the point that an extremely small probability of transmission did not exclude the possibility.

The trial exemplified a familiar narrative of the 1980s, as politically energized community members challenged the judgment, integrity, and conclusions of medical experts. Residents who perceived high rates of cancer in their neighborhoods, for example, repudiated the judgment of epidemiologists and public health officials who insisted that such "cancer clusters" were illusory.[126] In these controversies, mistrust of scientific authorities often dovetailed with suspicion of government bureaucrats. In his closing statement, Sullivan elided any distinction between the two categories when he declared that "big government is taking over."[127]

Although scientific evidence had accumulated about valid and invalid routes of transmission, widespread misunderstanding remained among the lay public. In part because mainstream media outlets would not use the terms "semen" or "vaginal secretions" when discussing transmission of the virus, preferring the euphemism "bodily fluids," many people harbored doubts about saliva, sweat, tears, urine, and vomit. Mayor Koch, often a loose cannon in his policy pronouncements, did not help matters when he publicly stated during the trial that he "would rather err on the side of caution" when considering whether to allow children with AIDS to attend school. Seeming to contradict both the CDC and the city's expert panel, he asked rhetorically, "You want to be bitten by someone with AIDS to be the guinea pig to determine whether it's transmittable?"[128] A national poll conducted at the time of the Queens lawsuit found that more than half of Americans believed that AIDS could be spread through casual contact such as sitting near an infected person. Another poll found that 47 percent believed that the virus could be contracted from a drinking glass, and 28 percent believed that it could be caught from a toilet seat.

The corollary of the belief that casual transmission was possible was that extreme measures to separate the infected were appropriate. A *Daily News* poll in October, when both the bathhouse and the schools controversies were garnering headline coverage in local newspapers and television broadcasts, found that 40 percent of New York City residents supported quarantining people with AIDS. At the news conference where she called for closing the bathhouses, mayoral candidate Diane McGrath had argued that people whose jobs entailed "intimate contact" with the public, such as doctors, nurses, teachers, food handlers, barbers, and beauticians, should be required to be tested for HIV, and those found to be positive should be fired. Such people were, she said, "a clear and evident menace to the health of their patrons."[129] In November, City Council member Noach Dear introduced a bill to bar any "carriers" of AIDS from schools. About one hundred demonstrators chanted and carried signs to protest what they saw as increasing hysteria about the disease.[130]

In February 1986, the court ruled that the plaintiffs had failed to show that the city should bar the child from school. Exclusion would, moreover, violate both the Rehabilitation Act, which prohibited agencies receiving federal funds from discriminating against the disabled, and the equal protection clause of the Fourteenth Amendment. "Although this court certainly empathizes with the fears and concerns of parents for the health and welfare of their children within the school setting," Judge Harold Hyman wrote, he was duty-bound "not to be influenced by unsubstantiated fears of catastrophe."[131]

The Limits of Public Health

By the end of 1985, more than 16,000 people had been diagnosed with AIDS in the United States, and about half had died. Although New York City's share of the epidemic had steadily declined as more cases were diagnosed around the country, the city was still the hardest-hit by far, accounting for approximately 4,000 cases.

Scientists eventually understood that HIV has an incubation period typically in the range of five to ten years. Since the first people diagnosed with AIDS had been infected with HIV in the 1970s, before the virus had been identified, there was nothing public health professionals could have done to prevent their becoming ill. By the time cases began to appear in hospitals and doctors' offices, it was already too late to stop the epidemic. There was clear if indirect evidence that gay men began to change their behavior as soon as the epidemic was recognized, before any prevention messages had been put forth. Between 1981 and 1983, the gonorrhea rate—a key indicator of unprotected intercourse—declined by 45 percent in the Lower West Side Health District, which included the gay enclaves of Greenwich Village and Chelsea, while rates of the disease in the rest of the city remained unchanged.[132]

The appearance of AIDS dramatically illustrated the difficulty of acting in a precautionary manner in the face of scientific uncertainty. Immediate, aggressive prevention efforts could have limited the number of new infections in the early 1980s, thus reducing the eventual sickness and death that would develop years later. Such efforts might well have had unintended consequences, however. Although he was often attacked for doing too little, David Sencer was concerned about the possibility of what might be called public health iatrogenesis—a situation in which interventions designed to prevent harm instead cause harm.[133] What might be the consequences of promulgating risk reduction guidelines if the virus could be transmitted in unforeseen ways? What human rights violations might be committed against the groups who carried (and spread) the new virus? Sencer's concerns about civil liberties and privacy rights were neither idle nor misguided, as some of his critics charged. Yet his methodical, cautious approach to educating the public was ill suited to the context of an emerging epidemic, which was often chaotic and marked by fear verging on hysteria. One of the greatest tools available to state and local health departments is the bully pulpit of the commissioner—a platform that Sencer was never entirely comfortable using. Sencer's successor, Stephen Joseph, would approach AIDS—and most other public health issues—with a very different style, but with no less controversy.

Chapter 5

City of Misfortune

IN MAY 1986, three weeks after being sworn in as the city's new health commissioner, Stephen Joseph appeared before a joint hearing of the City Council and the Board of Estimate to answer questions about the department's budget for the coming fiscal year. The event was largely ceremonial, but it gave Joseph the chance to advance his views of the city's most pressing health needs. After he gave a brief opening statement, the assembled politicians—thirty-five members on the council and eight on the board—peppered him with questions. Many of these, predictably, related to AIDS, which by a wide margin remained the most visible and contentious health issue in the city. The federal government doesn't seem to be doing much, one council member opined. How much money is it contributing to dealing with AIDS? Do we have enough funds for surveillance? Where can someone go to get free testing for the virus? Are placards and pamphlets effective tools for AIDS education?

But AIDS was not the only topic on the table that day. Joseph faced tough questions about many other health problems, representing politicians' pet concerns, the issues they had heard about from their constituents, and the stories getting the most attention in the media. What is the department going to do to improve the health of homeless people living in shelters and welfare hotels? How many children will be screened for lead poisoning in the coming year? Is there enough money in the department budget for tuberculosis control? Are we doing anything to monitor infant mortality?[1]

During the 1980s, AIDS competed for resources and attention with a set of interlocking public health problems rooted in poverty, social inequity, and racism. The city's economy turned around, but the gains were not evenly distributed across all classes; New York was increasingly polarized as the decade progressed, with extremes of wealth and hardship. For the already disadvantaged, it became a meaner, harsher place. The percentage of city residents living in poverty rose to one-quarter. After remaining stable for several years, rates of both drug use and violent crime began to spiral upward in 1985, swelling the city's jails and prompting the (largely ineffectual) expenditure of millions of dollars to stanch the problems. New Yorkers became desensitized to the sight of men, women, and children sleeping in doorways. Hospital emergency rooms overflowed with poor patients sick with the diseases of deprivation. "In this sea of New York's troubles," Joseph later wrote in his account of the epidemic, "AIDS was just one more rock dropped into the waves."[2]

Stephen Joseph was a native New Yorker whose career as a pediatrician had taken him far afield; he had worked as a Peace Corps doctor in Nepal and as a physician for the U.S. Agency for International Development in West Africa. He had risen to become the highest-ranking health official at USAID in the 1970s, when he became enmeshed in a controversy over the use of infant formula in developing nations. Activists charged that manufacturers such as Nestlé were aggressively promoting their products in spite of evidence that the failure to breast-feed was contributing to high infant mortality rates. Joseph fought for a World Health Organization (WHO) resolution that would create a voluntary code to curb the marketing of formula in poor countries. When the United States, alone among 118 nations, voted against the code, calling it a threat to free enterprise, Joseph resigned in protest. He promptly found himself unemployable in the world of international health, where U.S. funding dominated.[3] He had eventually been able to return to the field and was working as a special coordinator for child health at UNICEF when David Sencer resigned at the end of 1985. Local health care experts who admired Joseph's professional experience and political convictions recommended him to Koch's aides.

Both David Sencer, from 1982 through 1985, and Stephen Joseph, from 1986 through 1989, struggled to address health problems whose root causes remained outside the department's formal purview. Their task was complicated by unstable funding streams that made a coherent and sustained public health response difficult and by the involvement of advocacy groups, alternately supportive and critical, that undertook their own research and service initiatives and pressured the Health Department and other city agencies to do more.

The Politics of Poverty and Health

Homelessness in New York City had once been synonymous with "Skid Row," the mile-long stretch of flophouses on the Bowery where middle-aged alcoholic men eked out a precarious living. But large-scale shifts in the city's housing market and the local and national economies in the

1970s and 1980s changed the face of homelessness, which became far more demographically diverse and geographically dispersed than the city had seen before.

Between 1970 and 1980, the amount of low-income housing in the city shrank dramatically as residential stock in poor neighborhoods deteriorated and landlords found it cheaper to abandon properties than to maintain them. In some parts of the Bronx and Brooklyn, suspicious fires thought to be set by property owners seeking to collect insurance became epidemic. By some estimates, the city lost almost 90 percent of its low-cost residential hotel rooms.[4] During the same years, some 250,000 blue-collar jobs disappeared from the city. The fiscal crisis led to the slashing of jobs with city government, which had been an important source of low-skill, entry-level employment, especially for African Americans and Latinos. Beginning in 1981, the Reagan administration gutted federal housing assistance to the poor. All these factors combined to create a large population of homeless men, women, and children. Most were only episodically homeless, but some remained that way for years. Between 1960 and 1980, the average number of homeless families in the city's temporary shelters was about 600 per month; by the mid-1980s, the number had risen to around 5,000.[5]

A suit brought by the Legal Aid Society resulted in a 1981 consent decree declaring that the city had an obligation to provide emergency shelter for the homeless, and in 1982 the Coalition for the Homeless was founded in response to the growing crisis. Led by the combative attorney Robert Hayes, the coalition would prove to be a persistent thorn in the city's side, with litigation (or the threat of litigation) its preferred strategy for getting results. Alongside an older, more established charitable organization, the Community Service Society, the coalition began pressuring the city to take action on the increasingly visible numbers of people sleeping in doorways, parks, and subway and train stations because they had nowhere else to go.

A patchwork of temporary shelters run by the Department of Housing Preservation and Development and the Human Resources Administration grew up. Single people (mostly men) were directed to armories and other large buildings, such as vacant schools, where they slept on cots in large open areas, barracks-style. Families were sent to two types of temporary housing: hotels, which lacked stoves or refrigerators and often had shared bathrooms, and a smaller number of apartments with small kitchens and private baths. The hotels and apartments were privately owned and operated and received payments from the city. Families made up half of the city's homeless population; the typical homeless family was headed by a single woman with three children.[6]

The epithet "Dickensian" was often invoked to describe the squalor of homeless facilities: overcrowding and lack of privacy, peeling paint, threadbare mattresses, the ever-present threat of crime and violence. The facilities were a breeding ground for respiratory and gastrointestinal ailments such as measles, dysentery, and shigellosis. Because the hotels had no refrigerators, any food brought into them attracted rats and cockroaches. The department's Bureau of Environmental Health inspected each welfare hotel every six months for vermin infestations; when the Koch administration asked hotel owners to install small refrigerators in the rooms at city expense, the owners tried to bargain for a less-frequent inspection schedule in exchange. (The Health Department refused.)[7] Other common problems uncovered in the inspections included inadequate or nonfunctioning sinks and toilets, construction areas not properly sealed off from children, and insufficient emergency exits.

There were a few venues where homeless people could receive medical care. The Human Resources Administration contracted with the Health and Hospitals Corporation to provide limited clinical services at about half of the shelters run by the HRA. The Children's Aid Society set up an on-site medical clinic at one of the largest welfare hotels in 1983, and a group of physicians from St. Vincent's Hospital set up a clinic at the men's shelter on Wards Island. There was no systematic approach, however, to providing screening or other preventive services throughout the shelter system. As the problem continued to worsen—the number of families in temporary housing doubled during 1983, as did the average length of their stay—the Health Department, under David Sencer, established the Family Shelter Health Program. Seven full-time public health nurses were assigned to provide general preventive services, including health education, screening, and referrals to treatment. The program began in the city's three largest welfare hotels (one each in Manhattan, Brooklyn, and Queens); it soon expanded into the nine largest shelters, which together housed almost half of the city's homeless families.[8]

Infants and children, unlike homeless adult men, had a well-organized advocacy movement behind them, and it was concern about them that drove much of the public health response to the issue. The Citizens' Committee for Children, one of the most influential of the city's health advocacy groups, made the issue of homeless children a central focus; its support was critical in securing additional city funding for the department's Family Shelter Health Program.[9] In early 1983, New York governor Mario Cuomo commissioned Montefiore Hospital's Department of Social Medicine to study the health of homeless children in two of the city's largest shelters.

The issue of homelessness, like the fight over closing the bathhouses, became a symbolic weapon in the long-running political war between Mayor Koch and Governor Cuomo. In the 1977 mayoral contest, Koch had defeated Cuomo; the two men faced off again in the 1982 governor's race, with Cuomo emerging victorious.[10] Their personal animosity added an extra dimension to the inherent tension over home rule for New York City. When the Montefiore investigators hired by Cuomo found widespread malnutrition among homeless children, the finding was an embarrassment to Koch, who promptly ordered the Health Department to conduct its own survey.

In the summer of 1983, the department screened more than two thousand children under age thirteen in nineteen family shelters and hotels, focusing especially on their nutritional status. The study found no evidence of widespread malnutrition; overall the health status of the children was not significantly worse than that of a comparison group of nonshelter children. The discrepancy between these results and the Montefiore study was most likely due to the state's investigation having been limited to just two hotels, the Martinique in Manhattan and the Granada in Brooklyn, which were among the worst facilities in the system. The Health Department's report was careful to note that although no malnutrition had been found, "these findings should not be interpreted to mean that living conditions are ideal or desirable."[11]

The dueling studies of malnutrition illustrated the way in which public health research could serve as a lever to gain attention and resources for a social problem. Montefiore's Department of Social Medicine conducted rigorous scientific investigations, to be sure, but it was also a bastion of liberal politics whose members were committed to social justice as well as epidemiology. The documentation of some specific morbidity associated with homelessness could make a political impact in a way that a simple moral claim—that a civilized society provides basic habitation and subsistence for its most disadvantaged members—often did not. It seemed that thousands of children living in squalid temporary shelters was not enough to prick society's conscience, but if those children could be shown to be malnourished, then attention had to be paid.

A similar dynamic was at work in 1985 when Wendy Chavkin, a progressive young physician who headed the Health Department's Bureau of Maternity Services and Family Planning, collaborated with Alan Kristal, an epidemiologist with the Bureau of Preventable Diseases (who had done the calculation about the risk of AIDS in bathhouses) to study the birth outcomes of women in city-run homeless shelters. They found that the infant mortality rate for children born of women living in shelters was four times that of the city overall, and that homeless pregnant women were four times more likely than other city mothers to receive no prenatal care (see figure 5.1).[12] The potential for the study to embarrass the city was clear, and after the results were released to the press, Deputy Mayor Stanley Brezenoff summoned Chavkin, Kristal, and Commissioner David Sencer to his office to reprimand them, less for doing the research than for making the findings public.[13] But the study had the ef-

Figure 5.1   Children and Poverty

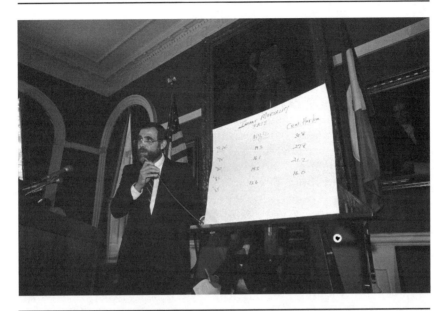

Source: Courtesy New York City Municipal Archives.
Note: Health Commissioner Stephen Joseph presents data on the city's infant mortality rates at a City Hall press conference in 1986. Concern among local politicians about child health was heightened by the rise in the city's homeless population and the cutbacks to federal safety-net programs during the Reagan administration.

fect that Chavkin and Kristal sought. After the study results were reported in the *Times*, the Koch administration announced a $1.6 million
increase in Health Department funding that enabled the number of public health nurses to be increased to nineteen from seven; pregnant women
and women with newborns were to be housed in a select group of shelters where special services would be available to them.[14]

Homelessness posed a particular problem for people with AIDS.
Their condition placed them at heightened risk for the contagions that
spread easily in barracks-style shelters; they also faced the threat of violence from hostile fellow residents should their condition become
known. Although the official policy of the Human Resources Administration was to provide people with AIDS with private rooms in welfare
hotels, in fact it was well known that there were hundreds of them in
shelters, either because they had not received an official diagnosis or
were afraid to come forth with their condition to a social worker, or because there were no private rooms available for them at the time of a
hospital discharge.[15]

Much of the Health Department's work with homelessness created new burdens for the city's Human Resources Administration, an agency that the *Times* dubbed an "empire of misfortune."[16] With 25,000 employees, an annual budget of $4.5 billion, and some 1.5 million clients, the HRA disbursed public assistance payments, conducted child abuse and neglect investigations, administered food stamps, and oversaw foster care and day care programs. Every health problem uncovered in the shelter system was another problem that the HRA had to deal with. Stephen Joseph's public outspokenness about the problems of the shelters—he made repeated statements to the press about issues facing people with AIDS in shelters, for example—created constant friction with his counterpart at HRA, William Grinker.

Health Department employees found HRA difficult to deal with because of its size and complexity. Simply finding a point of organizational entry and gaining the cooperation of someone well placed enough to make things happen was a challenge. After investigating several outbreaks of diarrheal disease, the Bureau of Epidemiology sought to conduct a study of shelter residents to better understand the prevalence and causes of the disease, but could not get anyone within HRA to approve the research.[17] After repeated outbreaks of diarrheal diseases in one shelter, Norman Scherzer, an assistant commissioner with the Health Department who worked on the homeless issue, asked that the HRA put soap and towels in all the bathrooms. HRA officials refused, saying that the clients would simply steal them. Replacing the soap and towels, Scherzer replied, would cost the city less money than continually chasing after the disease outbreaks.[18]

Perhaps the most serious epidemiological problem related to the city's shelter system was tuberculosis, an airborne disease that spread in enclosed spaces. In its congregate shelters for single men, with thousands of people suffering from poor nutrition and chronic health problems sleeping on closely spaced cots, the city could hardly have created a more successful environment for the transmission of tuberculosis. One hundred years earlier, the disease had spread in big cities in notorious "lung blocks," rows of tenements and lodging houses where the poor were packed into squalid rooms with little air or light. "Shelters," wrote two physicians who worked with the homeless, "are the lung blocks of the late 20th century."[19] As will be seen in the next chapter, the spread of tuberculosis among the homeless would eventually become the center of one of the worst public health calamities in the city's history.

The economic and social policies of the Reagan administration created an atmosphere of alarm, extending beyond the realm of homelessness, about the health of infants, children, and pregnant women. Federal cutbacks to Medicaid spending sent state legislatures around the country scrambling to find ways to provide health care for poor children.[20] Advocacy groups such as the Children's Defense Fund warned that cutbacks to safety net programs such as school lunches and day care and the block-granting of maternal and child health monies were endangering the welfare of disadvantaged youth.

When David Sencer issued a report on the city's health statistics in early 1984, local politicians, sensitized to the issues of child health and poverty because of the publicity around federal policies, seized on the infant mortality rates. Overall, infant mortality in the city declined slightly, reflecting several years of progress in medical care, but wide disparities remained among the health districts. The rate for the affluent east side neighborhood of Kips Bay was seven per one thousand births; in Harlem, some five miles north, the rate was twenty-one per one thousand. These disparities were hardly new—they had existed in some form for as long as statistics had been collected—but the political environment caused them to be viewed with fresh urgency. City Council president Carol Bellamy held hearings on the issue, and Mayor Koch, eager to repair the damage the hospital closings had done to his image among African American voters, devoted $2.4 million to a citywide initiative to lower the infant mortality rate.[21]

The Bureau of Maternity Services and Family Planning was one of the units of the Health Department that through years of attrition during the fiscal crisis had been reduced to practically nothing.[22] With the infusion of city money, the bureau established a pregnancy hotline to provide information and referrals on prenatal care and make appointments at facilities around the city (similar to the abortion referral hotline that had been established in 1970). The service, publicized with subway posters and radio and television public-service announcements, was soon receiving some two thousand calls per month. The money was also used to station public health nurses in six HHC hospitals to work closely with high-risk pregnant women.[23] A second phase of the infant mortality initiative was implemented in 1987, when the department received supplemental funding for a pre- and postnatal campaign in which public health nurses made home visits in the four neighborhoods with the highest rates of infant mortality: Central Harlem, Fort Greene and Brownsville in Brooklyn, and Mott Haven in the Bronx.[24]

The heightened concern about infant and child health called attention to the problems facing the Health Department's thirty-seven child health stations and eighteen pediatric treatment centers, most of which were located on the grounds of housing projects in the city's poorest neighborhoods. When Stephen Joseph became commissioner in 1986, he recruited Katherine Lobach as the new director for the Bureau of Child Health. For twenty years, Lobach, a pediatrician widely respected in local child health circles, had run a federally funded clinic in the Bronx affiliated with Montefiore Medical Center. She immediately undertook a comprehensive review of all fifty-five facilities and was dismayed by what she found: "techniques, equipment, facilities and systems which were becoming obsolete twenty years ago," she wrote in a report to Joseph.

> The facilities are usually shabby at best and at worst unsafe and/or uninhabitable, lacking heat in winter and air conditioning in summer, without fire exits or security, and repairs, painting, etc are long overdue. Out-of-order telephones, broken centrifuges, and non-functioning microscopes are daily frustrations.... The bad state of the physical plant discourages well-qualified physicians and other staff from taking positions . . . when they see where they will be assigned.[25]

The problems that Lobach found raised anew the old debate about whether the Health Department should provide ambulatory care and whether its clinical services were redundant with those delivered by the Health and Hospitals Corporation. Many of the child health stations were within a few blocks of HHC-run community health centers. A few weeks after Lobach began work at the Health Department, she was approached by Jo Ivey Boufford, a former colleague from Montefiore who was now the president of the HHC. Boufford was trying to enhance the corporation's primary care capacities and proposed that it take over operation of the child health stations. But Lobach resisted the suggestion, believing that the stations' unique preventive focus would be lost in the vast city hospital bureaucracy.[26] Even though the goal of eliminating redundancy and overlap seemed to argue in favor of Boufford's proposal, Lobach saw the provision of direct patient services as an important way for the Health Department to ensure that its programs were responsive to community needs. "If you're doing population-based public health, and your agency doesn't have any hands-on responsibility for [patient care], you become more and more divorced from the specific health care needs of your population," she later said. Providing clinical care "would continue to give us feedback about the status of children in ways that you couldn't get from just looking at cold data."[27]

Lobach undertook a massive, multi-year campaign of capital renovations to bring the facilities up to standard. But the department would eventually surrender the clinics to the Health and Hospitals Corporation in 1994 as part of a shake-up of city-run medical services. Mayor David Dinkins was under intense pressure to reduce the municipal payroll; the child health stations employed almost nine hundred people, and transferring them to the semiprivate HHC would move them off the city's books without actually reducing services or laying people off.[28] Lobach, who had devoted so much of her energy to renovating the facilities and improving the quality of care they provided, opposed the transfer to the end, as did the city's many child health advocates. But the health commissioner under Dinkins, Margaret Hamburg, took a more pragmatic stance and believed that the HHC's operation of all the public-sector medical services was a more rational way to organize care. Lobach would ultimately leave the Health Department and follow the child health stations to HHC.

An issue closely linked with both child health and homelessness was lead paint poisoning. The department's lead poisoning control program grew steadily after its creation in 1970. The program had been sustained through the city's fiscal crisis because most of its funding came from federal grants and the 1970s were a time of activism in the federal government on environmental issues in general and lead paint in particular. Agencies such as the National Institute for Occupational Safety and Health (NIOSH), the Occupational Safety and Health Administration (OSHA), the Environmental Protection Agency (EPA), and the Consumer Products Safety Commission (CPSC) all took on the issue of lead exposure.[29] After 1974, there were no deaths from lead poisoning in the city. The problem remained highly concentrated in the neighborhoods of Bushwick and Bedford-Stuyvesant, which together accounted for about one-quarter of all cases of lead poisoning uncovered in the city annually.[30]

When David Sencer became commissioner in 1982, the program faced several challenges. New scientific data had emerged suggesting that children could suffer harm from blood lead levels lower than previously suspected. The Board of Health had amended the health code to reflect the changed understanding of the problem by lowering the acceptable levels that would trigger mandatory abatement and removal of the child from the home—a change that dramatically increased the potential caseload of the program.[31] Almost two dozen of the child health stations, where most of the department's screening of blood lead levels was done, had been closed during and after the fiscal crisis. Because of cuts to the Bureau of Health Education, the department had no mass media programs to educate the public about the potential dangers of lead paint or continuing education programs for the city's medical professionals. The CDC's lead poisoning prevention program was one of the areas folded into the federal maternal and child health block grant and reduced by some 25 percent.

Faced with these constraints, and under constant pressure to increase operating revenue, the department's Bureau of Laboratories in 1981 had begun charging hospitals and private physicians to screen blood samples for lead. Members of the Mayor's Advisory Board on Lead Poisoning Control complained to Koch about the change, but the new fees led to only a slight drop in the number of specimens submitted for analysis;

an informal survey of eight major hospitals found no reduction in the amount of screenings performed.[32]

In his first year as commissioner, Sencer requested a special supplement of $300,000 in city funding for the lead program. The additional monies allowed the department to place twenty hematofluorometers (lead screening devices) in non–Health Department facilities such as hospitals and clinics to increase the number of children screened; eliminate the laboratory fees for lead poisoning testing; and increase outreach, including a new subway poster campaign, presentations to community groups, and a professional education seminar for nurses.[33]

Activists and politicians concerned with the lead paint issue pressured the department to do more. A particular source of discontent was the length of time it took—thirty-four days on average—for an apartment to be fully abated after a violation was discovered.[34] The Coalition to End Lead Poisoning, like the Coalition for the Homeless, found litigation to be an effective tool for forcing the city into action, and in the spring of 1984 the group filed a class-action suit on behalf of several lead-poisoned children and their parents. The suit named Koch, Sencer, and the commissioner of the Department of Housing Preservation and Development as defendants, charging that they had failed to adequately enforce the local laws and regulations designed to mitigate lead paint poisoning.[35] Like most litigation against the city, the case would go through years of appeals before being resolved in favor of the plaintiffs.

Funds to address the problem fluctuated widely during the 1980s. In the 1985 to 1986 fiscal year, the department's lead-control budget took another hit when the state reduced its contribution by about 20 percent, a result of cutbacks in the federal prevention block grant. Stephen Joseph convinced Mayor Koch to provide an additional $1 million of city funds for an expanded case-finding and abatement program. The Health Department received about one-third of the monies, with which it hired staff for five mobile screening teams who would conduct outreach in the highest-risk areas of the "lead belt" and additional laboratory personnel to process specimens; Housing Preservation and Development used the funds to increase inspections and improve its oversight of abatement work.[36]

At the same time, however, experts continued to disagree about the best procedures for abating a lead-contaminated environment. The Coalition to End Lead Poisoning pressed for the most stringent cleanup procedures, including sealing the area to prevent the spread of airborne contaminants, use of high-pressure vacuum pumps, sealing floors and nearby surfaces to avoid cross-contamination, and safety gear to protect workers performing the abatement.[37] But there was no universally accepted method. When Stephen Joseph made an informal survey of the local health departments in Baltimore, Cincinnati, and Boston and the state health departments in Maryland and Massachusetts, he found that all used significantly different methods.[38]

The increasing prevalence of homelessness, especially the rising numbers of homeless children, exacerbated the problems posed by lead paint as the city housed families in dilapidated welfare hotels and shelters. A survey by the Department of Housing Preservation and Development found that about one-seventh of the rooms in the largest hotels had lead paint violations.[39] In some facilities the problem was far worse: an inspection at one of the largest hotels in the Bronx found that seventy out of eighty-seven rooms had peeling lead paint that violated the health code; in three of the city's largest facilities, almost all of the rooms tested positive for lead exposure.[40] Homeless children were more than twice as likely as their nonhomeless counterparts to have elevated blood lead levels.[41] Ironically, the city found that compliance with abatement orders was much better among the hotel owners than among building owners in general, since the hotel owners derived so much of their business from the city's homeless caseload and thus had more to lose from noncompliance.[42]

The confluence of homelessness and lead paint poisoning placed the city in a double bind: adhering to the strictest standards of paint abatement would mean excluding some facilities from a scarce supply of temporary shelters. This dilemma was crystallized in the case of the Catherine Street Shelter, a 320-bed facility in a former school building in lower Manhattan. The city opened the shelter in late 1985 but continued renovations, including lead paint abatement, as families were moved in over the subsequent months. In the spring of 1986, the Legal Aid Society and the Coalition to End Lead Poisoning brought in several experts, including teams from the Montefiore Department of Social Medicine program and the Mount Sinai School of Medicine, to examine the sites. Their reports indicated that the ongoing painting, plastering, and other renovations were creating dust and fumes that produced hazardous exposures to lead. Health Department inspectors, however, believed that the possibility of unhealthy exposure was minimal and that, since it was unclear where else the families could go, removing them might cause even more harm than allowing them to stay.[43]

The standoff over differing interpretations of hazard levels continued for several weeks, during which time the state health department also sent inspectors. The Human Resources Administration eventually agreed to empty the facility and find other places for the families to stay; the Legal Aid Society, convinced that the HRA was not moving quickly enough, got a state supreme court judge to order the immediate removal of all the families remaining in the shelter. That summer, after the city had completed some $2 million worth of renovations, the judge allowed the families to come back.[44]

The episode exemplified the hard policy choices that were necessary at a time of both fiscal constraints and overwhelming need for human services, with many equally pressing health problems crying out for attention. It also underscored the difference between the accommodating approach of health officials and the insistence of activists that more be done. According to Assistant Commissioner Mark Rapoport, who was responsible for the Health Department's lead paint program, activists were "obdurate when they should have been flexible." Rapoport believed that groups such as the Legal Aid Society, the Coalition for the Homeless, and the Coalition to End Lead Poisoning had "the luxury of non-responsibility."[45] For their part, activists believed that they had ample reason to distrust the assurances of city government that problems would be taken care of. They resorted to litigation because they saw it as the only way to bring about desperately needed results in a municipal bureaucracy notorious for its glacial pace of change.

As scientific evidence continued to accumulate that lead could be harmful in amounts smaller than previously thought, it became apparent that a quick and inexpensive test for measuring blood lead levels that had been used for many years would no longer be adequate. "The need for resources will increase exponentially," an aide to Rapoport predicted when the CDC announced that it was considering lowering its acceptable threshold level.[46] The prospect of doing good public health with limited resources—of balancing competing demands for critical programs—continued to present intractable problems.

Drug abuse, even more than housing, was an area over which public health had only a tenuous reach, so there was little the department could do to directly address the problem of crack cocaine when it appeared in the city in the fall of 1985. Crack differed from powdered cocaine in that it was smoked rather than inhaled and was thus absorbed into the bloodstream more rapidly, resulting in an almost instant high. It was much cheaper than powdered cocaine—rocks sold for between $5 and $20, compared with $60 for a gram of powder—and the small rocks could be easily hidden and carried in small glass vials. Crack quickly displaced heroin as the drug of choice among young people.[47]

Within a year of the drug's first appearance in the United States, newspapers and magazines had run more than one thousand articles about the new threat, and for a time, crack competed with AIDS as the frightening plague that seemed on the verge of spreading into wholesome American communities. As was the case with most drug panics, it became difficult to disentangle fact from hyperbole and myth, but there was ample evidence that the drug had severe public health effects in the city, especially among poor youth of color in Harlem and Washington Heights, where its use was concentrated. Crack users, studies showed, were more likely than non-users or users of other drugs to have multiple sexual partners and to not use condoms; young women who were ad-dicted often had sex in exchange for the drug. The number of syphilis cases in the city increased 30 percent between 1985 and 1988, raising fears—later confirmed by epidemiologic research—that the drug would also fuel the spread of HIV.[48]

Crack also worsened the already troubled epidemiology of maternal and child health among the poor. In some hospitals in poor neighbor-hoods, between 10 and 20 percent of delivering women and their infants were positive for illicit drugs, mostly crack and cocaine.[49] From 1985 to 1986, the number of birth certificates in the city showing maternal sub-stance use rose by almost 70 percent.[50] Infants born to cocaine-using mothers were at heightened risk of being premature and having low birth weight.[51] Although the long-term prospects for "crack babies" did not turn out to be as grim as was feared at the time, the short-term con-sequences included a new burden on the city's already struggling child welfare system: the phenomenon of "boarder babies." A woman giving birth who was found to be a drug user was de facto suspected of child abuse, and her newborn was held in the hospital while the Human Resources Administration conducted a child-protection investigation.[52] These infants ended up living for months on end in hospitals because there was no place else for them to go. The problem peaked in early 1987, when there were 239 infants boarding in public hospitals.[53] The "boarder babies" phenomenon epitomized the social suffering that af-flicted many disadvantaged New Yorkers in the 1980s: about half of the babies boarding in city hospitals were there because of maternal sub-stance use; the other primary reasons were homelessness and parental death from AIDS.[54]

Under pressure from child welfare advocates who pointed out that the hospitals were not designed for such long-term care, the HRA ended the system of keeping the infants in hospitals and placed them instead in congregate care settings operated through private charitable organiza-tions known as agency-operated boarder homes. The facilities housed up to six infants and were staffed by HRA employees. A Health Depart-ment investigation found health and safety hazards in many of the homes, including outbreaks of diarrhea and other enteric and respira-tory diseases.[55] After an exposé of the conditions appeared in *Newsday*, the HRA was once again on the defensive, forced to remediate condi-tions in a program that was itself a reaction to a more deep-rooted set of social problems.

AIDS: Changing Faces?

The Health Department's response to AIDS changed markedly in 1986. This was partly because more money was devoted to the problem. Al-though federal AIDS funding to the city declined, both the Koch and

Cuomo administrations, after years of meager allocations, substantially increased their investments.[56] The Health Department's spending on AIDS programs, including surveillance and research, laboratory services, and health education, almost tripled in fiscal year 1986 over the previous year. Governor Cuomo's budget for fiscal year 1986 increased spending on AIDS by 60 percent, to $4.5 million from $2.8 million.[57] The city's total spending on AIDS, including both public health programs and treatment expenditures through the Health and Hospitals Corporation, increased to $250 million in fiscal year 1987 to 1988 and to $385 million in fiscal year 1988 to 1989.[58]

The change was also attributable to a new approach at the commissioner level. In temperament, Stephen Joseph could hardly have been more unlike his predecessor, David Sencer. Joseph was outspoken where Sencer was reserved, as headlong as Sencer was circumspect. It was in AIDS programming that the differences between the two men emerged most clearly. Joseph was determined to apply public health measures—even those that might be seen as intrusive or coercive—that had historically been used against other sexually transmitted infections. Like Sencer, Joseph's handling of AIDS would place him at the center of controversy and earn him both praise and invective.

One of Joseph's first moves was to dramatically expand HIV testing. In his first eighteen months, the department set up three sites where people could be tested anonymously; the number would grow to five in 1988 and eight in 1989.[59] Joseph was a strong believer in the value of the test, and he was facing external pressure from several quarters. There were persistent and growing demands from community members who wanted more settings where people could be tested. Private laboratories and clinics were seeking the department's permission to allow testing without the rigid counseling protocol that had been imposed under the city health code in April 1985.[60] The state was also moving ahead with its own plans for anonymous testing sites.[61]

Although state health commissioner David Axelrod believed that testing should be more widespread, he differed with Joseph over whether private laboratories should be allowed to perform the test to hasten turnaround time for results, typically two weeks. City- and state-run labs were the only ones doing the test, and although they performed it for free, their cumbersome procedures kept private physicians from using the service. (They would not provide a messenger service to pick up the blood draws at doctors' offices, for example.) Axelrod resisted the expansion out of concerns about quality control and the possibility that expanding the pool to commercial labs would endanger confidentiality.[62]

Joseph also sought to have the test performed more frequently in private medical settings. The department recommended that all physicians offer counseling and testing for their patients, but fewer than 3,000 of the city's 25,000 physicians sent in blood samples to be tested. Nevertheless, the increase in city test sites resulted in more than 108,000 tests being performed in fiscal year 1987 to 1988, more than thirteen times the number performed in the year before.[63]

Another major departure from the department's early approach to AIDS was aggressive use of mass media to disseminate prevention messages. Spending on AIDS education quadrupled in Joseph's first year as commissioner.[64] In the spring of 1987, the department partnered with the Madison Avenue agency Saatchi & Saatchi, which worked pro bono to produce a series of print and video public-service announcements encouraging condom use among heterosexuals.

Some of the ads, in explicitly attempting to link sex with death, reflected the deeply puritanical streak that had characterized venereal disease prevention messages since the Progressive Era.[65] One print ad depicted a man and woman embracing in bed over the tagline: "Bang, You're Dead!" (See figure 5.2.) Another warned of the risk that bisexual men might pose to their partners; it depicted wholesome-looking "Charlie" who "brought home a quart of milk, a loaf of bread and a case of AIDS" via his clandestine affairs with men. At the same time, however, the ads also broke ground in acknowledging that sex could be made safer. A print ad showing the contents of a woman's handbag, with a condom visible among the typical contents of comb, lipstick, and keys, carried the message: "Don't go out without your rubbers." (See figure 5.3.) The three television spots had a similar theme. In one, a middle-aged woman, looking into the camera, held up a condom and addressed her daughter: "If you're doing anything, you use one of these. You understand? 'Cause my baby is not getting AIDS."[66]

Given the polarized attitudes around sexuality, it was hardly surprising that everyone found something to dislike in the ads. Cultural and religious conservatives criticized them for condoning sexual activity. A spokesman for the Catholic Archdiocese of Brooklyn said that it was "offensive and inappropriate" that the city's AIDS messages failed to emphasize abstinence; City Council member Noach Dear, who had fought to close the bathhouses, called the ads "disgusting."[67] From the opposite end of the ideological spectrum, radical cultural critics slammed the ads as simplistic, sex-negative scare tactics that placed responsibility for the spread of the disease on individual behavior rather than political and social forces such as homophobia and racism.[68] When a subway poster appeared with the message "I got AIDS from the personals"—meant to discourage people from pursuing casual sex through classified ads—activists plastered the words "government inaction" over "the personals."[69] Some feminists wondered why the responsibility for men's use of condoms was being placed on women. But when it came to gender dynamics, pragmatism trumped idealism. "Few appeals to males engaged

Figure 5.2   AIDS Prevention Poster

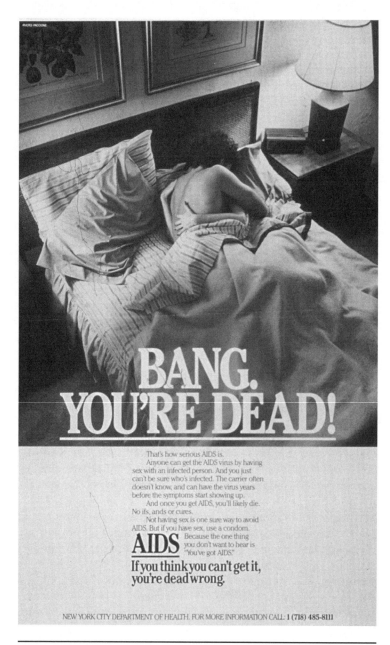

Source: Courtesy of the National Library of Medicine.
Note: One of a series of AIDS prevention posters that the department debuted in 1987. The poster's strong linkage of sex and death was typical of many public health messages about sexually transmitted diseases.

Figure 5.3   AIDS Prevention Poster

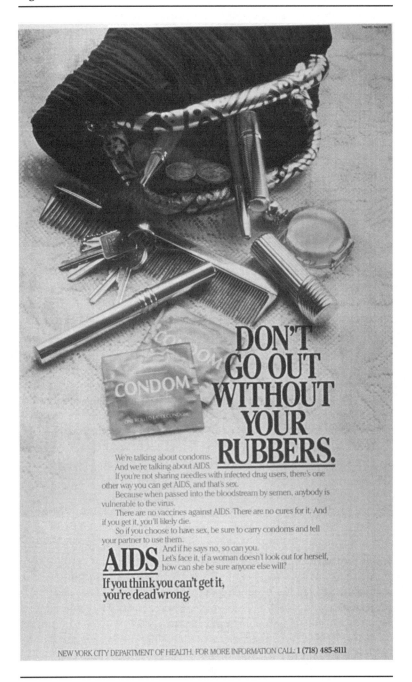

Source: Courtesy of the National Library of Medicine.
Note: One of the department's first AIDS prevention posters emphasized the importance of women's self-protection by depicting condoms among the contents of
a purse.

in the constant quest for sex will be helpful" was the blunt assessment of Assistant Commissioner Mark Rapoport, a close adviser to Joseph. "To quote a divorcee I know, 'Guys will do anything to get laid.' For that reason, 'self protection for women' needs to be the dominant theme."[70]

Although the print messages got fairly wide exposure—several businesses, including Metropolitan Life Insurance, underwrote the costs of ad space—the television spots were little-seen. Only WNYC, the city-owned public television station, agreed to run all three; the local NBC and CBS affiliates ran two of the three, but only after 11:00 PM.[71] At a time when the broadcast television networks refused to run condom advertising at any hour, the cultural barriers to AIDS education remained high.

Another reason for the department's evolving approach to AIDS was a changing epidemiologic picture. The public image of AIDS as a "gay disease" would persist for years, cemented by the initial *MMWR* reports and the early mobilization by gay rights activists, but this perception was always illusory. Retrospective studies showed that HIV entered the injection drug–using population around the same time that gay men began to become infected, and that cases of PCP, KS, and other opportunistic infections symptomatic of AIDS began occurring among users in 1978 and 1979. Women began to become infected at that time through drug use and through sex with drug-using partners.[72] But these men and women, generally poor and even more socially marginalized than gay men, did not come to the attention of private physicians, teaching hospitals, medical researchers, and federal health officials.[73]

Between 1982 and 1986, deaths among drug users in the city climbed sharply from conditions such as pneumonia, endocarditis, and tuberculosis, but because drug users were prone to a range of chronic health problems, underlying immune suppression was often missed as a cause of death and AIDS surveillance data underestimated the true incidence of disease in this population.[74] Even with underreporting, however, a new pattern became clear. In mid-1983, gay men accounted for 71 percent of New York City's AIDS cases and injection drug users for 17 percent; the following year, the corresponding figures were 61 percent and 25 percent.[75] The picture was even starker in poor neighborhoods in New Jersey, which had the nation's third-highest AIDS caseload. By March 1983, almost half of that state's AIDS cases were injection drug users, and two-thirds were black or Hispanic.[76] In 1988, newly diagnosed cases of the disease among drug users in New York City outnumbered those among gay men for the first time, and blacks and Hispanics accounted for half of the city's cumulative AIDS cases.[77]

The *City Sun*, a Brooklyn-based weekly newspaper covering African American issues, sounded an early alarm in the summer of 1985 with an editorial titled "Blacks Are Dying from AIDS, Too," which urged black political leaders to follow the example of gay community groups and pressure the city, state, and federal government to do more.[78] The Minority Task Force on AIDS was founded that fall, but for the most part prominent community figures—church leaders, politicians, activists on other social issues—were slow to mobilize around AIDS.[79]

Several interconnected social and cultural factors account for their hesitancy. The institutions that were traditional sources of support in African American communities, such as churches, social service organizations, and informal kinship networks, were strained to the breaking point from dealing with the long-standing problems of poverty and violence, exacerbated by the appearance of crack and the consequences of federal cutbacks in aid to the poor.[80] The proposition that AIDS was a more urgent threat than heroin or crack cocaine was not self-evident to many African American community leaders. They also viewed with justifiable suspicion the warnings of public health officials, whose technocratic approaches to disease control often seemed insensitive to the social inequities that underlay health problems in communities of color.

Many churches, which were central institutions in black communities, held negative views of homosexuality and were reluctant to speak openly about its existence among their congregations. Black gay activists, facing both racism within the gay community and homophobia within the African American community, were hesitant to acknowledge the risks of AIDS and inclined to see the condition as one affecting white gay men.[81] Moreover, blacks had long experienced racist denigration for their supposedly deviant drug use and sexual behavior, and they reasonably feared that "owning" AIDS within their community would provide another opportunity for whites to blame and stigmatize them.[82]

The issue of injection drug use was an especially painful one in poor communities such as Harlem and Bedford-Stuyvesant. "There is no empathy for intravenous drug users themselves," said one African American activist. "Intravenous drug users are seen as 'criminals' but their partners are viewed as 'victims.' So they and only they deserve compassion and care. But underlying social and economic conditions that lead people to and keep people in harmful or risky lifestyles are ignored."[83] This dynamic was captured in a graffito that appeared in Harlem during this period: "When will all the junkies die so the rest of us can go on living?"[84] Drug use was responsible for bringing crime, violence, and despair, yet drug users were also the family members, friends, and loved ones of the residents of those neighborhoods.

Open discussions of AIDS among blacks began to occur more frequently in the summer and fall of 1987, when a variety of local politicians and community groups sponsored conferences, forums, and other public gatherings. Congressional representative Charles Rangel held a hearing on pediatric AIDS in Harlem in July 1987; Manhattan borough president David Dinkins organized a community forum in Harlem a few months later. Several prominent black churches in Brooklyn held gatherings that drew large crowds. These local meetings coincided with similar events taking place around the country sponsored by national organizations such as the Southern Christian Leadership Conference, the National Coalition of Black Lesbians and Gays, and the Third World Advisory Task Force.[85]

One of the most common criticisms leveled by African American activists was that public health professionals too often imposed interventions on affected communities rather than attempting to help the existing sources of support within those communities mount a response themselves.[86] Mindful of these criticisms, the Health Department sought to establish partnerships to provide culturally appropriate materials produced by the affected communities. Between 1986 and 1988, the department contracted with twenty community-based organizations to provide AIDS education and prevention services.

One of the challenges of these arrangements was that most human services organizations operated on shoestring budgets and had full agendas already. Dealing with issues such as poverty, housing, and unemployment made it difficult for them to take on another area, especially one as complex and fraught with cultural meanings as AIDS.[87] Many needed extensive technical assistance in crafting prevention messages. "A constant refrain among the minority groups (whether social service organizations, advocacy groups or churches) with whom we have contact is the need for assistance in the development of agency-specific AIDS agendas and the design of appropriate services to meet the needs of their clients," a Health Department grants manager wrote to a CDC official. "Most organizations have a delineated scope of service and are not looking for ways to provide new, discrete AIDS education and prevention services, but are seeking ways to integrate the AIDS message into current service configurations."[88]

The most common route of HIV infection among African Americans was the sharing of blood-tainted syringes and other injection paraphernalia. As the increasing burden of the epidemic among drug users became apparent, reducing this risk emerged as the central challenge. An intervention that was gradually acknowledged to be among the most effective, however, would also prove most controversial.

"Get the Good Needles, Don't Get the Bad AIDS"

Needle exchange originated in Europe. When an outbreak of hepatitis B occurred among injection drug users in Amsterdam in 1984, a group of addicts—a "junkiebonden," or union of junkies—organized to pressure the municipal government to institute a program that would exchange clean, sterile syringes for used ones in order to eliminate the need for sharing. The realization around that time that the virus that caused AIDS was also blood-borne increased the urgency to expand this intervention, and needle exchanges were soon created in Australia, the United Kingdom, and other European countries.[89] These programs were part of a broader movement toward what became known as a harm reduction approach to drug use. According to this philosophy, governments should seek to minimize the potential harms—both medical and social—of use rather than attempting to stop people from using. At the same time that harm reduction was gaining popularity overseas, however, drug policy in the United States lurched sharply in the opposite direction, toward ever more draconian responses, as a renewed federal "war on drugs" emphasized interdiction and harsh criminal penalties.[90]

The possibility of a needle exchange in New York City had first been broached when David Sencer was commissioner. Sencer was initially skeptical that the availability of clean needles would stem the spread of AIDS among injectors. "I have had several discussions with professionals in the drug abuse field," he wrote in March 1985 in response to a local physician who had suggested that the city provide sterile equipment. "All agree that unless the needle or syringes can self destruct or be truly single use, the availability of free material would not be effective. Apparently the drug culture prefers to share paraphernalia."[91]

Over the next few months, however, Sencer's thinking on the issue evolved. He spoke with Don Des Jarlais, a researcher with the state Division of Substance Abuse Services. In collaboration with colleagues at the Narcotic and Drug Research Institute, Des Jarlais had done extensive interviews with injection drug users; as early as 1983, these studies had found that users were aware that AIDS could be transmitted via infected blood and were interested in obtaining new needles to avoid sharing.[92] The researchers had observed a dealer in Harlem making the pitch, "Get the good needles, don't get the bad AIDS."[93]

After talking with Des Jarlais, Sencer broached the subject in conversation with Koch, but the mayor was uncomfortable with the idea and initially rejected it out of hand. One night in the summer of 1985, however, Koch phoned Sencer at home. Although the mayor was still doubtful about the efficacy of the approach and its political feasibility, he was open to floating a trial balloon. "If you're willing to be the goat and write me a memo," Koch told Sencer, "I will leak that memo just to get things started."[94]

Sencer prepared a two-page memo summarizing the problems of injection drug use and their potential solutions. Users "have a desire to obtain sterile equipment," but they were unable to do so because several laws and policies stood in the way. "By forcing addicts to use each others' needles and syringes," Sencer wrote, "we are condemning large numbers of addicts to death from AIDS."[95] He made four recommendations: that the state repeal its law against the sale of syringes without a prescription (New York was one of only eleven states with such a restriction); that law enforcement agencies adopt a policy of not arresting people for possession of syringes; that drug treatment facilities be allowed to exchange sterile syringes for used ones; and that the sale of nonsterile syringes be made a violation of the health code. "These actions stop short," he stressed, "of the city actually providing the equipment." Koch nevertheless asked the Corporation Counsel (the city's law office) to examine the implications of the city itself assuming responsibility for the provision of needles. The city's lawyers determined that although there were potential complications in the courts from such a policy—the city might face tort liability or charges of criminal facilitation, for example—there appeared to be "no absolute legal bar" to a city-run syringe exchange.[96]

Koch also gave a copy of Sencer's memo to several criminal justice officials involved in drug abuse issues, including the district attorneys for each of the city's five boroughs and the special prosecutor for narcotics. The reaction here was predictably hostile. Special Assistant District Attorney for Narcotics Sterling Johnson scoffed at the notion that "slaves of addiction" in a "narcotic-induced stupor" cared about using clean syringes or could be taught to do so.[97]

Finally, Koch provided a copy to a reporter at the *Wall Street Journal* to gauge the response from local politicians and their constituents. After the *Journal* wrote about the proposal, the story was picked up by the *Times, Post,* and *Daily News.* The response was not entirely unfavorable. The *Times* opined that the proposal was "sensible and deserves a trial."[98] Surprisingly, a similar stance was taken by the *Staten Island Advance,* the daily serving the city's most politically conservative borough.[99] The attitudes of most local politicians, however, ranged from dubious to appalled. Noach Dear, a City Council member whose Brooklyn district included many socially conservative Italians and Orthodox Jews, expressed a common view when he argued, "We might as well begin selling the drugs the addicts shoot up with."[100] Koch's opponent in the mayoral contest, City Council president Carol Bellamy, called the idea "harebrained."[101] Within a month, Koch had gotten the information he needed: clean syringe programs were a political nonstarter. He announced in a City Hall news conference that the idea was one "whose time has not come and, based upon the response, will never come."[102]

Some of the resistance to needle exchange reflected moral judgments, such as the belief that because drug use was inherently harmful, the government should enact no policy to facilitate it. Other objections were based on empirical claims: that drug users would not take advantage of clean needles, that exchanges would lead to increased drug use, and that they would be ineffective at preventing the spread of AIDS. Research by Don Des Jarlais and others had already disproved the first of these claims at the time Sencer broached the idea to Koch, and by the time Stephen Joseph became commissioner, evidence was emerging that the other arguments were fallacious as well. The recommendations of official bodies began to reflect the emerging consensus. In 1986 both the World Health Organization and the Institute of Medicine recommended the adoption of policies to foster the use of clean needles.[103] Closer to home, the New York Bar Association recommended that the state legalize the sale of needles without a prescription. But the imprimatur of global and local expert bodies failed to shift public opinion, and a syringe legalization bill introduced in the state assembly won no support.[104]

One intervention that promised to reduce the risks of drug use but stopped short of needle provision was the distribution of small bottles of bleach that injectors could use to clean their syringes between uses. The idea was somewhat more politically palatable than needle exchange; U.S. Representative Bill Green, a Republican, suggested it to Koch during a congressional hearing after learning that Los Angeles and San Francisco had initiated such programs.[105] The costs would be modest, and the distribution could be done through existing venues serving users, such as methadone treatment clinics and the district health centers.[106] But African American community leaders and law enforcement professionals found the distribution of bleach no less objectionable than the provision of needles. In their eyes, it too seemed to legitimate and even encourage the use of drugs. Some staff members in the Health Department also harbored doubts about whether the improper use of bleach might pose health hazards to users.[107] One of the community-based organizations funded by the department, the Brooklyn-based ADAPT (Association for Drug Abuse Prevention and Treatment), did provide bleach along with condoms, safe sex kits, and instructions on cleaning "works."[108]

A critical underlying problem, everyone agreed, was the lack of drug treatment for users who wanted to quit. The waiting time to join a drug treatment program in the city averaged about six months. Joseph sought to address this issue with a plan to expand access to methadone maintenance therapy by making space available in sixteen of the district health centers. The clinics would operate after regular business hours and would be run by private methadone providers. Each program would have capacity for about 150 new treatment slots.[109] But local opposition to methadone maintenance facilities had not diminished since Robert Newman's initial efforts in 1970. City Council member Enoch Williams, for example, who represented Bedford-Stuyvesant, bitterly complained to Joseph when he learned about the proposal; Williams was especially upset because a four-hundred-bed shelter for homeless men had recently opened two blocks away from the district health center where the methadone program would be housed.[110] Community opposition ended up being moot, however, because Joseph's plan fell victim to city-state disputes over funding. When the deal had been struck in 1979 to transfer operation of the methadone clinics to the state health department, it was agreed that the state would henceforth provide drug treatment funds. Koch was adamant that the state be held to its word and that no city money would be used to expand treatment slots. The state made no funding available, and Joseph's proposal never went forward.[111]

Koch, who was not an ideologue on the issue of drug abuse, came around to the idea that a needle exchange program was at least worth trying, and with his green light, Joseph pressed ahead. Now a key hurdle was winning over state health commissioner David Axelrod, since the state health code regulated the sale of syringes and would have to be amended if a program were to go forward in New York City. Axelrod insisted that the only way he would allow the program to proceed was under the guise of research—a study that would evaluate the empirical claims about the potential benefits of needle exchange in preventing the spread of AIDS. Joseph had misgivings about this approach, since it would mean a delay in the creation of a full-scale program that could serve the entire population of drug users, but he ultimately accepted it because it seemed the only politically feasible approach.[112]

By insisting that proof of efficacy be established before a program was undertaken, Axelrod was holding needle exchange to a higher evidentiary standard than other interventions. As drug researcher Don Des Jarlais pointed out, public health professionals engaged in many activities, from creating pamphlets and subway advertising to distributing condoms, with no evidence that they actually worked.[113]

For months, the city and the state remained bogged down in methodological disputes. The needle exchange trial would have to be large enough to yield statistically significant results, but the larger the group of addicts enrolled, the greater the risk of public backlash; a trial small enough to fly under the political radar would be unable to detect the desired outcomes. When Axelrod insisted that the protocol be reviewed and approved by a state-hired biostatistician, it began to appear that the state was using scientific methodology to, in effect, calculate the study to death in order to avoid taking a politically unpopular step. "Please *get on with* this—we are losing precious time while we let the state drag their (and our) heels," an impatient Joseph wrote to one of his deputies after the state's biostatistics consultant made yet another round of suggestions for modifying the protocol.[114] The situation was exacerbated by the personal animosity between Joseph and Axelrod, both aggressive, stubborn physicians whose jobs routinely brought them into jurisdictional conflict.

While the city and state remained deadlocked, activists took matters into their own hands. ADAPT, the organization that the department funded to provide outreach to addicts, announced that it would begin passing out needles on its own in direct defiance of state law. Yolanda Serrano, the group's executive director, insisted that the action was necessary because of the magnitude and urgency of the health threat.[115] "She was right on the issue," Joseph later recalled, "but her tactic would have been disastrous because the state would have come down on her, the city would have come down on her, the mayor, the cops, the narcotics people. And goodbye our chance of getting anything done."[116] As soon as he learned of ADAPT's plan, Joseph telephoned Serrano to warn her of the risks the group was facing and the danger presented by their proposed action to the broader cause of expanding needle exchange; with a veiled threat to withdraw the department's funding from her group, he pleaded with her to back off.

Serrano did back off, and her threat turned out to be a spur to action on the part of the state. Six weeks later, Axelrod approved the protocol, and by the summer of 1988, the program seemed ready to be implemented, with the blessing of city and state lawyers and $250,000 of city funding. The trial would enroll four hundred participants, evenly divided between test subjects, who would be given a needle they could return at any time for a clean one, and controls, who would not. The exchange would be operated out of four district health centers. All participants in the program would receive a physical exam and be counseled about HIV risk reduction. They would receive an identification card with a photo and a fingerprint.

The *Times*, which had supported the idea when Koch floated it three years earlier, was once again supportive, but otherwise, public commentary was overwhelmingly negative.[117] "An insanity is about to be turned loose on the streets of New York," the *Daily News* warned, "unless reasonable men and women unite to smash it."[118] Particularly vociferous were the objections of black community leaders, who believed that drug addiction was an illness at least as damaging as AIDS. They saw the distribution of needles as a capitulation—a stopgap measure where justice demanded thoroughgoing reform. "Why do you offer addicts free needles," asked the legal scholar Harlan Dalton, "but not free health care?"[119] Many commentators saw barely concealed racism in the plan. Said police commissioner Benjamin Ward, "As a black person, I have a particular sensitivity to doctors conducting experiments, and they too frequently seemed to be conducted against black people."[120] Polls showed that substantial numbers of African Americans believed that the government allowed drugs to proliferate in poor neighborhoods in order to harm the residents there.[121] The *Amsterdam News* ratcheted up the rhetoric with numerous articles attacking the study, including a front-page editorial by the editor-in-chief calling for Koch to resign for his "arrogance, insensitivity and downright fatal reasoning."[122]

Joseph mounted a full-court press to counteract the criticism, writing detailed responses to the editors of the *Daily News* and the *Amsterdam News* and other outlets that attacked the plan and constantly reiterating his talking points to the print and television journalists covering the issue: that the program was driven by solid scientific evidence and would remain small-scale and tightly controlled. ("We are not dropping needles from helicopters," he helpfully explained to the *Times*.)[123]

Criticism intensified when the four sites were revealed. To avoid charges that he was bringing addicts into a neighborhood, Joseph selected four district health centers in neighborhoods with high levels of drug use, and he cleared the sites with Koch. But when the locations became public, community board members, City Council members, state legislators, and U.S. Congress members representing the neighborhoods all wrote to Joseph to demand that the exchanges be moved elsewhere.[124] (Methadone pioneer Robert Newman, who knew a fair amount about "not in my backyard," had predicted this reaction.[125]) Koch, despite the political pushback and his own misgivings about the efficacy of needle exchange, remained steadfast in his support. "We will come under great attack, as we already have, with respect to the implementation of the needle exchange program," he wrote to Joseph over the summer. "As you know, I am for it and will defend it even though my instincts tell me it will have little or no impact on the spread of AIDS."[126]

Koch was eventually forced into a partial retreat, however, when community leaders from Chelsea observed that the district health center there was across the street from an elementary school. As it turned out, all four of the proposed sites were near schools—indeed, every district health center in the city was within a few blocks of at least one school— and the prospect of innocent children being harmed was a political trump card even more powerful than the charge of racial genocide. In the ensuing uproar, Koch had to back down. He instructed Joseph to find other locations for the program. In desperation, with just days to go before the program was due to start, Joseph chose the only location he could control: 125 Worth Street. A large janitorial closet off the main lobby, near the room where birth and death certificates were distributed, was cleaned out and transformed.[127]

The location's chief political advantage—its distance from residential areas—was also its main weakness, since prospective clients would now have to trek to an unwelcoming site a few blocks from police headquarters (see figure 5.4). After just two people showed up to use the program on opening day, Joseph put the best face forward. "I think the enormous success of today," he said, "is that the program got off the ground at all."[128] The subsequent weeks were no more auspicious. A month after

Figure 5.4   Rally for Needle Exchange

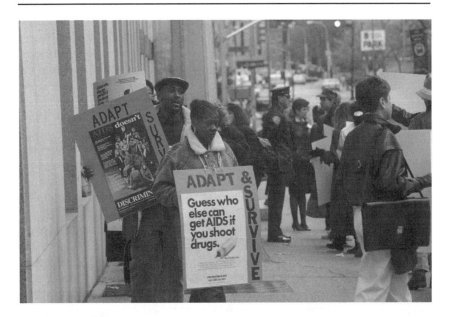

Source: Chester Higgins Jr./The New York Times/Redux, with permission.
Note: Demonstrators from community organization ADAPT (Association for Drug Abuse Prevention and Treatment) march in front of Health Department headquarters in support of the city's experimental needle exchange program in November 1988. The overwhelming public response to the program was negative, however.

the program began, the City Council voted overwhelmingly for a resolution calling for the program to be ended.[129] By that time just thirty-two people had enrolled.[130]

The program did grow steadily over the following year, and Joseph, committed to seeing it through, investigated the possibility of quietly expanding it to other sites. By mid-1989, however, the mayoral campaign was in full swing, and Koch requested that the expansion be delayed until after the election. The other five candidates for mayor opposed the program, and when Manhattan borough president David Dinkins, who had been outspoken in his criticism, defeated Koch in the Democratic primary, the demise of the city-run needle exchange was certain. Dinkins ended the program as soon as he took office in 1990.

This was not the end of needle exchange in the city, however. Activists began distributing clean needles illegally in the Bronx and Harlem and on the Lower East Side of Manhattan. Meanwhile, small-scale studies of the efficacy of syringe exchanges in other jurisdictions continued to be published. In the summer of 1991, researchers from Yale University announced the findings of a rigorous evaluation they had conducted of a program in New Haven, and Dinkins asked his new health commissioner, Margaret Hamburg, to review the issue. Hamburg, acutely aware of how politically explosive the issue remained, convened a working group of Dinkins administration officials to review all the scientific literature on the subject; she also held a series of intensive consultations with African American community leaders.[131] In the spring of 1992, Dinkins, on Hamburg's recommendation, announced that he would allow community organizations to use private and state funding to operate needle exchanges in the city.[132] It was a remarkable reversal given the firestorm that had surrounded Joseph's experimental program.

The controversies over needle exchange illustrated the complicated relationship between scientific evidence and public health policy. The lack of an extensive body of data supporting the efficacy of needle exchange impeded the ability of both David Sencer and Stephen Joseph to establish a program, but it is unlikely that a strong evidence base would have been sufficient to win over opponents, given the emotionally charged atmosphere surrounding the issue and the dire situation related to drugs in minority communities in the mid-1980s. Nor did the subsequent accumulation of evidence by the early 1990s guarantee that the policy would change. It was the political process skillfully negotiated by Hamburg, who was able to present the data convincingly to the mayor and skeptical community leaders, that enabled the science to drive policy.

"On Joseph's List": The Politics of AIDS Surveillance

Disease surveillance has provided the foundation of public health action since the nineteenth century, but it has never been a purely statistical undertaking. Social and political forces always influence which diseases get counted, how infected people are reported, and what actions are taken toward the ill. When health officials began collecting information about cases of syphilis during the Progressive Era, for example, two-tiered reporting was common. The physicians of middle-class or well-to-do patients reported cases by numerical code; only the poor who depended on public dispensaries had their names reported, and only prostitutes and lower-class patients were likely to face isolation or quarantine. Occupational diseases were largely excluded from health department record-keeping because of the opposition of industry and business, and as a result the incidence of conditions such as silicosis and asbestosis remained only dimly perceived for decades.[133]

AIDS reporting sparked some of the fiercest battles of the epidemic's first decade. Surveillance data could be used to either minimize or magnify the scope of the epidemic; personal information gathered via surveillance might be used to punish or coerce the infected. In New York City, these disputes pitted Joseph and the Health Department's epidemiologists, who sought to use long-standing public health measures to monitor and control the spread of HIV, against activists who viewed surveillance and the interventions it might trigger as threats to civil liberties and human rights.

The confidentiality procedures that had sprung up around AIDS in the epidemic's early years, such as the Health Department's decision not to forward the names of people with AIDS to the CDC, had often been ad hoc and reactive, formulated on the fly in an environment of fear and crisis. As the epidemic spread and it became clear that issues of privacy and confidentiality would only grow more complex, the need for a systematic and principled approach became apparent. Health officials and politicians at the local, state, and federal levels sought to craft policies to protect the confidentiality of AIDS-related information and, more controversially, debated whether there were situations in which confidentiality could be broken in the interest of protecting the public health.[134]

The backdrop to these discussions was the continued threat of stigma, discrimination, and violence against people with AIDS. In March 1986, William F. Buckley Jr., editor of the conservative journal the *National Review*, wrote in a *Times* op-ed column that all "carriers" of the virus should be "tattooed in the upper forearm, to protect common-needle users, and on the buttocks, to prevent the victimization of other homosexuals."[135] That such a proposal could be put forth by one of the country's leading public intellectuals in the "newspaper of record" was a measure of how threatening the policy environment was during the epidemic's first decade. That fall, California voters considered a ballot initiative that would allow the quarantine of people with HIV and the firing of anyone found to be HIV-positive from any job involving public contact, including waiter, flight attendant, police officer, and teacher. Although the proposal was soundly rejected, more than two million people in the nation's largest state voted for draconian measures that every public health and medical authority had condemned.[136] The specter of such actions hovered over debates about HIV policies in general and the privacy of HIV-related medical information in particular.

A few months after he became commissioner, Joseph began working with the department's general counsel, Irwin Davison, on a piece of legislation that would overhaul the confidentiality procedures surrounding HIV. He hoped to secure the support of Mayor Koch and Governor

Cuomo and the sponsorship of one or more state legislators. After more than a year of delicate negotiations with AIDS and civil rights organizations such as the Lambda Legal Defense and Education Fund, a bill was prepared, and at a legislative hearing in the fall of 1987 Joseph publicly declared his intent to seek a modification of state law.[137] The bill included several highly sensitive provisions. Minors would be able to be tested and treated for AIDS and their providers forbidden to disclose the procedures to the parent or guardian without the minor's consent (similar to provisions in place for abortion and treatment of sexually transmitted diseases). Health care providers would be able to disclose HIV-related medical information to other medical personnel involved in the treatment of a patient. The most controversial provision involved physicians' breaking confidentiality to warn the sex and drug-using partners of people with HIV.[138]

A health care provider's duty to warn had long represented a thorny ethical dilemma, with two values—protecting a patient's privacy and preventing harm to a third party—in competition. In the best-known legal decision on the issue, the California Supreme Court had held in 1976 that a psychologist whose patient revealed an intention to harm another person had an obligation to break confidentiality and warn the potential target. "The protective privilege ends," the court declared, "where the public peril begins."[139] Although the duty existed in common law, there was no statutory requirement in New York State. Doctors could warn third parties who had been exposed to a communicable disease, but AIDS had never been defined under law as communicable.

The positions of public health officials and AIDS activists on the issue tended toward ambivalence and caution. Most gay and civil rights groups viewed with great suspicion any crack in the wall of privacy surrounding HIV-related medical information, yet they also recognized the morally troubling implications of an HIV-positive person's failure to disclose his or her status to partners. Representatives of both Gay Men's Health Crisis and the Lambda Legal Defense and Education Fund warily conceded the need for narrow exceptions to strict confidentiality procedures in cases where an unknowing partner was at risk. Public health officials were not monolithic in their views. The director of community health for the New York State health department opposed Joseph's proposal on the ground that the specter of confidentiality breaches would discourage people from seeking testing.[140]

A bill ultimately found bipartisan support in the state legislature and passed in the summer of 1988. It gave the state the strongest privacy protections for AIDS-related information in the country. Under the law, anyone tested for HIV had to give written informed consent and receive counseling before and after the test. One of Joseph's key goals was weakened in the process, however. The duty to warn became permission to warn; doctors could choose to break confidentiality to advise the sexual or drug-using partners of HIV-positive people and would be protected from liability if they did, but they were not legally required to do so.[141]

It was during the debate over confidentiality that the Health Department first came into conflict with the AIDS Coalition to Unleash Power, or ACT UP. The group was founded in March 1987 out of a belief that existing AIDS organizations, especially GMHC, were being insufficiently aggressive in the fight to bring money and attention to the epidemic. In its peak years of activity, between 1987 and 1992, ACT UP numbered around five hundred; its membership was mostly white, male, and well educated.[142] The group drew on techniques of civil disobedience and radical street theater, and it quickly became known for flamboyant, media-friendly events that skillfully exploited the power of images. In their first action, several hundred demonstrators staged a sit-in at the foot of Wall Street in front of Trinity Church to demand faster Food and Drug Administration approval of experimental AIDS drugs. The protest was widely covered in the press and set a tone for future events. Subsequent demonstrations targeted panels at the International AIDS Conference, the headquarters of the FDA, the trading floor of the New York Stock Exchange, and the White House. ACT UP actions were loud, colorful, and dramatic, designed to upend what the group saw as the intransigence and complacency of those who should have been leading the fight against AIDS. Medical researchers, government officials, politicians, and journalists all faced the group's wrath.

The group met with Joseph in October 1987 to discuss the city's response to AIDS.[143] Since many of their concerns, such as inadequate hospital beds and home care services, were matters over which the Health Department had no sway, Joseph could not have satisfied their demands, and it was not surprising that he would eventually become a target of their protests. When he did, it was over the issue of surveillance, and the situation grew even uglier than might have been expected.

Although AIDS cases had been counted with a high level of completeness since the beginning of the epidemic, the number of people infected with HIV could only be guessed at. A back-of-the-envelope calculation by department epidemiologists in 1985 estimated that there were 400,000 people with HIV in the city. After being cited publicly on several occasions, that number took on a life of its own, even though the AIDS surveillance staff privately doubted the figure's accuracy and were uncomfortable with its use. The number of new AIDS cases that were actually being diagnosed in the city did not support that high an estimate of HIV-positive people. In 1987 Joseph ordered the calculation of a new estimate. With no systematic reporting of HIV cases, however, and no hard figures on the numbers of gay men and injecting drug users, the necessary numerators and denominators in the calculation would have to combine statistics with some amounts of ideology and educated guessing. Joseph told Mayor Koch that the task of estimating the size of the HIV-positive population was like "navigating from New York to Tahiti in the old days of sail: based on scientific principles, inevitably subject to a range of error (which can be minimized), needing constant course checking, and requiring alteration when necessary."[144]

Over the next year, Rand Stoneburner and the rest of the AIDS surveillance staff recalculated the numbers in each of the CDC's risk categories, resulting in a downward revision of the overall estimate by about one-half, to about 200,000. The largest adjustment occurred in the estimated number of HIV-positive gay men. The previous figure had been derived in part from Alfred Kinsey's 1948 estimate that one in ten men was exclusively homosexual, a number that critics had long charged had no solid foundation. In the new calculation, the number of infected gay men was revised downward, from the range of 150,000 to 300,000 to a range of 46,000 to 70,000. The surveillance group was careful to state that they were making no claims about the overall size of the gay male population in New York City, only about the proportion of that group that was HIV-positive.[145]

The revised estimate of 200,000 HIV-positive people was not released publicly, but the issue was forced in July 1988. The Health Systems Agency (HSA), a private, city-funded planning organization, had convened a task force, which included some of the department's AIDS surveillance staff, to identify the resources that would be needed for AIDS treatment and prevention in the coming years. The task force had prepared its own estimate, also in the range of 200,000, which it planned to release as part of a larger report it had prepared for the Koch administration. The publication of the new HSA figures would raise questions about the discrepancy with the Health Department's official estimate, still on the record as 400,000, so Joseph scheduled a press conference to present the department's revised figure before the release of the HSA report. He gave a heads-up to Koch, deputy mayor Stanley Brezenoff, and HHC president Jo Ivey Boufford about the planned announcement, which, he predicted, would stir controversy.[146] Joseph did not, however, alert GMHC to the planned announcement. The night before the press conference, GMHC's executive director, Richard Dunne, learned about the report when a *Times* reporter called him for comment; his deputy director, Tim Sweeney, phoned Joseph asking him to delay the conference, but Joseph declined. The failure to consult with community figures, Dunne later charged, "has impaired the credibility of public health officials and has damaged relations among all of us working the fight against AIDS."[147]

The press conference at City Hall on July 19 did not go well. Protesters, already alerted to the key findings of the report by an article in that morning's *Times*—the headline was "New York Estimate for AIDS Infection Cut Almost in Half"—showed up with signs that read HALF-COUNTS BY HALF-WITS. At one point Joseph misspoke and implied that the recalculation posited fewer gay men in New York City than previously thought, which it explicitly did not do.[148] But even if the event had gone precisely according to script, that would not have contained the fury that erupted. To gay activists, it appeared that the Health Department was attempting to downplay the severity of the epidemic in order to devote fewer resources to it. Their suspicions were shaped by the longstanding perception that the city had failed to respond to AIDS with sufficient urgency. Joseph's press conference came three months after the state comptroller had released a report predicting that the city would have only half the number of hospital beds it would need for AIDS patients over the next several years. The timing of the announcement reinforced activists' belief that the HIV prevalence numbers had been manipulated in order to justify the Koch administration's inadequate health spending.[149]

The issue of HIV estimates permanently poisoned the Health Department's already prickly relationship with ACT UP. Within weeks of the announcement of the new figures, several ACT UP members had begun an escalating campaign of harassment designed to drive Joseph from office (see figure 5.5). Some of their actions were relatively peaceful—they released dozens of helium-filled pink balloons into the vaulted ceiling of the 125 Worth Street lobby—but others were violent and threatening. A month after the press conference on the estimates, a group of a dozen protesters twice occupied Joseph's office, disrupting meetings, shouting demands, and refusing to leave; they were arrested for trespassing and removed by police. At public forums they attempted to shout him down, comparing him to the Nazi doctor Josef Mengele. Flyers appeared around town with a bloody handprint and the slogan "Stephen Joseph has blood on his hands." Protesters began shadowing Joseph on his extensive speaking and meeting schedule, causing him to travel with two bodyguards. ACT UP members obtained his home telephone number and began phoning anonymous death threats against Joseph and his wife in the middle of the night. Protesters surrounded his home on the Upper West Side and plastered his front door with flyers and red paint.[150] ACT UP's protests extended beyond the group's vendetta against Stephen Joseph. The department was forced to cancel its long-standing monthly forums where invited researchers presented their findings to the public because the gatherings repeatedly degenerated into ugly confrontations as ACT UP members shouted down the speaker.[151]

Throughout these events, Joseph continued to enjoy strong support from Koch, who praised Joseph's "great courage under very difficult

Figure 5.5   Controversy over Numbers

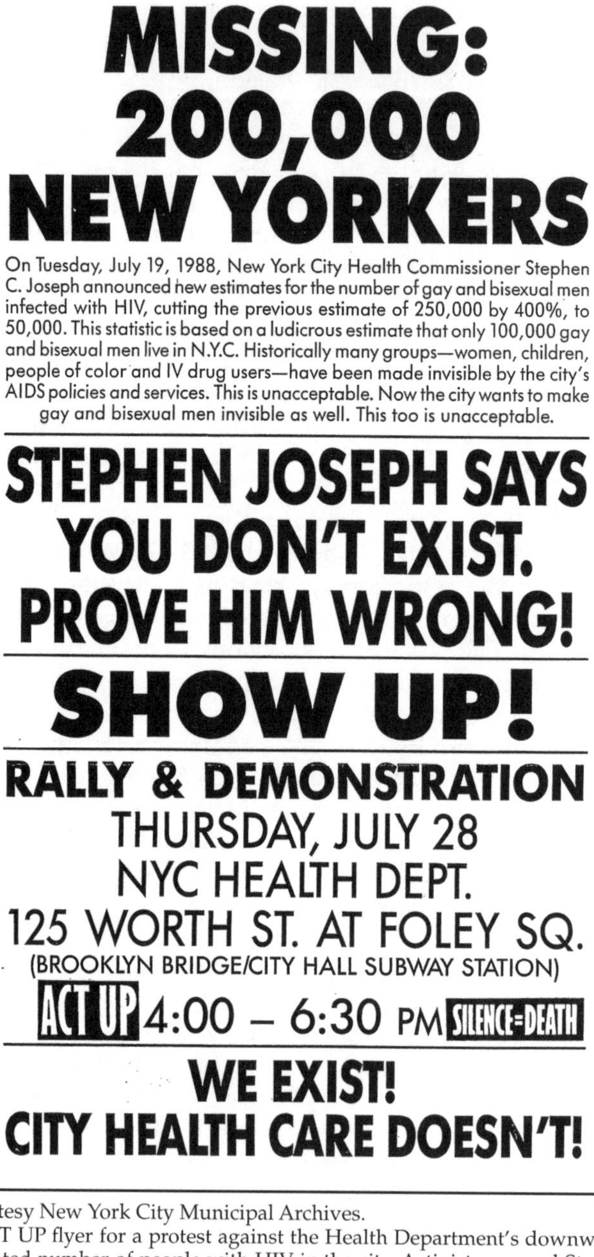

MISSING: 200,000 NEW YORKERS

On Tuesday, July 19, 1988, New York City Health Commissioner Stephen C. Joseph announced new estimates for the number of gay and bisexual men infected with HIV, cutting the previous estimate of 250,000 by 400%, to 50,000. This statistic is based on a ludicrous estimate that only 100,000 gay and bisexual men live in N.Y.C. Historically many groups—women, children, people of color and IV drug users—have been made invisible by the city's AIDS policies and services. This is unacceptable. Now the city wants to make gay and bisexual men invisible as well. This too is unacceptable.

STEPHEN JOSEPH SAYS YOU DON'T EXIST. PROVE HIM WRONG!

SHOW UP!

RALLY & DEMONSTRATION
THURSDAY, JULY 28
NYC HEALTH DEPT.
125 WORTH ST. AT FOLEY SQ.
(BROOKLYN BRIDGE/CITY HALL SUBWAY STATION)

ACT UP 4:00 – 6:30 PM **SILENCE=DEATH**

WE EXIST!
CITY HEALTH CARE DOESN'T!

Source: Courtesy New York City Municipal Archives.
Note: An ACT UP flyer for a protest against the Health Department's downward revision of the estimated number of people with HIV in the city. Activists accused Stephen Joseph of manipulating the numbers in order to justify what they saw as the city's inadequate spending.

conditions."[152] But the mayor's support was about to be tested during an even more contentious debate over surveillance.

Public health officials at the local and state levels had begun calling for name-based reporting of HIV cases as soon as the antibody test was licensed in 1985. In their view, the value of such reporting was obvious. Since HIV-positive people could go for years without developing clinical symptoms, statistics on AIDS cases presented an out-of-date epidemiological picture—the people who had been infected several years earlier. Information about current HIV infections was necessary for planning prevention efforts that responded to current trends in the epidemic. Further, knowing the names of infected people could enable health departments to provide counseling about risk reduction and preventing transmission and could facilitate follow-up with them should new treatments became available. But AIDS and civil rights activists, mindful of the threatening social, political, and legal environment, successfully fought most such efforts. Colorado, which had an interventionist health commissioner and a relatively small epidemic, was the first to require reporting of HIV-positive people by name, but by 1988 only thirteen other states had followed suit; these did not include New York, California, New Jersey, or Florida, which together accounted for the large majority of the nation's AIDS cases.[153]

It was not surprising that Joseph, who believed strongly in applying traditional public health methods to the control of HIV, would push for name reporting, especially after the first antiretroviral medication, AZT, was licensed in 1987. In his view, the changing clinical picture of AIDS lent new urgency to the task of identifying those infected so that treatment and care could be made available to them and their partners. The vituperation he had received from ACT UP did not deter him from this course. On the contrary, political opposition simply increased Joseph's stubborn and principled determination to press ahead with actions he believed to be justified by the demands of public health. When he was invited to give a plenary address at the International AIDS Conference, an annual gathering of researchers, clinicians, and policymakers, he thought it would be an ideal forum for making his proposal. The conference, which was to be held in June 1989 in Montreal, would be a high-impact venue where he could communicate his views to the most influential audience and gain maximum press attention.[154]

When Joseph revealed this plan for the Montreal address at a meeting of his senior staff members that spring, the group was stunned. "You're crazy," said one assistant commissioner. "You think you're being tortured now. Just imagine." Said another, "If you want to take six months and bring people along to your point of view, have some community consultations. You make some cogent arguments here." The department's AIDS staff knew that regardless of the public health merits of the plan, the community reception would be overwhelmingly negative.[155] In March, some three thousand protesters, in the city's largest AIDS demonstration ever, had surrounded City Hall for more than three hours demanding that the city devote more resources to AIDS prevention and care.[156] This was not a propitious moment to present an inflammatory policy proposal.

The scene at the Montreal conference, where Joseph addressed an audience of one thousand, was no surprise given the pattern of protests that had been established over the previous months. When Joseph came to the podium, several dozen members of ACT UP rose, turned their backs to the stage, unfastened their watches, and held them in the air to signify time passing and people dying (a gesture they had made toward other speakers at the conference). As he spoke, the group repeatedly interrupted him with shouts, including, "Commissioner of death!" and "Shame!" At a press conference later that day, activists once again attempted to shout down Joseph's comments.[157]

Back home, the reaction was equally predictable. Protesters marched on 125 Worth Street carrying signs that read "FIRST YOU DON'T EXIST, NOW YOU'RE ON JOSEPH'S LIST."[158] A new round of flyers denouncing Joseph appeared around the city. Koch, locked in a tight reelection fight and under intense scrutiny over his administration's handling of AIDS, looked for a way to defuse the controversy. He convened a meeting at Gracie Mansion (the mayoral residence) with twenty physicians, scientists, activists, and representatives of AIDS service organizations to discuss the proposal for mandatory named reporting of HIV cases. The meeting's outcome was never in doubt: the plan was off the table. Joseph, who would later dub the event "the Saturday morning massacre," felt stung by the failure of his colleagues to speak out on behalf of a proposal that he believed was clearly defensible on public health grounds, as well as by what he saw as Koch's caving into political pressure on this issue after having backed him during the controversies over needle exchange and the HIV prevalence estimates. In the wake of the City Hall protest and the Gracie Mansion meeting, Koch made a further concession to activists: he added $1 million to the Health Department budget to expand the counseling and testing program and to provide public education about it; about twenty counselors were hired who would be stationed in public hospitals and drug treatment programs to encourage people to be tested.[159]

By the time the HIV testing program began, Ed Koch had been defeated in the Democratic mayoral primary, and it was clear that Joseph's days as commissioner were numbered. He had been a polarizing figure. The vilification he had received from community leaders and activists was unprecedented for a health commissioner, eclipsing both the populist anger that had been directed at Lowell Bellin during the hospital wars and the dissatisfaction that health professionals felt toward Reinaldo Ferrer in the aftermath of the fiscal crisis. Yet Joseph had also won plaudits from experts in the field as diverse as Alex Wodak, the Australian researcher who was an internationally recognized expert in harm reduction, and Daniel Callahan, the president of the Hastings Center, a bioethics think tank.[160] The *Times* praised Joseph's leadership when he resigned, saying, "On all or most issues, he has been right, and prescient."[161]

There was one issue on which Joseph had not been prescient, however. Reflecting on his experiences years later, Joseph identified the major shortcoming of his time as health commissioner as his failure to deal effectively with tuberculosis. An ancient disease that experienced a modern-day resurgence amid HIV, homelessness, poverty, and the other social pathologies that marked New York City in the 1980s, TB reached epidemic proportions—with new, deadlier strains—at a time when it should have been long eliminated. This resurgence should have come as no surprise. Experts inside and outside of 125 Worth Street had seen it coming for years.

Chapter 6

Chronicle of an Epidemic Foretold

LEO MAKER—THIRTY-EIGHT years old, homeless, drug addicted, and sick with tuberculosis—seemed to personify the social disorder engulfing New York City when the *Post* ran a full-page photo of him on its cover next to the headline "One Man's Trail of TB." The exposé, the first of a series of articles on the disease in the fall of 1990, described how Maker "roamed the city for eight months spreading tuberculosis."[1] Once headed toward elimination in the United States, tuberculosis resurged in the 1980s among the city's poorest and most troubled residents. The rate of disease among welfare recipients who abused alcohol or drugs was seventy times as high as the rate for the U.S. population overall; the problem was most severe in Harlem, a neighborhood that had long epitomized deprivation in the midst of affluence.[2] To many readers of the *Post*—a tabloid given to sensationalist warnings of doom—the return of the disease was one more sign of the city's deterioration. When a headline later in the series declared that "Homeless Contaminate Public Areas in City," the editors plainly meant more than the spread of bacteria.

The resurgence of tuberculosis after a long period of decline and the subsequent efforts to control it followed a pattern that one physician called "the U-shaped curve of concern." In this model, attention to a public health problem decreases over time as it becomes less prevalent and generates less fear. Eventually the problem begins to worsen again as a consequence of the diminished resources. At some point, the situation is once again perceived as urgent, and funding rises. Attention to the problem thus follows a "U" shape, falling, bottoming out, then rising again.[3] Federal, state, and local resources to control tuberculosis hit their nadir in the 1970s and remained low throughout the 1980s—the bottom of the "U"—before turning upward in 1992.

Why did the problem fester for more than a decade, even as a handful of experts warned of looming disaster? Why did the level of concern remain flat for so long and turn upward when it did, and not earlier? That the disease was neglected until it threatened to spread beyond concentrated pockets of poverty—"no one is safe" was the *Post*'s warning—is a valid explanation but an insufficient one. Many other factors influenced the shape of the curve: failures of vision and commitment on the part of health officials at all levels; the patchwork nature of private and public medical care; the bureaucratic inefficiencies inherent in city government; and the difficulty of addressing health problems that were the product of seemingly intractable social conditions. The eventual control of resurgent tuberculosis, accomplished with remarkable swiftness beginning in 1992, turned out to be one of the greatest triumphs in the Health Department's history and would be widely held up as a model of effective public health intervention. The failures that preceded the effort are also instructive.

From Commitment to Complacency

Tuberculosis is one of history's deadliest scourges and remains a leading cause of death globally. The mycobacterium that causes the disease spreads via airborne droplets and most often attacks the lungs, though it can infect other parts of the body. In the majority of infected people, the illness remains latent and asymptomatic. Patients have a roughly 10 percent lifetime risk of progressing to active illness, which is characterized by cough, fever, fatigue, and weight loss. Infected people are especially at risk of becoming symptomatic when their immune systems are weakened. The mortality rate for untreated illness is about 50 percent.

The struggle to control tuberculosis was one of the crucibles through which the Health Department established itself as a strong presence in the city at the turn of the twentieth century. Hermann Biggs, head of the Bureau of Laboratories, successfully fought to require physicians to report cases of TB to a central registry in 1896—a move that the local medical societies viewed as an unprecedented intrusion into the doctor-patient relationship—and this pioneering surveillance enabled the department to track patients and oversee their care. Public health nurses visited patients' homes to conduct "sanitary supervision," helping them to lead healthier lives and avoid infecting others.[4] In the 1930s, the department established a network of chest clinics to provide diagnostic services and referrals to medical care. This multifaceted control program contributed to the decline of the disease.[5]

Tuberculosis thrived in crowded, poorly ventilated housing, and as the disease became rarer it was increasingly concentrated among the poor. By midcentury, the four health districts in the city with the worst rates of tuberculosis also had high levels of poverty, unemployment, dilapidated housing, and juvenile delinquency. The prevalence of the illness in Central Harlem, where the population was 93 percent black and 3 percent Puerto Rican, was roughly three and a half times that of the city overall.[6]

The development of antibiotics transformed the medical management of the disease. The first anti-TB medication, streptomycin, was introduced in 1947; two more drugs, isoniazid and para-aminosalicylic acid (PAS), soon followed. A four-month hospital stay had once been standard, but now new drugs allowed patients to return to the community. The Health Department's chest clinics began an innovative program dispensing oral antibiotics in 1953, and the number of hospital beds devoted to tuberculosis shrank from more than 6,600 in 1950 to around 1,000 in 1960 as fewer patients required bed rest and observation. The shift from an inpatient to an outpatient model of care brought a new set of challenges, however. A full course of therapy could take from nine months to two years, but the acute symptoms of the disease generally subsided after a few weeks—at which time many patients, no longer feeling ill, stopped taking their medication. Failure to complete therapy led to the development of resistant strains of the bacillus.[7]

During the Great Society era, federal funding enabled the Health Department to set up a program of "combined chest clinics" in eight hospitals that augmented the department's older facilities. The rationale behind the combined clinics was that since so many TB patients had additional health problems, they would be better cared for in settings where other medical services were readily available rather than in a clinic devoted exclusively to TB. The combined clinics were soon serving around 6,300 patients, almost half of the unhospitalized active cases of TB in the city.[8]

The declining incidence of the disease and its changing medical management prompted a mayoral task force in 1968 to recommend restructuring the city's control and treatment programs. The group urged the elimination of the remaining inpatient tuberculosis beds. In place of institutional treatment, they called for a system of outpatient care that included comprehensive social services, new clinics with flexible hours located in poor neighborhoods, and housing programs for patients who lacked a stable residence.[9]

Over the next decade, just one of these recommendations was carried out: the elimination of inpatient beds. Concern about tuberculosis—which had long since dropped off the list of the nation's leading causes of death—dwindled as medical and public health professionals grew convinced that infectious diseases no longer presented a significant threat in the United States. At the same time, there was a waning of the Great Society ideal that the government should play an activist role in ameliorating the problems of the inner-city poor. The federal and state governments withdrew virtually all their support for New York City's TB control activities during the 1970s, a time when the city could ill afford to compensate for the losses. In 1972 the federal TB monies were block-granted, and the funds for New York City declined from $1.4 million to $283,000.[10] Between 1974 and 1978, the state cut its TB funding to the city from $500,000 to $200,000. During those years, the Bureau of Tuberculosis Control lost eighty-three employees, more than half of its staff.[11] During the city's 1975 fiscal crisis, five of the department's fourteen chest clinics were closed.

In 1979, the state withdrew the last of its funding for TB, and with it went twenty-eight positions, half of the staff of the combined chest clinics, including record-keeping personnel, public health nurses, and field investigators who were the key to ensuring treatment completion. The outreach staff who monitored patients fell from twenty to two.[12] In the early 1970s, the federal government had paid for about 70 percent of the city's TB control activities; a decade later, local tax revenues supported virtually all of the city's efforts.[13] None of the components of the community-based system that Lindsay's task force had recommended in 1968 to alleviate the difficult life circumstances of people with the disease or to support them in completing their treatment regimens was put in place.

The abandonment of tuberculosis patients bore striking similarities to the deinstitutionalization of people with mental illness in the 1960s and 1970s. That movement was spurred by treatment advances, concern about poor conditions in state asylums, and the increasing recognition of the right of the mentally ill to live under less restrictive conditions in the community. The outpatient counseling centers and supportive services that had been envisioned when mental hospitals began debouching patients by the thousands never materialized, and by the 1980s a large population of people with psychiatric disorders were scraping by in squalid housing, not taking needed medication, and living in increasing numbers on the streets.[14]

The head of the Health Department's Bureau of Tuberculosis Control during this period was Alje Vennema, a Canadian physician who had spent several years during the 1960s as a volunteer at a small hospital in rural Vietnam. Vennema was experienced at dealing with health care provision in straitened circumstances and foresaw what would happen as resources were whittled away. When the state halved its financial contribution in 1978, he prepared a report titled "Tuberculosis Control, an Impending Crisis" for commissioner Reinaldo Ferrer. "Tuberculosis cases will go unreported and unsupervised," Vennema predicted. "Tuberculosis contacts will go undetected. The untreated cases will walk in the streets of New York."[15] Vennema was an indefatigable advocate for increased resources, but he had a brusque, often impolitic manner that won little support for his cause. He was able to plug staffing holes with employees reassigned from other areas of the department, but he believed that their suitability for TB outreach work was "questionable."[16] With a characteristic lack of diplomacy, Vennema described his replacement staff as "inadequately trained, incompetent, unmotivated, and insufficient."[17]

It did not take long for the effects of the cuts to be seen. In 1979 the tuberculosis rate rose for the first time since 1962. The number of new cases, 1,530, was an increase of 17 percent over the previous year. Central Harlem led the city in its death rate from the illness, which was now more than quadruple the city average.[18] About half of all new cases were black, and about 10 percent were Puerto Rican.[19] The uptick in cases prompted a small infusion of resources. Twenty-one new public health advisers were hired in 1980 to monitor patients. The following year, however, several staff members whose salaries were paid by the CDC had to be let go because of cuts to public health spending in the Reagan administration's first budget.[20]

In 1980 the Council of Lung Associations of New York set up a task force to evaluate the spike in cases. "It must be strongly suspected," the report claimed, "that the increase in newly reported cases in New York City is in part the result of fiscal neglect. At federal, state and local levels, public health funds allocated to TB are inadequate, in some instances so grievously inadequate as nearly to amount to dereliction and default on legal mandates."[21] The group's report underscored the poor clinical management of people with the disease. Fewer than six in ten patients in the city completed their full course of treatment; around one in five was lost to follow-up entirely. The report also noted a troubling increase in drug resistance. Nine drugs made up the antituberculosis armamentarium by 1980, and a survey that year of almost three hundred patients in the city found resistance in at least some patients to six of them.[22]

When the Health Department began reducing funds for tuberculosis in 1970, Mayor Lindsay had received dozens of letters from physicians, hospitals, and charitable organizations protesting the cuts.[23] A decade later, however, the urgency surrounding the disease having waned and more critical problems having overtaken the city, only a handful of people were still speaking out. After cuts in state funding forced the elimination of outreach staff from the chest clinic at Harlem Hospital, Charles Felton, the head of pulmonology, warned commissioner Reinaldo Ferrer about "the devastating effect this measure is having on field work among contacts of tuberculosis patients and preventive treatment of such contacts."[24] The U.S. congressman who represented the Bronx complained to Mayor Koch about staff cutbacks at the chest clinic there.[25] But in the midst of the widespread social and economic devastation that afflicted Harlem and the Bronx during these years, the loss of tuberculosis services did not rise to the level of a crisis.

Although the people advocating for more resources were few in number, the systemic problems were amply documented. Between 1982 and 1984, the city's tuberculosis control infrastructure was the subject of three detailed and highly critical reviews. In early 1982, comptroller Harrison Goldin, whose office had recently probed the city's response to the deinstitutionalized mentally ill, investigated the TB situation. Shortly after that, David Sencer asked his former colleagues at the CDC to evaluate the department's program. And during 1983 and 1984, Sencer convened a task force of prominent local physicians that met nine times to determine how to best respond to the deficits identified in the CDC review.

All three of these reviews described a litany of clinical and administrative problems that resulted in the systematic failure of patients to receive adequate care. Tuberculosis treatment in the city was a hodge-podge of public and private, with about 40 percent of patients receiving care in the private sector and about 60 percent being seen by the Health Department or one of the public hospitals. Patients were often lost to follow-up upon discharge from their initial hospitalization because no one at either end followed through to ensure continuity from inpatient to ambulatory care. Private physicians did an inadequate job of monitoring their patients' compliance with treatment and failed to report to the Health Department when a patient "broke supervision" and stopped showing up for routine monthly appointments.

Given the Health Department's long history of tuberculosis control, one might have expected that patients seen in the chest clinics would be better cared for than those in the private sector, but this was not always the case. Because the department could not offer salaries that would attract top-caliber physicians, much of the clinical care was substandard, with patients placed on TB medications to which they had documented resistance.[26] Alje Vennema tried to convince the local medical schools to support a portion of the salary of residents who would receive training in the chest clinics, but he was unable to arouse any interest in the idea.[27] Patients drifted away from care because of lax administrative procedures. "Even for very high risk patients, 2, 3, or even 4 appointment letters are sent to patients before the outreach worker is called," the CDC review found. "Often 4 to 6 weeks elapse before a field followup by outreach workers is initiated."[28] There was no computer database to track patients; civil service rules limited the ability of outreach workers to follow up with patients after hours; and the department lacked staff who spoke Spanish, Haitian Creole, and Chinese.[29] The combined chest clinics that had been set up in city hospitals in the 1960s were "combined" in name only, with virtually no assistance or input from the Health Department. Vennema recommended that the department withdraw its remaining personnel stationed there. "I do not believe either the patient or the respective facilities would suffer," he said, because the department's presence had become so negligible. The money saved, he believed, would be better redirected into centralized control activities, such as outreach workers for monitoring ambulatory treatment.[30]

The inadequate clinical management of the disease was evident in the department's statistics on patient outcomes. Only 40 percent of patients converted to negative sputum status—indicating that they were no longer infectious—after three months of treatment, and only 50 percent converted after six months, compared to the recommended rates of 75 and 90 percent, respectively.

There was a small bright spot amid the many failures. In 1980 the department received a $150,000 grant from the CDC to undertake a two-year pilot called the Supervised Therapy Program (STP). Four field-workers were hired to provide supervision to about eighty patients thought to be at risk of noncompliance because of a history of not taking medication, mental illness, alcoholism, or drug abuse. After eighteen months, the STP patients had a treatment completion rate of 81 percent.[31] The prospects for additional funds to expand the program were dim, however. "Virtually all of [the CDC's] budget is being used to maintain basic essential functions," David Sencer explained to city comptroller Harrison Goldin. "Monies for special projects are simply not available."[32] Over the objections of the Reagan administration, Congress revived federal categorical funding for tuberculosis in 1981, but no monies were appropriated until 1986, and then appropriations were far under the amount authorized.[33] Although the department did manage to sustain the supervised therapy program beyond its initial two-year pilot, it remained small-scale, with the staff never exceeding ten and their caseload representing a tiny fraction of the patient base. Critically, the program did not include homeless patients.

A handful of experts foretold an impending crisis. The increases in tuberculosis case rates still remained modest, however; indeed, the rate dipped slightly in 1984, though it remained well above what it had been in the 1970s. It was possible in the mid-1980s to believe—or at least hope—that tuberculosis might resume its downward trend.

Pouring Oil on the Coals

In 1986, several months after Stephen Joseph became health commissioner, the mayor's Office of Management and Budget asked him to group Health Department programs into high, medium, and low priority. Joseph placed the chest clinics in the low-priority category—programs that, having "less public health impact . . . could be reduced proportionately more than the programs in either the high or medium priority categories"—alongside activities such as regulating mobile food vendors and operating orthopedic clinics for handicapped children.[34] A year later, Ed Koch wrote to Joseph, "I am told the rising rate of tuberculosis constitutes a danger just short of AIDS."[35] Joseph was still confident that the disease could be controlled. "I would definitely not classify TB as a public health danger of anywhere near the same magnitude as AIDS," he replied. "Although incidence of TB is rising, it is a *curable* disease through public health efforts and advances in chemotherapy."[36]

As he would later admit, Joseph was lulled into thinking that the long-standing availability of a wide range of antibiotic treatments against tuberculosis would translate into control of the disease. He was also distracted throughout his tenure by newer and more high-profile concerns such as AIDS and homelessness. Most critically, Joseph underestimated the synergistic effect that these emergent problems would have on the incidence of TB.

Tuberculosis had long been recognized as a particular problem of the homeless, especially alcoholic homeless men, whose weakened immune systems made them vulnerable to reactivation of latent infection.[37] The transient, disordered lifestyle of people on the streets made taking pills and keeping appointments difficult, and the dormitory-style shelters that became commonplace in the city in the 1980s were an ideal setting for the spread of airborne contagions (see figure 6.1). As New York City began to warehouse thousands of people in these environments, the number of TB cases diagnosed among shelter residents climbed steadily, from 65 in 1982 to 158 in 1986.[38] A widely publicized outbreak of drug-resistant TB that struck the residents and staff of a six-hundred-bed shelter in Boston was an object lesson about the problems of managing the disease among the homeless.[39]

In response to the growing shelter population, Alje Vennema requested city funds to hire eight new public health advisers to follow up on homeless TB patients and observe them taking their medications, an initiative modeled on the successful CDC-funded Supervised Therapy Program that had begun in 1980. The Office of Management and Budget granted the request, but with a restriction: the funds could be used to monitor patients only while they were homeless; once a patient secured a permanent residence, he was to be transferred to another caseworker not paid for with the new funds. Stephen Joseph balked at the OMB's condition. "This goes against our current concept of [supervised therapy]," Joseph attempted to explain, "namely, engaging non-compliant patients in a relationship with the same field worker to encourage and ensure compliance for duration of treatment."[40] Joseph lost this fight with the mayor's office, and another window opened in which a patient could be lost.

As it turned out, the new outreach workers, hired in the fall of 1986, could not duplicate the success that STP had achieved. They were unable to consistently locate most of the people enrolled in the program; of 500 patients, only around 180 were under regular supervision a year later. One in four was lost to follow-up entirely. The advisers assigned to the program, having been inadequately trained, believed that it was better for the patient to take a few days of medication per month than no medication at all. In this way, they contributed to the development of drug-resistant strains.[41]

As concern was rising about the effect of homelessness on tuberculo-

Figure 6.1   Homeless Shelter

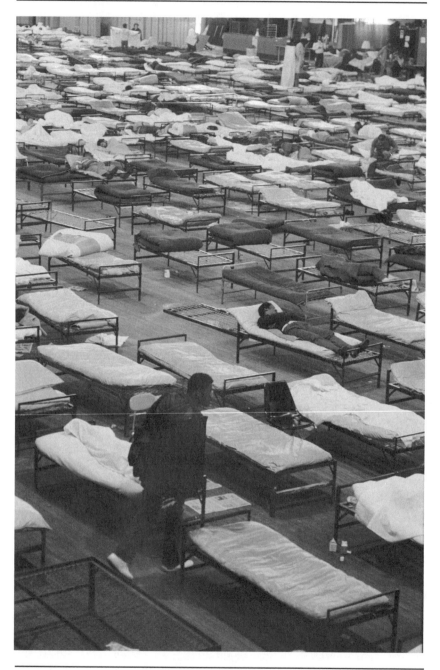

Source: Keith Meyers/The New York Times/Redux, with permission.
Note: The barracks-style shelters in which the city housed thousands of men on narrowly spaced cots in the 1980s were ideal settings for the spread of airborne contagions such as tuberculosis.

sis rates, there was also a growing realization about the impact of AIDS on TB rates. A report from the New York Lung Association in 1985 noted that the groups most affected by AIDS and TB were the same—black and Hispanic males age twenty-five to forty-four—and a diagnosis of one disease in this group closely preceded or followed the other. "Traditionally, compromised immunity among those infected with TB has resulted in disease," the report observed. "It is plausible to suggest that epidemic immune deficiency may be associated with the increased TB incidence."[42]

Rand Stoneburner of the AIDS Surveillance Unit used the Health Department's AIDS and TB registries to confirm the observations made in the Lung Association report. There was a significant overlap between the two lists. The patients in common were 87 percent male, 81 percent black or Hispanic, and much more likely than other AIDS patients to be injecting drug users. Stoneburner's findings joined a spate of other studies published in 1986 and 1987 linking the two diseases. People with AIDS were far more likely to progress to active TB than those who were not immune-compromised; people who were co-infected progressed to active disease at a rate of 10 percent per year, compared to a 10 percent lifetime risk for those who were not HIV-positive.[43] The effects of HIV on the TB problem began to be seen in 1986; rates continued to creep steadily upward the rest of the decade. As Karen Brudney, a physician who treated homeless patients at Harlem Hospital, put it in a subsequent article, "The advent of HIV in the 1980s poured oil on the smoldering coals of TB among the homeless."[44]

In the fall of 1987, Joseph asked officials with the Centers for Disease Control to once again evaluate the city's tuberculosis control efforts. In the five years since the CDC had done its last review, the problems documented in the prior report had only worsened. Management and staffing problems continued to plague the Bureau of Tuberculosis Control. With few career advancement opportunities, there was high staff turnover among outreach workers. They had no access to cars to conduct follow-up appointments outside Manhattan, which limited the number of patients they could have under their care; the department budget provided no money for incentives such as fast-food meals, toiletries, and subway or bus tokens that might increase patients' adherence to medication, so outreach workers paid out of pocket for these items. Caseloads far exceeded what each worker could reasonably carry. There was little coordination between the staff working with the housed patients and those tracking the homeless.[45]

The CDC's report also underscored the failure of the Health Department, the Health and Hospitals Corporation, and the Human Resources Administration to work collaboratively. The very structure of city government, with health, welfare, and social service functions dispersed among separate agencies competing for scarce resources, inhibited the kind of coordinated care that tuberculosis patients required. This segmentation was especially apparent in the case of homeless people who had special clinical needs. William Grinker, the head of the Human Resources Administration, was already under pressure from the Health and Hospitals Corporation to establish a shelter for people with chronic mental illness when Stephen Joseph asked HRA to do more to segregate tuberculosis patients within shelters.[46] Grinker argued that such suggestions erroneously viewed the shelter system "as the answer for clients with health related problems for which we have no current feasible alternatives; rather than as a short-term alternative to other more appropriate long-term solutions. The shelter becomes the path of least resistance because of our need for a longer-term health-related facility."[47] Grinker assured deputy mayor Stanley Brezenoff that "HRA is not trying to shirk its duty here," but he insisted that the Health and Hospitals Corporation should shoulder the burden of operating the homeless TB ward. Advocates outside city government took a dim view of the three agencies' failure to work together. Karen Brudney, who was one of the harshest critics of the city's efforts, accused them of "ostrich-like behavior" and of having "outdone one another in fingerpointing."[48]

After protracted negotiations, the Health and Hospitals Corporation opened an eighty-six-bed shelter at Bellevue for homeless tuberculosis patients in late 1988. The ward had partitioned sleeping areas, special diets, and more amenities than other shelters; the Health Department provided staffing.[49] Once again, however, the mayor's office attempted to cut budgetary corners by refusing to approve new hiring. When the Health Department presented its budget plan, the Office of Management and Budget insisted that the department staff the new shelter with current outreach workers, reasoning that the shelter's inhabitants would be drawn from the existing TB caseload.[50]

Meanwhile, the Coalition for the Homeless took up the issue of homeless HIV-positive people, who were at risk of contracting tuberculosis in shelters. Homeless people with AIDS were—at least in theory—given shelter in private rooms, where their weakened immune systems were less exposed to contagions. No such accommodation policy existed, however, for people who had tested HIV-positive but had not yet become symptomatic, even though they were also at increased risk for disease. The coalition sued the city in 1988, demanding that the Human Resources Administration provide private rooms for HIV-positive people. After protracted negotiations with the state Department of Social Services, which regulated shelters in the city, the HRA devised a plan for segregated areas in several shelters. Although the plan called for HIV-positive people to be segregated from the broader shelter population, they would nevertheless be housed twelve to a room—an arrangement that did not, advocates argued, protect them from the threat of tuberculosis. Litigation over the issue would continue for years.[51]

Following the tack taken by the Coalition for the Homeless, the Legal Aid Society sued over another congregate setting that was highly risky for the spread of tuberculosis: the city jail on Rikers Island. The institution's contagious disease unit did not have adequate ventilation to prevent the spread of airborne diseases, which posed a special risk to the numerous inmates—as many as one in five, the city estimated—who were infected with HIV. A court ordered the city to provide appropriate isolation facilities at Rikers Island for patients with tuberculosis and other infectious diseases. As with the issue of HIV-positive people in homeless shelters, it would take many more years of legal maneuvering to resolve the problems on Rikers Island.[52]

As other city agencies were mounting a slow and piecemeal response to the interlocking problems of tuberculosis, AIDS, and homelessness, the Health Department continued to struggle with internal difficulties. In the wake of the CDC's 1987 review, the Bureau of Tuberculosis Control added twenty new staff members.[53] A critical vacancy remained, however. After thirteen years as director of the bureau, Alje Vennema resigned in early 1987. The department recruited extensively for months but could not find a suitable candidate. After the post had been vacant for almost a year, Joseph was able to bring on Jack Adler, the chief of pulmonary medicine at Brookdale Medical Center in Brooklyn. But Adler was available to do the job on a part-time basis only. In a sign of growing concern within the Koch administration about the tuberculosis situation, deputy mayor Stanley Brezenoff protested the hiring. "While I am sympathetic to the fact that this has been a difficult position to fill," Brezenoff wrote to Stephen Joseph, "I am concerned that this major program area does not have a full time director."[54] Joseph insisted that there was "little hope of recruiting someone else"—the position was a demanding one requiring specialized background and skills, and the department could not offer a salary that was competitive with the private sector.[55]

Joseph also approved an ill-advised plan to increase screening among schoolchildren. Foreign-born children, especially those from Latin America, the Caribbean, Africa, and Southeast Asia, were at heightened risk of tuberculosis. Although the most recent CDC reviewers had expressed concern about this population, they commented in their report that "it may not be wise to undertake widespread screening programs while large numbers of patients needing supervised therapy are not receiving it."[56] Like any mass screening program in a low-prevalence population, testing close to one million schoolchildren consumed great resources in exchange for a relatively meager return. Katherine Lobach, who headed the Bureau of Child Health, which included the school health program, was strongly opposed. The program ended up being "a nightmare," she said. "From the standpoint of finding active tuberculosis in children it was like looking for a needle in a haystack. The resources that were put into that were just outrageous."[57]

In the late 1980s, there was increasing awareness of the problem outside a small circle of advocates, and public pressure built on the city to act more forcefully. Joseph received complaints from the City Council member representing Brooklyn's Flatbush neighborhood, which had a high concentration of Caribbean immigrants, among whom rates of tuberculosis were high.[58] The City Council member and state assembly member representing the Washington Heights neighborhood in northern Manhattan expressed concern about the Fort Washington Armory, one of the largest and most notorious of the city's barracks-style shelters. They had been alerted to potential problems there by staff at New York Presbyterian Hospital, the teaching hospital for Columbia University's medical school, which was directly across the street.[59] Ed Koch grew increasingly worried about the situation; in early 1988, he asked Joseph whether the city had the authority to detain noncompliant patients.[60] But the city's response remained incoherent and inadequate, and the Health Department's programs continued to be insufficiently funded and poorly managed.

The inauguration of a new mayor and the appointment of a new health commissioner in 1990 might have been a turning point for bold action against the disease. A series of crises in the first months of the new administration, however, repeatedly drew attention and resources away from tuberculosis.

Imminent Perils

Manhattan borough president David Dinkins was elected the city's first African American mayor in the fall of 1989, edging out U.S. attorney Rudolph Giuliani in one of the closest races in the city's history. That Giuliani, a Republican, could attract so much support in a city where four out of five voters were Democrats was a measure of the significance of race, especially among the relatively conservative white ethnic residents of Brooklyn, Queens, and Staten Island.[61]

Dinkins pledged publicly to appoint a cabinet that reflected the city's diversity. The position of health commissioner, traditionally not one of the most high-profile jobs in the mayor's administration, was more sensitive than at any time in recent memory because of the controversies sparked by programs such as needle exchange and HIV case reporting. Dinkins's search committee for the job was carefully selected to include representation from the major constituencies concerned with AIDS and minority health; the chair was Mathilde Krim, cofounder of the American Foundation for AIDS Research (AmFAR) and one of the city's most influential AIDS advocates and philanthropists.

Woodrow Myers, the Indiana health commissioner, seemed an ideal choice for the post. Thirty-five years old and African American, Myers was a driven personality who seemed to combine medical expertise with management acumen. He had gotten his undergraduate degree from Stanford when he was nineteen years old and his medical degree from Harvard when he was twenty-three.[62] Unlike most health officials, who augmented their training in medicine with a public health degree, Myers had returned to Stanford to earn a master's in business administration, a degree that he believed would be better preparation for effecting change in the world of health care. One of his first challenges in Indiana had been the controversy over Ryan White in Kokomo; he had supported White's attending school and had won praise for his stance and his effective handling of the situation. The search committee enthusiastically recommended that Dinkins hire Myers.

In preparation for the move from Indiana, Myers read Tom Wolfe's best-selling novel *The Bonfire of the Vanities*.[63] The caustic satire of fin-de-siècle New York could have been a cautionary tale for Myers, who soon found himself caught in a scrum of interest-group politics. The trouble began when a reporter from the gay magazine *Outweek* reported that in Indiana Myers had supported mandatory name reporting and contact tracing for people with HIV and the quarantine of people with the disease who knowingly infected others. Such measures were not outside the public health mainstream in some parts of the country, but in New York City—where the AIDS caseload was the highest, advocacy groups were most influential, and the orthodoxy of protecting civil liberties was strongest—they were anathema. Some activists faulted the search committee for not having looked into Myers's background more thoroughly.[64]

After a hastily arranged conference call on which Myers assured the committee that he would enact policies appropriate for the political and epidemiological context of New York, the group reaffirmed their recommendation. A week later, however, Mathilde Krim and the representatives of Gay Men's Health Crisis and the Lambda Legal Defense and Education Fund abruptly withdrew their support after the *Post* ran an article in which Myers appeared to support both mandatory named reporting and quarantine. The article did not quote Myers, and he claimed that it distorted his views. ACT UP, quick to see threats from public health officials, responded with a series of protests outside of Gracie Mansion and City Hall.[65] An official announcement of the appointment was repeatedly put off. At Dinkins's request, Myers maintained public silence throughout the affair, but in the midst of the accusations he wrote to the mayor reaffirming his "dedication to the individual rights of all

Figure 6.2   Protesting the New Commissioner

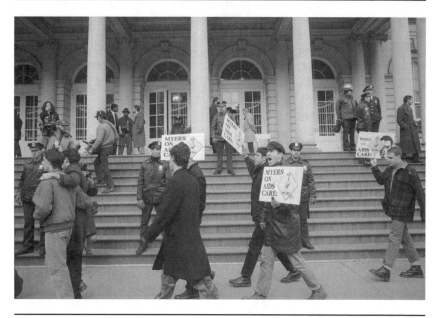

Note: ACT UP members protest in front of City Hall in January 1990, after Mayor David Dinkins announced the appointment of Woodrow Myers to the post of health commissioner. They were angered by AIDS policies Myers had reportedly endorsed during his tenure as Indiana state health commissioner.

human beings and to the importance of implementing sensitive, community based and effective programs to manage this epidemic."[66]

The controversy exposed divisions within the AIDS advocacy community between gay activists, for whom civil liberties trumped other concerns, and groups representing people of color, for whom the symbolic significance of the city's first African American health commissioner was paramount. For weeks, the episode played out in an embarrassingly public way and put Myers on the defensive before he had set foot in 125 Worth Street. When Dinkins finally announced the appointment at City Hall, two hundred ACT UP protesters carried signs and chanted, "Woody Myers, just you try it, we'll go out and start a riot" (see figure 6.2).[67]

Once on the job, Myers sought to shake up the Health Department with business school thinking. He salted his memos with phrases like "asset basis" and "return on investment"; he proposed developing a new Health Department logo that would anchor a publicity campaign for the agency to include coffee mugs and T-shirts.[68] He adhered to a hierarchical management style, rarely consulting with those who did not report directly to him.[69] Myers's blunt determination to put in place his own management team—at his first staff meeting he announced, "Half of you won't be here in six months"—set off an exodus of experienced deputies. Among those who left were Ellen Rautenberg, who had been the department's chief liaison with AIDS activists and had often smoothed over tensions during Stephen Joseph's stormy tenure, and Mark Rapoport, who had helmed critical program areas such as lead poisoning and homelessness. As longtime employees exited in large numbers, morale dropped among those who remained.

Whatever hopes Myers may have had for patching up relations with AIDS advocacy organizations were quickly dashed over the inflammatory issue of injection drug use. In his first news conference, in April 1990, Myers said that he favored expanding drug treatment but was "ideologically opposed" to needle exchange and could not imagine any empirical evidence that would change his mind.[70] Myers considered needle exchange "shortsighted and wrong. It absolved the government of the bigger problem, which was figuring out what to do about drug abuse."[71] A month after taking office, he was reviewing the department's contract with the Brooklyn-based community organization ADAPT, which had received city funds since 1986 to provide outreach, education, and safe injecting supplies such as cotton balls, alcohol pads for skin cleaning, and "cookers," small containers used to heat and purify drugs. The proposed contract was for $861,000. Myers instructed his staff to maintain the amount of the contract but to disallow any funds to be used for safe injection programs. ADAPT could continue to conduct these activities, Myers said, but the group would have to find non-city money to do it.[72]

When news of the decision became public, the AIDS advocacy community was once again split. On one side were white activists, who generally lined up in favor of safe injection programs; on the other were groups representing the interests of people of color, who saw such efforts as undermining the more important struggle to treat addiction and end drug abuse. Several AIDS organizations, led by GMHC and AmFAR, held a press conference to urge Myers to reconsider, and ACT UP held a protest rally.[73] The Black Leadership Commission on AIDS, a sixty-five-member association of medical professionals, politicians, businesspeople, and clergy, backed Myers's decision. The group likened bleach distribution to "a Trojan horse for the African American community in that it is superficially attractive but contains a grave element of risk."[74] Views on harm reduction did not map consistently onto race and ethnicity, however. ADAPT's director, Yolanda Serrano, was Latina; Billy Jones, the African American psychiatrist who headed the city's Department of Mental Health, Mental Retardation, and Alcoholism Services, favored bleach distribution, as did Emilio Carrillo, the Cuban American physician who headed the Health and Hospitals Corporation.[75]

A month after Myers's decision, the Board of Estimate held a special hearing on the defunding of ADAPT's safe injection outreach. Twenty organizations offered emotional testimony against the move; Mathilde Krim compared the decision to disallow safe injection supplies to the withholding of antibiotics in the U.S. Public Health Service's Tuskegee syphilis study.[76] The comparison to Tuskegee was a reliable rhetorical bludgeon wielded on both sides of the clean needles debate; two years earlier, police commissioner Benjamin Ward had implicitly likened syringe exchange to Tuskegee.[77] In Krim's case, however, the argument proved ineffective: Myers's decision stood.

That the issues of drug use and HIV prevention would prove divisive was no surprise. At the same time the episode with ADAPT was unfolding, however, the department was engulfed in another controversy that was wholly unexpected—and far more damaging to its reputation.

On May 6, 1990, an article headlined "Cancer Outrage" filled the front page of the *Daily News*. "More than 2,000 pap smears languished in a city health department laboratory," the article began, "leaving hundreds of women at high risk for cervical cancer without knowing it."[78] Front-page stories on the scandal continued for the following week. The department's Bureau of Laboratories, which had performed essential if unglamorous work largely hidden from public view for almost a century, was thrust into an unprecedented and unwelcome spotlight. The episode, one of the most embarrassing in the department's history, temporarily displaced all other health issues from the political agenda.

The Bureau of Laboratories in the 1980s employed about 360 people and each year conducted testing on about one million specimens submitted by Health Department clinics, hospitals, and private physicians. The bureau included a cytology laboratory with a staff of nine who processed some 28,000 pap smears per year. The tests came from two sources. About 80 percent were sent in by the ten maternity and infant care clinics, which provided prenatal care for low-income women; the remainder came from the department's thirteen sexually transmitted disease (STD) clinics. Ideally, pap smears were read within forty-eight hours of receipt.[79]

In May 1988, the Bureau of STD Control, concerned that the STD clinics were seeing women at heightened risk of cervical cancer, changed its policy to recommend more frequent testing. Women would be routinely offered a pap test if they had not had one in the previous six months rather than in the previous year. Participants at the meeting where this decision was made would later disagree on a critical point: did anyone ask the staff of the cytology laboratory whether they would be able to handle the increase in slides that could be anticipated from the new screening policy?

The answer to that question soon became apparent. In the first month after the new policy went into effect, the number of slides submitted by the STD clinics more than tripled, and turnaround time steadily increased—first to about ten days, then to about three weeks. The director of cytology, Lucy Feiner, requested additional staff, and ads were posted for a part-time cytotechnologist. But qualified cytotechnologists were in high demand, and the Health Department pay scale was considerably lower than what they could earn in the private sector. By February 1989, the backlog of slides totaled around 4,300 and turnaround time had grown to as long as five weeks. At the end of that month, the Bureau of STD Control decided to return to its old policy of annual pap screening because of the excessive turnaround time. In March, the Bureau of Laboratories prepared a new needs proposal requesting $154,000 to hire two cytotechnologists and provide nine hundred hours of overtime for a cytopathologist. The mayor's Office of Management and Budget rejected the proposal; Stephen Joseph, not realizing the severity of the situation, chose not to appeal the OMB's decision.

For several months, Lucy Feiner repeatedly asked for more staff, and her relationship with the director of the Bureau of Laboratories, Kenneth Dressler, grew strained. Meanwhile, employees of the Bureau of STD Control had become increasingly troubled by the situation. The clinics continued to send in a total of about three hundred slides per month, and the turnaround time had lengthened to about five months. In May 1989, the bureau changed the recommended screening policy to once every two years. Stephen Schultz, the deputy commissioner responsible for both Laboratories and STD Control, spoke to Joseph about the problem. Neither was aware, however, of how bad the situation had grown.

By late 1989, some three thousand unread pap smear slides were stacked up in the Bureau of Laboratories. The Bureau of STD Control decided that all the STD clinics would stop doing pap smears. A handout was prepared in English and in Spanish to be given to patients informing them that a pap smear had not been part of their care and that if they had not had a normal one within the last year they should get one at another facility.

Lucy Feiner resigned in September 1989. Her replacement, Elena Estuita, began in December after a three-month delay while the city processed her paperwork. Estuita immediately made technical changes that allowed more slides to be read more quickly. As cytotechnologists made their way through the backlog and started returning results to the clinics, John Miles, the director of the Bureau of STD Control, realized that they were returning smears with signs of cancer that were a year old. He notified his boss and the department's legal counsel.

In early 1990, Estuita decided to send the remaining unread slides, numbering about two thousand, to a private laboratory for review. City purchasing rules required that all contracts over $10,000 be competitively bid, a process that could take at least six months. To get around this barrier, she divided the unread slides into smaller lots, each costing under $10,000. Three batches, each with approximately six hundred slides, were sent to an outside lab between March and May 1990. The third batch of slides, submitted by the clinics about a year earlier, was sitting in the Bureau of Laboratories waiting to be sent when the *Post* broke the story.

City Council members declared that they were "shocked and outraged" at the affair, and Myers was forced to hold a news conference where he concurred that the events constituted a "betrayal of the public trust."[80] To lead an internal investigation into what had gone wrong, Myers turned to Katherine Lobach, the director of the Bureau of Child Health. Lobach was seen within the department as someone of great integrity and competence; more important, she had no connection to any of the events in question. Kenneth Dressler, the director of the Bureau of Laboratories, and John Miles, the director of the Bureau of STD Control, lost their jobs, as did their boss, deputy commissioner Stephen Schultz. To track down the women whose abnormal results were months old, the Bureau of STD Control put together a team of the most experienced field-workers, who launched a massive search and located women as far away as Alaska and Panama. The vast majority of the women were contacted, but a few remained permanently lost to follow-up.

Some of the problems identified in the investigation of the pap smear scandal had clear relevance to the ongoing saga of tuberculosis: the failure to recognize the potential magnitude of a steadily worsening situation, the difficulty of attracting competent professionals to work for meager public-sector salaries, and the roadblocks that city bureaucracy could place in the way of efforts to mount an effective public health response. Whatever wisdom might have been gained from these lessons would not prove easy to apply, however, since the city was teetering on the verge of a fiscal crisis that threatened to be as severe as the one that struck in the 1970s.

In 1990 rates of tuberculosis continued their seemingly inexorable upward spiral. By the end of the year, the city had recorded 3,520 cases of the disease, an increase of almost 40 percent over the previous year, and more than triple the number of cases in 1978. New York City, which held 3 percent of the country's population, accounted for 15 percent of its TB cases.[81] In November, shortly after the *Post*'s sensational weeklong exposé, the City Council held hearings into the problem. Council members asked for a complete listing of all the city's facilities in predominantly

African American and Latino neighborhoods and their hours of operation; several members, predictably, tried to pin down Myers on the number of undetected cases in the city and the risks that these people might pose to the "general public."[82] Myers reassured the council that people in good health were unlikely to become infected from riding on the subway or in an elevator.[83]

A few weeks later, Myers pleaded with the mayor's office to allow the hiring of forty grant-funded candidates whose positions had been frozen for months.[84] At the same time, he asked Emilio Carrillo, head of the Health and Hospitals Corporation, about the possibility of dedicating beds in one of the municipal hospitals to a closed TB ward for persistently noncompliant patients. Carrillo resisted the idea. "Given our overcrowded facilities and at a time when HHC is reeling under the need to maintain vital services in the context of a rapidly shrinking financial base," he wrote, "dedicating a cohort of beds to provide medical care for these patients, with the concomitant security requirements and support services, would severely stress our fiscal reserves."[85]

Both the unwillingness of the mayor's office to release money for new employees and Carillo's concern about a "shrinking financial base" were symptomatic of the city's grim, and worsening, economic situation. From the moment David Dinkins stepped into City Hall, dire budgetary predictions hung ominously over his administration. Municipal expenses had steadily risen during the 1980s in response to social ills such as homelessness, AIDS, and drug-related crime. In the wake of the 1987 stock market crash, the city lost many jobs in the financial sector and the economic outlook darkened. Federal funds had provided about one-fifth of the city's budget in 1980; by 1990 that support accounted for only 9 percent.[86] Just weeks into his term, Dinkins had sent a memo to all his agency heads warning that the city faced a potential budget shortfall of as much as $1.3 billion over the next two years. Several months later, he instituted a salary freeze and a 5 percent pay cut for all city employees making more than $70,000 per year.[87]

In the first budget reduction request to the Health Department, Dinkins asked Woodrow Myers to cut almost $4.6 million from the agency's budget. Myers, eager to demonstrate both his loyalty to the mayor and the fiscal prudence he had honed in business school, responded by suggesting $7.2 million in cuts, exceeding the target by 85 percent. When the Office of Management and Budget submitted a follow-up request, Myers obliged by suggesting two additional programs for elimination—the window guards program and school health counselors—for a further savings of $2.9 million.[88]

In early May 1991, Dinkins unveiled what quickly became known as the "doomsday budget," which proposed devastating cuts to municipal services; the already grim picture for the city's disadvantaged residents promised to get worse with the elimination of homeless shelters, clinics, and social programs. At the end of the month, Woodrow Myers testified before the City Council committees on finance and health about what he called "incredibly difficult and extremely painful actions" that the Health Department would have to take because of the city's financial situation.[89] The cuts he proposed to the department budget were deep and wide, exceeding at one stroke the reductions that had taken place over the course of two years during the depths of the city's 1975 to 1976 fiscal crisis. The annual budget would be cut by 26 percent, to $243 million from $327 million. Virtually all maternity and family planning services would be eliminated, including the infant mortality initiative, adolescent parent education, and pregnancy testing; $7.1 million and 250 staff positions would be cut. The Chelsea district health center, which housed clinics for TB, AIDS counseling and testing, child health, and immunization, would be closed. The sexually transmitted diseases program would reduce by one-third the number of patients treated and contacts traced. The Bureau of Laboratories budget would be cut by half; 1.5 million fewer specimens would be analyzed for lead, syphilis, HIV, and TB. Most sweeping, the entire school health program, which employed dozens of school nurses throughout the city, would be eliminated, for a savings of $7.5 million.[90]

Myers would not remain to preside over the cuts. The day before he outlined the department's budget for the City Council, Myers submitted his resignation to Dinkins, citing his desire to return to Indiana to be closer to his ailing father and mother-in-law.[91] He had been on the job for just over a year. Rumors had been circulating for months that he was unhappy in New York City and frustrated over the numerous bureaucratic and budgetary obstacles to implementing his vision for the department.[92]

As acting commissioner, Dinkins appointed Margaret Hamburg, an assistant commissioner whom Myers had recruited to the department the previous year (see figure 6.3). As Hamburg reviewed the budget that was due to be adopted in less than a month, she grew alarmed, not simply by the probable consequences of the drastic reductions, but because she believed that many of the cuts were illegal. The city health code obligated the department to fulfill a wide variety of functions, and Hamburg recognized that many of the cuts that Myers had directed would place the department in default of legal mandates. She turned for guidance to members of the Board of Health, who in turn notified Dinkins's office. In a series of emergency meetings, Hamburg worked with the mayor's staff, the president of the City Council, and the corporation counsel to craft a budget that was within the law.

The situation was so dire that in the fall Kevin Cahill, the chair of the Board of Health, convened a symposium of the city's medical, business, and political leaders to draw attention to the need to protect vital public

Figure 6.3   Hamburg Is Appointed

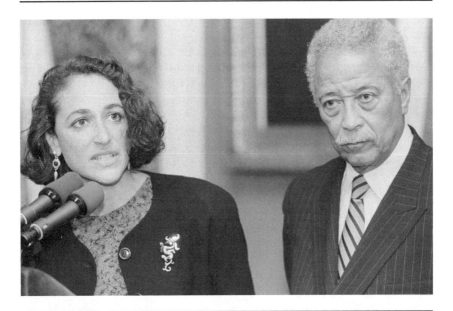

Source: Courtesy New York City Municipal Archives.
Note: Margaret Hamburg answers questions from reporters at the press conference at which Mayor David Dinkins announced her appointment to the post of health commissioner in a permanent capacity.

health functions even in fiscal crises; a volume of cautionary essays titled *Imminent Peril* was the result.[93] By that time, several unions had brought suit against the city seeking temporary injunctions that would prevent the elimination of programs such as school health, correctional health, and day care regulation.[94] The budget that Hamburg ultimately negotiated with the mayor's office was 15 percent below the prior year, rather than 25 percent below as in the budget Myers had submitted; the revised version rescinded the cuts that would have violated legal mandates and most endangered public health.[95]

The department's budget crisis was a trial by fire that by all accounts Hamburg handled ably. Although her experience in public health was thin, Hamburg had an impressive background, both personal and professional, in medicine. Her parents were nationally known physicians. Her father, David Hamburg, had been chair of the psychiatry department at Stanford and president of the Institute of Medicine; her mother, Beatrix Hamburg, had been the first African American admitted to Yale Medical School. Margaret Hamburg had received her medical degree from Harvard; before joining the Health Department, she had done neuroscience research at The Rockefeller University and served as special adviser to Anthony Fauci, the head of the National Institute of Allergy and Infectious Diseases.

As much as her professional accomplishments, it was Hamburg's accessibility, even temper, and steady management style that made her an effective leader for the department at a time when it was buffeted by fiscal constraints, bad press, and low morale. A minor controversy over the fact that she did not hold an MPH or other master's degree, as required by the health code, did not derail her appointment, and Dinkins named her to the position in a permanent capacity in December 1991. At age thirty-six, she was the youngest health commissioner in the city's history.

By the time she assumed the job, Hamburg had begun to move aggressively against tuberculosis. A new and frightening element had been added to the mix: lethal strains of the disease resistant to multiple drugs.

The U-Shaped Curve

One reason the resurgence of tuberculosis struck a nerve with the public and politicians was that it reinforced the narrative of a city that was spinning out of control. New York's quality of life seemed to reach a nadir in the early 1990s, surpassing even the depths of filth, crime, and violence of the late 1970s in the aftermath of the fiscal crisis. The homicide rate peaked in 1990, when the city recorded 2,262 murders; especially horrifying were high-profile cases of bystanders and children being shot in drug dealers' turf battles.[96] That fall, a *Time* magazine cover story lamented "the rotting of the Big Apple."[97] The *Post*, whose headlines were a reliable barometer of middle-class opinion, demanded of the mayor, "Dave, Do Something!"[98]

It was against this backdrop that outbreaks of multi-drug-resistant tuberculosis (MDR-TB) began to strike in institutional settings in 1990 and 1991. A dozen inmates and one guard died of MDR-TB in jails in Queens and upstate in Syracuse.[99] Around the same time, hospitals began reporting outbreaks of MDR-TB among their patients.[100] The CDC, convinced that drug-resistant strains of tuberculosis were no longer a significant problem in the United States, had stopped nationwide surveillance for them in 1985, so it was impossible to know whether these clusters were aberrations or harbingers of a wider epidemic. The public health implications of the outbreaks were grave. The case fatality rate for TB resistant to two or more drugs was 40 to 60 percent.[101] Treating drug-resistant strains involved a complicated treatment regimen that could take as long as two years to complete.

Karen Brudney, who had observed abysmally low treatment completion rates at Harlem Hospital, was convinced that MDR-TB was on the rise in New York City; she shared her concerns with Thomas Frieden, a young physician who was on assignment as an Epidemic Intelligence Service officer at the Health Department. Frieden responded quickly. He enlisted the help of three public health advisers from the TB control program and trekked to seventy-two hospitals around the city, collecting sputum samples of 466 patients who had had positive TB cultures in April 1991. He then sent the isolates for drug-susceptibility testing and also used a sophisticated new DNA analysis.

The results were even worse than what Brudney and others had feared. One-third of the patients were infected with strains of TB resistant to at least one of the standard drugs; one-quarter were resistant to isoniazid, the first-line treatment, and one-fifth were resistant to both isoniazid and rifampin. Although the strongest predictor of having a drug-resistant strain was a history of prior treatment, the majority of these patients were initially infected with drug-resistant strains.[102] Officials at the CDC were alarmed by the high rates that Frieden and his team had uncovered and responded by undertaking a national survey. Their study determined that New York City accounted for more than half of the cases of drug-resistant TB in the country.[103]

The emergence of widespread drug resistance and the danger that the new strains posed to hospital employees, police officers, child welfare workers, prison guards, and other people in occupational settings was a critical factor in the turning upward of the "U"-shaped curve of concern. Margaret Hamburg wrote to members of the state's congressional delegation in hopes that they could obtain additional federal appropriations. She also drafted a letter for Mayor Dinkins to send to U.S. Secretary of Health and Human Services Louis Sullivan requesting an emergency appropriation to the city of $15 million. Ted Weiss, the congressional representative from Manhattan who had held early hearings into the government's response to AIDS, took up the issue of TB a week before Christmas 1991.

At the hearings, a stream of witnesses testified to the severity of the problem.[104] A representative of DC 37, the health care workers' union, warned of the threat that TB posed to hospital employees. Harlem-based physicians Charles Felton and Karen Brudney told of their experiences struggling to treat difficult patients with paltry resources in a fragmented system; Felton charged that the dire situation was "the culmination of years of habitual neglect of the health needs of this inner city population" and that government at all levels had been "sluggish in reacting to a persistent health menace."[105] When Hamburg's turn came to testify, she hammered home the enormous commitment of federal money that would be necessary to bring the disease under control. "Although this monetary investment may be large," she told the committee, "I can assure you that it does not compare to the financial cost we will surely face later on if we do not take decisive action now."[106] She noted that although Congress had authorized the CDC to spend $36 million nationwide to fight tuberculosis, only $15 million had been appropriated. In the wake of the hearing, Congress made an emergency appropriation of about $100 million to the CDC's budget for TB control. Of that amount, New York City received $40 million.

Hamburg named Thomas Frieden, whose documentation of MDR-TB had played a key role in securing the new funds, as the new director of the Bureau of Tuberculosis Control in May 1992. Only thirty-one years old, Frieden had a youthful appearance that made him easy to underestimate. (Arriving in Bangladesh to give a keynote speech at a conference a few years later, he was greeted by the organizer's startled exclamation, "But you are a boy!"[107]) This impression did not last long. As he set about transforming the way the city managed tuberculosis, people throughout the health care system discovered in Frieden an aggressiveness and a steely resolve to get results.

One of the most urgent priorities was to gain control of outbreaks in hospitals. Frieden and his staff spent many hours working with infection control staffs across the city, emphasizing the need to do more aggressive laboratory work to diagnose drug-resistant strains and to comply with the CDC guidelines for isolation and air filtration. Isolation rooms were supposed to be maintained at negative air pressure relative to hallways so that airborne droplets would not escape the rooms; since most hospitals' ventilation systems could not accomplish this, special fans were needed that would suck air into filters fitted with ultraviolet lights, which had been shown to kill the bacillus. Health care workers and visitors were supposed to wear masks in TB patients' rooms.

In spite of the department's efforts, the outbreaks proved difficult to keep under control, not only because of technological barriers but because of poor management within the hospitals. In one instance, a patient's chest X-ray showing clear signs of advanced disease was never placed in his file or given to his doctor; he was assigned a room with four other patients, where he stayed for four days before a sputum test came back positive and he was transferred. Within ten weeks, three of the roommates had developed MDR-TB; the fourth was diagnosed fourteen months later.[108] Doors to hospital rooms were often left open; patients were removed from isolation without laboratory confirmation that they were no longer infectious.[109] Even though hospitals were aware of the danger posed by noncompliant patients, some were reluctant to seek orders of detention because they would have to bear the additional costs of posting a guard and would lose patient beds from converting shared rooms to single-patient occupancy.[110]

Elmhurst Hospital in Queens, which had experienced one of the first and most severe outbreaks of MDR-TB, reported additional cases during 1993, including a cluster of six infants infected in the nursery and maternity ward. The hospital had spent thousands of dollars to equip twenty-seven isolation rooms with state-of-the-art air filters—but only four of the rooms had private toilets, so patients in isolation had to walk down the hall past half a dozen rooms to a shared bathroom, potentially spreading disease along the way.[111] The situation at St. Clare's Hospital in Manhattan proved the most severe and difficult to control. Frieden later called the institution "the Broad Street pump of MDR-TB," a reference to the infamous source of cholera-tainted water in nineteenth-century London. "They had dozens and dozens and dozens of cases," he recalled, "and the hospital was in denial, and the administration was in denial, and finally I remember we had a meeting, kind of a knock-down-drag-out meeting where we just rubbed their noses in the data."[112]

At the same time, the city's Department of Corrections was finally taking action to bring the outbreaks at Rikers Island under control after years of delay. At the beginning of 1992, a federal district court judge ordered the city to declare a state of emergency, which would allow the city's comptroller to waive bidding requirements for the construction of a new tuberculosis wing in the infirmary.[113] The first forty-two units were completed four months later. Each isolation cell cost $450,000, for a total renovation cost of some $60 million.[114]

As the institutional outbreaks were being addressed, Hamburg and Frieden put in place a plan to ensure that the thousands of ambulatory patients in the city would complete their treatment. Given the debilitated state of the city's tuberculosis control infrastructure, however, the influx of federal money was only the beginning of a solution. A series of legal and bureaucratic obstacles had to be overcome.

The first and in some respects most important step was to expedite hiring. In October 1992, representatives came together from all the city agencies that would have to work together in the TB control effort, including the Health and Hospitals Corporation, the Human Resources Administration, the Office of Management and Budget, the Department of Corrections, and the Mayor's Office of Operations. At the meeting, everyone was asked to state what he or she believed was the most important thing the city could do to control tuberculosis. Frieden's answer was that newly hired employees in the tuberculosis program should be expedited through the city's cumbersome administrative procedures, which could delay hiring for months. The mayor's office granted Frieden's request.[115]

The other critical challenge was addressing the legal and ethical implications of coercive measures to control the disease. Because non-adherence to medication had played such an important role in the emergence of drug-resistant strains, it was clear that the city would have to adopt more aggressive means of increasing treatment completion rates. Directly observed therapy (DOT) and detention would be central to this effort.

Directly observed therapy had emerged as a response to a problem that became evident in the therapeutic boom of the postwar era: people are not good at taking their medication. For patients young and old, male and female, well-to-do and indigent, in the developing world as well as in economically advanced nations, non-adherence to doctors' medication orders appears to be a universal tendency. "The individual who uses new drugs on a routine basis without help and encouragement from others," wrote one expert on compliance, "is probably the abnormal one."[116] TB presented a more difficult problem than most diseases. It was treated with multiple pills that could have unpleasant gastrointestinal side effects; symptoms abated soon after the regimen was begun, but several more months of medication were necessary before the patient was cured. Directly observed therapy, in which outreach workers monitored the patients as they swallowed the pills, was an attempt to address this problem. Public health officials in Hong Kong and Madras, India, had achieved high treatment completion rates with DOT, but only a few local and state health officials in the United States embraced the approach because the costs were seen as unjustified given that TB was on the decline.[117] Baltimore was one of the few communities to use DOT, beginning in 1981; over the next decade, the city recorded a major decline in cases, even as rates crept upward in other major cities.[118]

DOT raised a thicket of ethical and practical questions. Was it a helpful service or a burdensome intrusion on patient privacy? What criteria should determine a patient's need for DOT? Although homeless patients and injection drug users were more likely than others to be non-adherent, the problem was by no means limited to these groups: one study found that about half of all TB patients stopped taking their medication for at least two months.[119] Should DOT be offered to—or required of—every patient as a default? Would putting all patients on observation waste scarce resources on people who would take their pills without assistance? Would it send a stigmatizing message that health officials did not believe that patients could be trusted, or would universal application reduce stigma by normalizing the process?

An even more sensitive issue than DOT was involuntary confinement of noncompliant patients. Detention had a longer history than DOT and a more checkered one, having often been used against the disadvantaged of society. In the early twentieth century, a ward at Riverside Hospital in Manhattan had been set aside for patients considered by doctors to be a danger to the community because of their perceived likelihood of spreading disease—a determination influenced by social judgments as well as scientific ones.[120] With the advent of antibiotic therapies, more than thirty states used involuntary hospitalization for patients deemed unlikely to complete treatment, especially alcoholics and the homeless living on skid row.[121]

During the 1960s and 1970s, courts around the country expanded protections for individuals against government coercion, ruling that commitment statutes for people with mental illness, drug addiction, and alcoholism had to ensure that those detained were able to contest their confinement before a judge. It was only a matter of time before coercive measures to control infectious diseases would be similarly called into question. In 1980 the West Virginia Supreme Court struck down a statute for the detention of TB patients, ruling that patients could not be held without written notice and right to counsel.[122]

As Hamburg and Frieden contemplated what was likely to be a dramatic expansion of the use of DOT and detention, the need for a legal framework that could withstand scrutiny in the courts was obvious. The health code granted broad discretion—it allowed the commissioner to detain a person with tuberculosis "upon determining that the health of others is endangered"—and provided no standards for making such a judgment and no guarantee of due process for the detainee.[123] Although the constitutionality of that section of the code had never been challenged, it would clearly not pass muster with a court in 1993.[124] Over the course of 1992, the department carefully crafted the legal apparatus necessary for the widespread use of such measures and built political support for them through community consultations.

The potential use of DOT and detention was especially sensitive because of the overlap in the epidemics of HIV and TB. Advocates for people with AIDS had spent the epidemic's first decade arguing—mostly successfully—that because of the intimate nature of HIV transmission, coercive approaches would be ineffective and counterproductive. Because tuberculosis spread via the air and could pose a risk to casual contacts, however, there was widespread agreement, at least in principle, that health officials should be able to limit the liberty of patients who might put others at risk. This prospect was alarming to groups such as Gay Men's Health Crisis and the Lambda Legal Defense and Education Fund, whose members worried that people with AIDS might be unduly subject to civil liberties violations.[125] The Health Department's legal counsel, Ron Bogard, convened a series of broad-based consultations with AIDS advocacy, gay rights, and civil liberties groups to solicit input into proposed changes to the health code.[126] Seeking their buy-in was partly an effort to craft the best possible law, but it also served the politically strategic purpose of preempting the objections of likely opponents.

Although discussions with community members often centered on the potential abuse of government authority, not all groups shared these concerns. At a community meeting at a church in Harlem, where Frieden was seeking support for the department's authority to detain noncompliant patients, African American residents voiced a very different sentiment from the ones raised by civil liberties groups. "Why the hell didn't you do this before?" the residents asked Frieden. "You white folks are just getting worried about TB because it's affecting you. It's been devastating our community for years. We know about these people. They should be on their medicine."[127]

In October 1992, Frieden made a presentation to the Board of Health on the need to amend the health code. He insisted that the department had to have the authority to detain the small number of patients whose persistent noncompliance endangered the public.[128] Frieden did not dispute the claims of advocates for the homeless and people with HIV that societal inequities lay at the root of the TB problem, nor did he deny that the people most likely to be targets of coercive measures were already disadvantaged in many other ways. "Although society is, in part, responsible for the situation, this doesn't mean no action should be taken," he told the board members. "To continue to allow these individuals to infect others compounds social injustice with deplorable inaction."[129]

Two months later, representatives of community organizations had additional opportunities to weigh in on the proposed health code amendments at a public hearing.[130] Many health professionals turned out to testify in favor of them, including representatives of academic medical centers and hospital administrators who spoke about the threat that MDR-TB posed to health care workers and the broader patient population. Much of the vocal support was due to the efforts of Mark Barnes, the energetic young lawyer who served as Hamburg's assistant commissioner for policy. He had called prominent members of the medical community to make sure that they would come to speak at the hearing; in some cases, he wrote or edited their testimony for them to ensure that the compelling reasons for the Health Department's proposals were clearly articulated.[131]

Advocacy groups such as the Commission on Human Rights, the Lambda Legal Defense and Education Fund, and the New York Civil Liberties Union viewed the proposed changes warily. They argued that not only should the department have to prove that every person to be detained posed a substantial risk to the health of others, but that less restrictive options should be tried before the most severe deprivation of liberty was ordered. In a formal response to the public comments, however, the department insisted that health officials "cannot and should not be required to exhaust a rigid, pre-set hierarchy of alternative measures that would ostensibly encourage voluntary compliance, but then be compelled to wait for the patient to fail each of them."[132]

In April 1993, the Board of Health approved the amendments to the health code that allowed patients to be ordered to take their medications under direct observation. If patients failed to comply with DOT, they could be detained involuntarily in an inpatient facility—not just until they were non-infectious, but until they were completely cured. Under the new provisions, the Health Department had to inform the patient of the right to be represented by an attorney and to provide an attorney if the patient asked for one. If the patient requested release, the commissioner had to respond before a court within seventy-two hours. Each order for detention had to be reviewed by the court within sixty days and every ninety days after that, regardless of whether or not the patient asked to be released.[133] On the critical issue of whether less coercive measures had to precede an order of detention, the department prevailed. The commissioner was required to set forth "the less restrictive treatment alternatives that were attempted and were unsuccessful *and/or the less restrictive alternatives that were considered and rejected, and the reasons such alternatives were rejected.*"[134]

With a solid legal structure in place and a massive hiring of new outreach workers under way—the staff working on TB would eventually grow to more than six hundred—the department moved ahead with a strengthened program in which directly observed therapy became the standard of care. Frieden undertook an education campaign throughout the city's public and private hospitals and an equally ambitious staff training effort in the department's own chest clinics about the critical importance of ensuring treatment compliance through universal DOT. In June 1992, he publicly announced that the Bureau of Tuberculosis Control would seek to increase the number of patients receiving DOT, then about 50, to 500 by year's end. That goal was exceeded. By the end of 1994, some 1,200 patients in the city were receiving DOT.[135] Patients were told that taking their pills under observation was the best way to control the spread of the disease. They could opt out of observation for various reasons (for example, if their workplace could not accommodate a DOT outreach worker), but the standard explanation given to patients was: "This is how we do it."[136]

About one-third of patients were seen by providers in the private medical community, and two-thirds received their therapy from Health Department workers. Patients under Health Department supervision received one of two types of DOT. One was clinic-based, in which patients came daily or twice weekly and were seen by an interdisciplinary team of medical and social service providers. The other consisted of community-based appointments at sites chosen by patients. Homes and workplaces were the most common venues for receiving DOT, but outreach workers went to every conceivable location: street corners, crack dens, train stations, homeless camps under bridges. In some cases the places were chosen because patients did not want their families, friends, or coworkers to know that they were being treated for TB; in other cases, it was because they had no stable residence or employment.[137]

As the DOT program expanded, Frieden spearheaded a campaign to upgrade the quality of care in the department's nine chest clinics. He re-

ceived a commitment from the mayor's office to provide funds to renovate the buildings (a process that would take a decade) and began a
painstaking effort to bring higher-caliber physicians onto the staff. He
was able to set up the type of residency program that Alje Vennema had
sought in the 1980s, in which infectious disease residents rotated through
the clinics. He tirelessly recruited new doctors and at the same time
forced out the worst-performing of the department's deadwood—sometimes with a veiled or explicit threat to expose a physician's poor treatment decisions to the state licensing board.[138]

The final piece of the department's control effort was the detention of
persistently non-adherent patients. The city paid half a million dollars to
renovate a twenty-five-bed ward in Goldwater Memorial Hospital on
Roosevelt Island in the East River, and in the third week of September
1993, Rafael Serrano was admitted as the first patient. Serrano had been
diagnosed with MDR-TB the previous year and had persistently failed
to take his full course of medications; when hospitalized in isolation, he
repeatedly left his room to visit with other patients, even after an attendant was posted at his door to keep him in. A dozen other patients soon
joined Serrano in the Goldwater ward.[139] A few months later, Bellevue
Hospital opened a twenty-one-bed locked ward.[140] The Bellevue ward
was eventually designated as the facility for patients who were infectious; patients who had completed enough of their treatment to convert
to non-infectious status were admitted to Goldwater to finish out their
course of medication.

In the first two years after the health code was changed, 304 patients
were served with a "commissioner's order"—either to be examined, to
complete treatment, to undergo DOT, or to submit to detention, either
until non-infectious or until cured. Orders were issued for fewer than 4
percent of the total number of TB patients during that period. Compared
with other TB patients, those subject to regulatory orders were much
more likely to be alcoholics, crack users, homeless, or former prisoners.[141]

In the mid-1980s, fewer than a dozen patients had been detained each
year for persistent non-compliance.[142] In the two years following the re-
visions to the health code, 139 patients were detained. For those with
drug-susceptible TB, the median stay was twenty-one weeks; those with
MDR-TB stayed an average of just under one year in detention. Everyone associated with the tuberculosis control program agreed that a credible threat of detention was key to the success of DOT.[143]

A Triumph of the Technocratic?

Dixie Snider, who had led the Centers for Disease Control's 1987 review
of tuberculosis in New York, had predicted that it would take ten to fifteen years to control the disease in the city.[144] By the end of 1993, some

Figure 6.4   Announcing a Drop in Tuberculosis

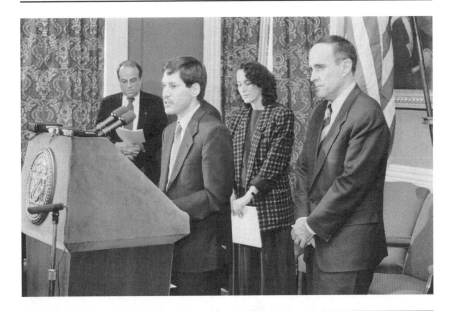

Source: Courtesy New York City Municipal Archives.
Note: At a City Hall news conference, Thomas Frieden (at lectern), director of the Bureau of Tuberculosis Control, announces a sharp drop in the number of tuberculosis cases. Frieden is accompanied by Health Commissioner Margaret Hamburg and Mayor Rudy Giuliani.

eighteen months after the strengthened program began to be put in place, the number of tuberculosis cases in the city had declined by 15 percent from the previous year—to 3,235 from 3,811 (see figure 6.4). Frieden and his colleagues were stunned at the results that their efforts seemed to be producing. "I just couldn't believe how quickly cases came down," Frieden later recalled. "We looked at the data. Was it wrong? Had we made a mistake? But we had actually improved surveillance— we had better surveillance but many fewer cases."[145] They wrote up a report and sent it to the *New England Journal of Medicine,* but the editors, skeptical that such a dramatic decrease could occur in so short a time, told them to wait another year to see if the trend continued and then re-submit their article. The following year, new cases dropped even further, to 2,995, for a two-year decline of more than 20 percent.[146] The portion of patients completing their treatment rose from about half to 90 percent; the percentage of cases that were drug-resistant declined from one-third to one-quarter.[147] The journal accepted the paper.

Although the swiftness of the decline drew widespread comment, another important aspect of the control effort was less noted: the department's approach had left untouched the deeply entrenched social conditions that gave rise to the epidemic. The program of directly observed therapy worked within structures of poverty and deprivation—welfare hotels, homeless encampments, crack dens, jails, neighborhoods devastated by the war on drugs—rather than attempting to reform them. Homelessness did not decrease in New York City during the 1990s; punitive narcotics laws were not repealed; drug treatment was not expanded. New York City's economy boomed in the 1990s, but these gains did not accrue equally to all city residents. Instead, economic polarization reached unprecedented levels over the decade.[148]

It was an article of faith among public health professionals in the post–World War II era that social problems were at the root of tuberculosis and that, as a corollary, the best way to fight the disease was to address these underlying issues. "Probably the most important preventive measure in tuberculosis," the director of the Bureau of Tuberculosis Control wrote in 1967, "is improvement of the socio-economic conditions of the population most at risk. This requires improved housing, education and job opportunities, and stabilization of the family. Such activities are not within the framework of the Bureau of Tuberculosis, but, increasingly, we should concern ourselves with these social aspects of health maintenance."[149] The urgency of the situation in 1991 tested the Health Department's commitment to that belief. Commenting on the tension between the need to attack the root causes of disease and the imperative to act quickly to prevent sickness and death, Margaret Hamburg put the matter bluntly: "We cannot afford to hold off on TB control efforts and wait until a damaged society is repaired."[150]

The control of drug-resistant TB in New York City was undoubtedly a triumph, one that has since been widely cited in academic and popular journals as a case study of what can be accomplished when basic tools of public health are applied with sufficient funding, commitment, and skill. That it was an essentially technocratic solution is not necessarily inconsistent with a commitment to social change. Working in the context of profound injustice, Hamburg, Frieden, and their colleagues saw the Health Department's tuberculosis control effort as a form of justice, to the extent that it relieved the disproportionate burdens that illness places on the disadvantaged.

Chapter 7

Threat Levels

ONE MONDAY in late August 1999, Marcelle Layton, the Health Department's assistant commissioner for communicable disease, received a call from Deborah Asnis, a physician at Flushing Hospital in Queens, about two elderly patients there with unexplained and baffling symptoms. They were feverish, weak, and confused; in one the weakness was so severe that it verged on paralysis. After discussing several possible diagnoses, including polio, Guillain-Barré syndrome, and botulism, Layton and Asnis agreed that these were most likely cases of viral encephalitis. Layton arranged to have samples of their cerebrospinal fluid shipped to the state laboratory for testing and sent two staff members to the hospital to review the patients' charts. At the end of the week, Asnis called back to tell Layton that she had a third patient with the same symptoms. While they were on the phone, a colleague of Asnis's happened to walk by and mention a similar case at a nearby hospital. Since the city normally recorded fewer than ten cases of viral encephalitis in an entire year, the possible occurrence of four cases around the same time and place was cause for concern and investigation.[1]

Two classes of virus, enteroviruses and arboviruses, were known to cause clusters of encephalitis in the summer. Enteroviruses, which included polio and Coxsackie virus, spread via the saliva or feces of infected people. Arboviruses, such as yellow fever, dengue, and malaria, were transmitted by mosquitoes and other insects. New York City had not seen arbovirus illnesses since the yellow fever epidemics of the eighteenth century.

On Saturday, Layton and Annie Fine, an epidemiologist on her staff, drove to Queens to review the cases, including a fifth patient who had just been admitted to a nearby hospital. The patients were too ill to be interviewed, so Layton and Fine spoke to their family members about the patients' daily routines, recent travel, diet, and possible exposures to other illnesses in the family. The only thing the patients seemed to have in common was that they lived within a few miles of each other (but did not know each other) and were in the habit of spending time outdoors in the evening. On Sunday, Layton discussed the cases with experts in enteroviruses and arboviruses at the CDC; she and her staff spent the rest of the day phoning hospitals in Queens, Brooklyn, and surrounding counties looking for reports of similar illnesses. Their inquiries yielded three more possible cases, bringing the total to eight. All of the patients were between fifty-eight and eighty-seven years old and lived in Whitestone, a middle-class neighborhood of detached houses, neatly kept yards, and many swimming pools.

On Monday morning, the investigation shifted into high gear. Layton and her staff called all seventy-two hospitals in the city asking if they had seen any encephalitis of unknown origin. Even though an arbovirus outbreak in New York City would be highly unusual, Layton wanted to get a better sense of the mosquito situation around the patients' homes. The department had no entomologists on staff, so she enlisted the help of one from the American Museum of Natural History, who went with an epidemiologist to Whitestone. They walked from house to house observing mosquito activity and reinterviewed the families of the victims about their routines in the weeks before they fell ill. One, a smoker who lived with a nonsmoker, had been in the habit of having a cigarette on his front porch in the evening; another was an avid gardener; another had been helping a neighbor put in a new swimming pool. At the home of one of the patients, his wife described how her husband, who suffered from insomnia, often went outside around four o'clock in the morning to rest in a lawn chair. As she talked with the investigators, she took them out to the backyard, where they noticed several barrels partially filled with water. It had been a relatively dry summer, the woman explained, so to conserve city water, they were collecting rainwater for their garden. Looking in one of the barrels, the entomologist saw that it was filled with the larvae of *culex* mosquitoes, a common vector for arboviruses.

As the week went on, the department's calls to city hospitals uncovered more suspected cases of encephalitis. Two of Deborah Asnis's patients, an eighty-year-old man and an eighty-seven-year-old woman, died. Layton contacted the Mayor's Office of Emergency Management about the possibility of pesticide spraying; since the department's mosquito control program had just two employees and no equipment for spraying, it would need outside help. The department's communications staff began planning media alerts and a public information strategy in case the CDC's tests confirmed that a mosquito-borne virus was the cause of the outbreak. Concerned about a run on pharmacies for insect repellent, the department bought 500,000 cans of DEET for possible distribution in the affected areas. If the lab results came back positive, the department would have to move quickly.

If the swift yet methodical preparations that week had the practiced air of an emergency drill, it was partly because there had been heightened awareness within the department for several years about the importance of planning for outbreaks—both naturally occurring and humanly instigated—of unusual illnesses. Enhancing the capacity to respond to health emergencies became a top priority during the 1990s under Commissioner Margaret Hamburg. She was among a growing number of public health professionals and government officials concerned about the threat of emerging infectious diseases. The city's outbreak of drug-resistant tuberculosis had been an early warning about these dangers. Scientific journals and the popular media began calling attention to the risks of new and resurgent pathogens such as Ebola, Marburg virus, plague, anthrax, and smallpox that might be introduced into the United States through international travel or a terrorist act.[2]

The risks were clearly demonstrated in the fall of 1994 when an outbreak of pneumonic plague struck Surat, India. The department had recently instituted a broadcast fax system and used it to alert New York City hospitals to be on the lookout for possible cases. Hamburg worked with the CDC quarantine station at Kennedy Airport to ensure that protocols were in place for triage and isolation should a case be detected on any of the more than thirty flights that arrived in New York City from India every day. She then made sure that Mayor Rudy Giuliani knew about the department's efforts.[3]

Hamburg had been one of the few commissioners from the Dinkins administration who had been asked to stay on when Giuliani took office at the beginning of 1994. She had impressed the mayor's transition team with her comprehensive knowledge of the department and her ability to forcefully articulate its mission and importance. It also did not hurt that she was able to announce a sharp drop in tuberculosis cases three months after Giuliani took office, allowing the mayor to bask in the reflected glow of a public health triumph.

Hamburg's focus on emerging infections was good public health, but it was also politically strategic—a way to demonstrate the importance of the Health Department to a mayor who was inclined to undervalue it. Rudy Giuliani had a neoliberal hostility to the public sector, and he came into office in 1994 with a clearly stated intent to reduce the size of city government and privatize as many of its functions as possible. In his first month in office, he announced plans to eliminate up to 18,000 city jobs.[4] He derided the public hospital system as a "politically mandated jobs program" and announced that he would attempt to sell or lease several institutions of the Health and Hospitals Corporation.[5] The Health Department was clearly at risk for sharp cuts in budget and personnel.

Having made public safety and quality of life the centerpiece of his mayoralty, Giuliani insisted that police and fire would be insulated from cuts. To protect the Health Department, Hamburg shrewdly positioned it as a kind of uniformed service. This conception was, of course, historically rooted; not for nothing did the U.S. Public Health Service have an officer corps. As Hamburg sought to enhance the department's capacity to respond to emerging infections, she also took every opportunity to remind the mayor and his advisers that public health was a form of public safety.

In 1995, not long after the India plague outbreak, Hamburg invited Joshua Lederberg, the Nobel Prize–winning scientist and authority on biological weapons and emerging infections, to brief the mayor about anthrax and bioterrorism. A few weeks later, members of a religious cult released poison gas in the Tokyo subway system, and Giuliani was able to tell the public that he had already been advised on bioterrorism by a leading expert in the field. Later that year, Hamburg and several department staff members participated in a preparedness exercise coordinated by the Federal Emergency Management Agency (FEMA) that simulated the release of anthrax in the city.[6]

Hamburg's initiatives dovetailed with efforts throughout city government to prepare for crises of all kinds. Giuliani created the Mayor's Office of Emergency Management in 1996 to coordinate these efforts. The office conducted drills such as one in which hundreds of participants came together from across city government to simulate responses to chemical attacks like the one in Tokyo.[7] These exercises tested the city's capacity to monitor developing situations in hospital emergency rooms, handle sudden influxes of patients needing acute care, distribute vaccines and treatments to large numbers of ill or wounded people, and control contamination in the air and water.

Hamburg left the department in early 1997 to take a high-ranking position in the Department of Health and Human Services in Washington, D.C. Preparedness efforts continued under her successor, Neal Cohen, even though he brought a very different set of interests and skills to the job. Cohen was the first psychiatrist to serve as health commissioner. The circumstances of his appointment were also unique. When Rudy Giuliani named him to the post in January 1998, Cohen was already serving as the commissioner of the Department of Mental Health, Mental Retardation, and Alcoholism Services; the mayor announced that he would seek to merge the two departments. (The move would require amending the city charter either by City Council action or popular vote.) In the meantime, Cohen served jointly as the commissioner of both agencies.

Most observers agreed that a closer linkage of public health and mental health was highly desirable, and experts in both fields had broached the possibility of such a merger over the years. Cohen had been one of the strongest proponents of bringing together the two fields. He believed that the preventive orientation of public health, especially the use of surveillance and epidemiological analysis, could strengthen the delivery of mental health services; conversely, the neighborhoods with the highest rates of poverty-related health problems, such as tuberculosis, infant mortality, and asthma, were also those most at risk for mental disorders and could benefit from enhanced mental health services.[8]

The mayor's appointment of a health commissioner who lacked a traditional public health background raised some eyebrows, especially since concern about infectious diseases was running high. But Cohen also had many supporters in the city's health care establishment, who praised his administrative abilities and his years of experience as a prominent practitioner and advocate for community mental health services. During the 1980s, he had served as the director of psychiatry at Gouverneur Hospital, where he had done pioneering work on mental health services for the homeless.[9]

Voters would eventually approve the merger of the two departments in November 2001. Before that, however, Cohen presided over two of the most challenging episodes in the Health Department's history: the unexpected outbreak of a disease that had never been seen in New York City, and the unprecedented trauma of the September 11, 2001, terrorist attacks. Cohen would be a frequent presence at press conferences, often flanking the mayor and officials from law enforcement and emergency management. The department's communicable disease and communications staffs would be placed on the firing line as well as they sought to investigate threats and to simultaneously warn and reassure a confused and anxious public.

Disease Without Borders

Neal Cohen briefed Mayor Giuliani on the mysterious outbreak in Queens as the department's communicable disease and communications staff were waiting to hear whether the CDC would confirm a mosquito-borne illness in the last week of summer in 1999. The results finally came back from the CDC's arbovirus lab in Fort Collins, Colorado, at 2:00 PM on the Friday before Labor Day weekend. Epidemiologist Annie Fine took the call from the lab and then ran through the halls of 125 Worth Street—like Paul Revere, her colleagues recalled—shouting, "It's positive!" The lab had identified the illnesses in Queens as St. Louis encephalitis, an arbovirus closely related to yellow fever. Mild cases of the disease looked like the flu; only rarely did it progress to severe symptoms requiring hospitalization. The United States typically recorded several dozen cases of St. Louis encephalitis each year, mostly in the South and the Midwest, but the virus had never been seen in New York City.

That evening, at a hurriedly assembled press conference in Queens next to Powell's Cove, a marshy area on Long Island Sound, Giuliani and Cohen stepped before the cameras to announce that an outbreak of mosquito-borne encephalitis was occurring and that the city would begin pesticide spraying. The mayor asked for residents' cooperation with the effort; Cohen reassured people that the probability of becoming infected with the disease was "very, very low" and urged people who were bitten by a mosquito not to panic. Within a few hours, helicopters from the Office of Emergency Management began spraying the chemical malathion over Whitestone and adjacent areas in Queens. Aerial and ground spraying continued over the Labor Day weekend in northern Queens and in Bronx neighborhoods just across the narrow stretch of Long Island Sound that separated the two boroughs.

Correctly anticipating that the announcement of the outbreak and the spraying would spark a wave of public concern, the department set up a hotline with seventy-five people taking calls around the clock, as well as a separate line staffed by doctors to answer queries from health care providers. Staff members began going door to door to talk about mosquito control and distributed brochures in eight languages. For the first time in its history, the department was responsible for a daily press briefing to satisfy reporters' constant demands for updates on the situation. The appearance in the city of a new, insect-borne disease—even one that was so far responsible for only two fatalities—was sensational news.

The following Wednesday, around thirty senior Health Department staff members and officials from the Office of Emergency Management gathered for a conference call with the CDC. A large batch of specimens had come back from the Fort Collins laboratory, and the news was not good: suspected cases in the Bronx, Brooklyn, and Manhattan were positive. A pall fell over the room as it became clear that the epidemic was wider than had been feared and that spraying would have to be done not just in pockets but throughout the city. As soon as they grasped the significance of the news, everyone in the 125 Worth Street conference room stood up with a shared sense of urgency and filed out, even as their CDC colleagues continued talking on the other end of the speaker phone. They hurried into Marcelle Layton's office to locate the new cases on the large map of the city that was posted on the wall, dotted with colored pins representing confirmed and possible cases. Two days later, Giuliani announced that spraying would expand to all five boroughs (see figure 7.1).

In Manhattan, where tall buildings made helicopter flight risky, spraying was done mostly by trucks. Each night in selected neighborhoods, trucks made the rounds in the evening and early morning hours accompanied by two police cars broadcasting a warning over loudspeakers to stay out of the way. In other boroughs, spraying was mostly done by air. Residents were warned to close their windows and turn off air conditioners when the spraying was scheduled and not to leave children's toys outside.

From the perspective of the Health Department, the citywide spraying was a responsible course of action. There was no vaccine or treatment for St. Louis encephalitis, and the epidemic curve was still on its way up, with no peak in sight. The autumn was turning out to be warm and wet, ideal for mosquito breeding and ongoing disease transmission. Although direct contact with malathion could cause minor irritation of the skin and eyes, most scientists considered it very safe for mass spraying, and entomologists at both the CDC and the state health department had recommended it for use in New York City. Nevertheless, pesticides had acquired a bad name in the post–*Silent Spring* era, and the expanded spraying enflamed the concerns that callers were already expressing on the Health Department's hotline.

To be sure, many residents supported the city's actions. Some claimed angrily that the city had been delinquent in its mosquito control efforts and felt that the spraying was long overdue. Bronx borough president Fernando Ferrer took the opportunity to lambaste his longtime rival Giuliani for having devoted insufficient city resources to reducing the mosquito population. For many other New Yorkers, however, the prospect of being exposed to an airborne chemical was far more alarming than the risk of contracting encephalitis from a mosquito. The department's hotline was receiving thousands of calls per day, and the majority were from people expressing concern about the effects of the pesticide, not about the virus. People were especially alarmed about the risks to children, pets, and vegetable gardens. At community meetings in neighborhoods where spraying was scheduled, angry residents shouted down Health Department staff who were attempting to explain the city's response and allay fears; at one meeting in Queens, two department epidemiologists were called Nazis. In some neighborhoods, residents attempted to block the spraying trucks on their rounds. The Queens Green Party organized protests. "The spraying of New York City with pesticides," said a spokesperson for the group, "is much worse than the problem it is intended to cure."[10]

Ideally, the areas subject to spraying would have been determined by the location of infected mosquitoes. The department had just begun mosquito surveillance and lacked extensive data, however, so the city's response had to be guided by where the human cases were being found. This imperative added pressure to what would have been an intense outbreak investigation under the best of circumstances. Health Department staff called hospitals daily and heard about hundreds of potential

Figure 7.1   Press Conference on Mosquito Spraying

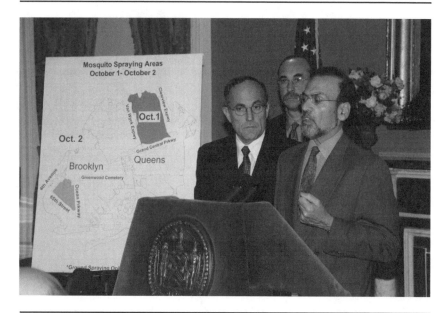

Source: Courtesy New York City Municipal Archives.
Note: Health Commissioner Neal Cohen (right), flanked by Mayor Rudy Giuliani and Jerome Hauer, director of the Office of Emergency Management, describes the areas designated for mosquito spraying in the fall of 1999.

cases. (The symptoms of St. Louis encephalitis mimicked those of the flu, and most of these cases would turn out to be unrelated to the outbreak.) The epidemiologists needed to obtain samples from suspected cases rapidly so that the mosquito control efforts could be better targeted. They aimed to collect samples within a day of receiving a case report; because the department's own laboratory did not have the capacity to test for St. Louis encephalitis, fluids had to be shipped using commercial express mail services to the state laboratory in Albany and the CDC's arbovirus lab in Colorado. More than two thousand specimens would ultimately be collected and shipped that fall.

As more potential cases were discovered, puzzling aspects of the epidemic nagged at Layton and her colleagues. Some cases that seemed to show all the telltale symptoms were coming back negative on lab tests. In contrast to the CDC's results, the state laboratory was reporting that it could not find St. Louis encephalitis in the samples of cerebrospinal fluid it was receiving. On the hotline, meanwhile, callers kept mentioning dead birds.

Unknown to the Health Department, large numbers of birds, especially crows, had begun to die in the area several weeks earlier. Veterinary scientists with the state Department of Environmental Conservation had examined hundreds of crows to try to determine the cause of the mysterious deaths, but their work had been independent of the investigation of the cases of human encephalitis. Over the Labor Day weekend, three flamingos, a pheasant, a cormorant, and a bald eagle died at the Bronx Zoo. Tracey McNamara, a veterinary pathologist at the zoo, conducted autopsies on the birds and found signs of encephalitis. Struck by the coincidence of the deaths with the outbreak of St. Louis encephalitis, she reported her concerns to the CDC. The outbreaks could not be related, McNamara was told: St. Louis encephalitis did not kill birds.

McNamara pursued the lead, sending samples to other laboratories and continuing to press CDC officials to consider the possibility that they had misidentified the viral culprit. Eventually, the CDC lab conceded that it had erred in attributing the outbreak to St. Louis encephalitis. On Friday, September 24, three weeks after the first news conference, the CDC notified the Health Department that the Fort Collins lab had isolated West Nile virus, a close relative of St. Louis encephalitis that was often cross-reactive on laboratory tests. West Nile virus was endemic in Africa; in recent years outbreaks had occurred in eastern Europe, Russia, and the Middle East. But it had never been seen in the Western Hemisphere before.

The Health Department was quick to emphasize that the change in diagnosis did not affect the city's response: control measures were the same for both viruses. The new information did have important ramifications, however. The CDC's misidentification of the virus cost public health officials credibility at a time when many residents were doubting the wisdom of pesticide spraying. The epidemiological picture worsened. Many suspected cases that had tested negative for St. Louis encephalitis had to be retested for West Nile, and many came back positive. The size of the outbreak roughly doubled, from around fifteen confirmed cases to around thirty, with a much larger number of potential cases; new cases turned up north and east of the city in Westchester and Nassau Counties. Members of the communicable disease staff already struggling to keep up with the investigation of the human cases had to begin collecting dead birds and sending tissue samples for laboratory testing.

The identification of West Nile virus also required additional consultations with law enforcement. Marcelle Layton had met with the FBI earlier in the month about the possibility that the outbreak of St. Louis encephalitis was bioterrorism. The revelation that the outbreak was due to an even more unusual pathogen raised new fears that it had been deliberately introduced. The concerns increased when it came to light that in the 1980s the Centers for Disease Control had provided samples of West

Nile virus to researchers in Iraq who were later found to be developing a bioweapons program. The possibility that the outbreak was the work of terrorists was eventually discounted; the most likely scenario, CDC officials concluded, was that an infected mosquito or an infected person had brought the virus to the United States on an airplane. This explanation was hardly less troubling, however, because of its implications for the spread to the United States of diseases not previously seen here.

Ultimately, sixty-two people were diagnosed with West Nile virus in four states during the 1999 outbreak; fifty-nine of these patients required hospitalization, and seven died. New York City accounted for forty-five of the cases and five of the fatalities. It was estimated that around 1,900 people were exposed to the virus that fall. Most cases of the disease were asymptomatic, but about one-fifth of those infected developed fever, headache, and fatigue. Fewer than 1 percent of those infected progressed to the encephalitis that had put Deborah Asnis's patients in the hospital. During the two months in which the department's hotline operated, it received more than 150,000 calls. The spraying continued through early October, and no new cases were found to have occurred after late September.

Planning for a potential return of West Nile virus was a major focus throughout the spring of 2000. The department's communications team prepared educational materials and planned meetings with community groups to try to preempt a reemergence of controversy should pesticide spraying once again prove necessary. Speakers from the department gave more than two hundred presentations in settings such as community centers, senior centers, and schools. In April, the Board of Health passed a resolution giving the department new powers to abate mosquito breeding sites. Inspectors were authorized to gain access to private property to search for water accumulations, conduct tests for larvae, apply larvicide, or order the source of the accumulation removed.[11]

After two dead crows were discovered on Staten Island in July 2000, the city began spraying again. The next day, several individuals and environmental groups operating under the umbrella of the No Spray Coalition asked a judge to issue an emergency injunction to stop the spraying. The judge denied the motion, and the coalition sued the city, arguing that the use of pesticides violated federal and state environmental laws. That fall, a U.S. district court dismissed all their claims except one: that the city's actions violated the federal Clean Water Act. The dispute ultimately hinged on the question of whether the helicopter spraying had discharged pesticides directly into waterways, which would have violated the act; the city's lawyers insisted that it had not.[12] The No Spray Coalition would continue its battle against the city's use of pesticides for several more years, ultimately dropping the suit in 2007.[13] Ironically, in Nassau County, immediately east of the city on Long Island, two wrongful death lawsuits were filed against the county, claiming that the county's failure to spray pesticides had resulted in deaths from West Nile virus.[14]

Subsequent outbreaks of West Nile virus were more widespread but less deadly. In 2000 cases were detected in twelve states and the District of Columbia, but there were fewer patients with severe illness and fewer fatalities.[15] New York City recorded twenty-one cases and two deaths from the disease. The outbreak was centered on Staten Island, which had almost three-quarters of the cases. Although West Nile virus did not turn out to be the calamity that many had feared, its appearance in New York City was, in its own way, as unsettling to public health professionals as the emergence of AIDS had been almost two decades earlier. West Nile was a jarring reminder that infectious diseases, though no longer the leading causes of death, could still pose a grave threat. As microbes increasingly crossed international boundaries, the world was becoming smaller and more dangerous.

Terror and Its Aftermath

The airplane attacks on the twin towers of the World Trade Center on September 11, 2001, and the spread of anthrax spores through the U.S. mail shortly afterward had profound and lasting effects on the physical and mental health of many New Yorkers. For the Health Department, the terrorist acts presented challenges that were logistical, scientific, and political. These challenges came on the day of the attacks as department employees swung into action amid destruction and chaos; in the following weeks as they sought to carry out essential functions in an environment of fear and uncertainty; and in the subsequent months and years as they adopted new policies and procedures to deal with future terrorist threats.

Health Department employees were arriving for work at 125 Worth Street, just nine blocks from the towers, when the first hijacked airliner hit the north tower at 8:46 AM. The second plane hit the south tower seventeen minutes later. Drawing on procedures honed during tabletop exercises and preparation drills over the prior years, they immediately assembled in the third-floor conference room and activated emergency committees devoted to issues such as surveillance, environmental health, laboratory services, and information systems.[16] Commissioner Neal Cohen headed to the Office of Emergency Management's command bunker at Seven World Trade Center, across the street from the towers, where top city officials were to gather in the event of crisis. The building was clearly unsafe (it would collapse several hours later), so

Mayor Giuliani and an entourage of officials trekked uptown in search of a base of operation, eventually setting up temporary shop at a fire station on Houston Street a mile north.[17]

By 10:30 AM, both towers had collapsed and toxic clouds of smoke, dust, and chemicals had settled over lower Manhattan. As shell-shocked, ash-covered workers and residents of downtown neighborhoods streamed north, Health Department staff quickly transformed their building lobby into an informal triage center. Although there were no clinical facilities available there, staff with medical training assisted people in treating dust inhalation, eye irritation, and scrapes and abrasions.[18]

That afternoon, a surreal scene unfolded in Thomas Paine Park across from 125 Worth Street. Trucks pulled up and workers began unloading hundreds of wooden planks, which they started hammering together into gurneys that would carry the wounded and the dead from the towers. Some of the people heading out of lower Manhattan stopped at the park, picked up hammers and nails, and began helping with the grim task. The sound of hammering provided an eerie soundtrack to the work at the Health Department that day.[19] The gurneys would prove unnecessary, however. When Health Department employees contacted emergency rooms around the city to assess their capacity to treat the expected influx of wounded people, they learned that those coming in were suffering from only minor wounds. Most of those who escaped the disaster were uninjured; those who did not were buried in the rubble of the collapsed towers. Approximately 2,750 people died in the attacks; the exact number would remain disputed for years.

That night, hobbled by the lack of phones and computers—telecommunications and electricity had been knocked out in most of lower Manhattan—and uncertain whether further attacks might be coming, Health Department employees began leaving 125 Worth Street. They relocated to the building that housed the department's Bureau of Laboratories, two and a half miles north on First Avenue, which would serve as their headquarters until November. One of the last to leave was Marcelle Layton. Long after midnight, several exhausted employees gathered in her office to discuss what they believed would be a danger in the coming weeks: acts of bioterrorism.[20] Thousands of doses of antibiotics from the National Pharmaceutical Stockpile had already been flown into New York to be ready for mass distribution in case an infectious agent had been released in the plane crashes.[21]

In the days after the attack, the most immediate concerns were related to environmental hazards at the sixteen-acre site of the collapsed towers and the surrounding neighborhoods.[22] As thousands of firefighters, police officers, and rescue workers began sifting through the rubble looking for survivors and clearing away more than a million tons of debris, the Health Department was responsible for procuring and distributing respirators at the site. More than two hundred restaurants and groceries in lower Manhattan had been abandoned by their owners and managers when they fled after the attack, leaving behind tons of perishable food that could have led to massive rodent infestations. The department dispatched teams of inspectors to collect and dispose of decaying food, a task that would take almost three weeks. Inspectors from the department also examined the area around the site with Geiger counters to determine if radiation had been released from the airplanes during the crash or from destroyed equipment in medical or dental offices. Fires smoldered at the site for months after the collapse of the towers, and firefighters pumped millions of gallons of water onto them. With the threat of West Nile virus on everyone's mind, the department applied larvicide to any standing water it found on the site.[23]

The most contentious environmental concern in the months after the attacks was the air quality in lower Manhattan. The collapse of the towers created a miasma of pulverized concrete, wallboard, glass, paper, fiberglass, silica, and asbestos.[24] Such materials could irritate airways and exacerbate respiratory conditions such as asthma, but the effects of long-term exposure were unclear. The Health Department followed the lead of the Environmental Protection Agency, which had primary responsibility for taking air quality measurements and issuing safety guidelines. Days after the collapse, the EPA issued a statement that the air in lower Manhattan was safe to breathe; taking their cue from federal officials, the Health Department issued a statement that the risk of long-term health effects from the fallout was "extremely low."[25]

But as the 20,000 people who lived in lower Manhattan gradually moved back into the apartments they had left, they questioned, with increasing bitterness, the assurances that government officials were giving. The Health Department was widely ridiculed when it advised, based on EPA recommendations, that residents clean the dust from the surfaces in their apartments by wiping them down with a damp cloth or mop and vacuuming with high-efficiency particulate air filters. These methods may have been appropriate, but to people who had recently witnessed a horrific disaster that they were convinced had unleashed potentially deadly toxins, the advice seemed absurdly inadequate.[26] A central point of contention became the EPA's measurements of toxic chemicals that were thought to have been released during the building collapse, including dioxins, benzene, lead, and chromium. The official pronouncements contradicted people's experience. As proof of the danger, residents of the affected neighborhoods offered their own symptoms, including sore throats, coughs, wheezes, and irritated eyes.[27]

In the weeks after the attack, the department continued to track emergency room visits and the adequacy of hospital staffing and equipment and sent out fax and email alerts to health care providers about potential health problems related to the attack, such as psychological trauma and asbestos exposure.[28] Within days, the CDC had sent some fifty epidemiologists who were stationed in the emergency rooms of fifteen hospitals in the five boroughs to monitor the appearance of illnesses that might be the result of bioterrorism.[29] Most experts believed that the intense heat from the burning jet fuel would have incinerated any potential biological agents on the planes that crashed. Nevertheless, the department was in constant contact with local hospitals, academic medical centers, and private physicians, urging them to be on the lookout for unusual clusters of illness.[30]

On October 1, Joel Ackelsberg, a member of the department's communicable disease staff, got a call from a physician about a thirty-eight-year-old woman with an inch-long lesion on her chest and swollen lymph nodes in her neck. The woman, Erin O'Connor, worked as an assistant to NBC news anchor Tom Brokaw at the network's offices in Rockefeller Center in midtown Manhattan. The doctor initially thought that the lesion was the result of a spider bite, but O'Connor told him that two weeks earlier she had opened a threatening letter addressed to Brokaw that contained two suspicious powders. Ackelsberg got the letter from the FBI and had it tested along with a skin sample in the Health Department's laboratory. Both tested negative for anthrax. Since the case seemed to be a false alarm—there had been numerous hoaxes in the prior weeks—no one at the Health Department notified the mayor's office.[31]

Anthrax, caused by a bacillus found in livestock and soil, was one of the diseases that federal officials had been most concerned about when they began preparing for bioterrorism in the 1990s. The cutaneous form of the illness, caused by skin contact with anthrax, took the form of a lesion that developed into a black ulcerated sore. It was treatable with antibiotics and rarely lethal. Much more fearsome was the disease's inhaled form, which attacked the lungs and spread unchecked through internal organs. After a period of rapidly worsening flu-like symptoms, inhalation anthrax was almost universally fatal.

When a man in Boca Raton, Florida, was diagnosed with inhalation anthrax in early October, federal health officials at first sought to assure the country that the case was an isolated incident unrelated to terrorism. Within a few days, however, one of the man's coworkers at American Media, the company that published the tabloid newspapers the *National Enquirer* and *The Sun*, was also diagnosed with the disease, and the FBI took over the investigation and sealed the company's offices.[32] On October 9, the Health Department sent out a special fax alert to the city's 65,000 physicians reminding them to watch for "non-specific flu-like symptoms" that might indicate a case of anthrax.[33] That day, Erin O'Connor went to another doctor about her symptoms, which had worsened, and the doctor notified the Health Department. This time a tissue sample and the letter were sent to the CDC for testing.

At 3:00 AM on October 12, CDC director Jeffrey Koplan phoned Marcelle Layton to tell her that the letter had tested negative for anthrax but the tissue sample was positive. (Eventually, a second threatening letter that O'Connor had handled was found in a file at NBC; it tested positive for anthrax.) Layton immediately called Neal Cohen, who met with Mayor Giuliani a few hours later and had another call with Koplan.[34] That morning, police cordoned off Rockefeller Center, and Cohen joined Giuliani at a press conference announcing the case. The department's communicable disease staff began interviewing hundreds of employees at the center, doing nasal swab testing for exposure to anthrax and distributing a fourteen-day course of the antibiotic Cipro as prophylactic. Over the next four days, more than 1,300 people were interviewed, tested, and given antibiotics.[35]

In quick succession over the next week, three more cases of cutaneous anthrax were diagnosed in the city, in employees of CBS and the *New York Post* and in the infant son of a producer at ABC; all were thought to have been infected by contaminated letters. Working with investigators from the CDC, the FBI, and the New York Police Department, epidemiologists interviewed employees at the sites, conducted nasal swab testing, and dispensed prophylactic antibiotics to another 1,300 people. Another site was set up at a U.S. Postal Service processing and distribution center on the west side of Manhattan after mail-sorting machines there were found to be contaminated with anthrax spores.[36]

The anthrax scare broadened as the month went on. Congressional offices were shut down after anthrax-tainted letters were sent to the office of Senator Tom Daschle, and cases of inhalation anthrax were diagnosed in workers at postal facilities in New Jersey and Washington, D.C. In spite of the bioterrorism preparedness exercises that had been conducted in the prior years at the federal level and in New York City, the investigation of the attacks did not go as smoothly or as effectively as might have been hoped. A New York police detective improperly handled one of the NBC letters and was exposed to anthrax. It was revealed that the FBI had failed to notify Giuliani's office about the letter sent to Tom Brokaw, which they had learned about on September 25.[37] Tensions flared between the CDC and the FBI, with health officials accusing law enforcement of not sharing critical information, especially the fact that the anthrax sent to Daschle's office was far more finely cut—and therefore more likely to disperse through the air and be inhaled—than the material that had been sent to the New York media companies. Union leaders representing postal workers charged that the FBI's failure to share what they knew led to the preventable deaths of two employees at a mail facility in Washington, D.C.[38]

Meanwhile, anxious New Yorkers began to see suspicious white powders everywhere they looked: on subway platforms, in apartment lobbies, in stores, on sidewalks. Doctors reported that panicked residents were flooding into emergency rooms asking to be tested for anthrax or to be given Cipro because they had come in contact with some kind of powder they believed to be deadly spores.[39] The episode once again highlighted the difficulties of public communication in an environment of fear and uncertainty.[40] Giuliani was widely praised for his daily press conferences, which were matter-of-fact and reassuring without being patronizing. His task was complex: getting people to be alert but not panicked, worried but not too worried; conveying the gravity of the situation and the need for ongoing vigilance, while also making clear that for most New Yorkers the likelihood of coming in contact with anthrax was remote. In late October, Giuliani and Cohen sought to redirect health concerns when they encouraged people to get a flu shot—not only because the flu posed a greater risk than anthrax to far more people, but because reducing cases of the flu would decrease the prevalence of flu-like symptoms that so many people were mistaking for anthrax. Cohen said in a press conference, "If we can just transfer some of the anxiety that people feel unnecessarily about their possible exposure to anthrax or bioterrorism and do something very health preventive and positive, such as getting a flu shot, we'll see a lot of value in New York City."[41]

Such statements, however, could not tamp down the anxiety unleashed by the anthrax attacks. The demand for testing of suspicious powders quickly swamped the Health Department's laboratory capabilities. Within the department's Public Health Laboratory was a four-hundred-square-foot bioterrorism lab that, before October 2001, had two employees who processed one or two samples per month. On the day after the announcement of the NBC case, the lab received thirty-four samples that were deemed high priority for immediate testing; over the next two months, some 3,200 specimens arrived. The lab became contaminated with anthrax spores, and three laboratory technicians whose protective gear was not properly in place were exposed to anthrax and had to take prophylactic antibiotics (none went on to develop the disease).[42] As the samples flowed in, the lab prioritized them according to the likelihood of the threat based on the circumstances. Several politically connected people called Neal Cohen on behalf of a friend or relative asking that a certain specimen be given priority testing.[43]

The CDC quickly offered to help the department conduct a massive upgrade. The building was reconfigured to accommodate additional staff, equipment, and security. Within a few days, the facility was converted into a twenty-four-hour, seven-day operation with seventy-five employees, with Health Department workers being joined by additional staff from the CDC and the Department of Defense.[44]

Ultimately, seven cases of cutaneous anthrax would be diagnosed in the city, all of them related to contact with powder sent through the mail.[45] The last case to be diagnosed was the city's sole case of inhalation anthrax. The case seemed inexplicable and troubling. Kathy Nguyen was a sixty-one-year-old stockroom clerk at the New York Eye, Ear, and Throat Hospital on the Upper East Side. She went to an emergency room on October 28 with fever, muscle aches, and severe shortness of breath and tested positive for anthrax. She died three days later.[46] The hospital where she worked was immediately shut down, and the Health Department's epidemiologists once again joined the CDC and law enforcement in investigating.

A Vietnamese immigrant who had been in the United States for two decades, Nguyen lived a solitary life in the Bronx, had no connection to the media companies that had been targeted, and did not handle mail in her job; there was no evidence that she had been involved in terrorist activity. Investigators searched her apartment, reviewed her phone and bank records, and interviewed her neighbors, coworkers, acquaintances, and employees at businesses she patronized. Using data stored on her Metrocard transit pass, they retraced her subway journeys and tested every station she had passed through for anthrax. How Nguyen contracted the disease was never determined; the most likely explanation, investigators concluded, was that she had come in contact with a piece of mail that had been cross-contaminated in one of the postal facilities through which the anthrax-tainted letters had passed.[47]

As it was dealing with the immediate crises of environmental contamination and acts of bioterrorism, the department was also laying the foundation for addressing the longer-term damage to New Yorkers' physical and mental health from the traumatic events of that fall.

The department partnered with the state Office of Mental Health on Project Liberty, an initiative funded by the Federal Emergency Management Agency to address the mental health problems related to the World Trade Center attacks. The program offered telephone support and individual and group counseling sessions. In November 2001, the Health Department undertook a media campaign to promote use of the counseling services with the slogan "New York Needs Us Strong." The services were promoted through radio and television spots and subway posters; more than a million copies of a brochure were distributed in English, Spanish, and Chinese. Within the first six months of the program, more than 90,000 people had received counseling; the program operated through the end of 2003 and provided services to more than one million New Yorkers. Calls to the hotline spiked sharply around the first anniversary of the attacks.[48]

In 2002, in partnership with the federal Agency for Toxic Substances and Disease Registry, the department created a database to track the health status of people who had been affected by the disaster. Four categories of people were identified for inclusion: people who were south of Chambers Street on September 11, residents below Canal Street, workers who had been involved in the rescue and recovery at the site, and the students and staff of schools south of Canal Street. More than 71,000 people enrolled in the registry and completed thirty-minute interviews between September 2003 and November 2004.[49] Data from the World Trade Center Health Registry would confirm that the survivors who were most directly affected by the attacks suffered a range of persistent health problems, especially respiratory symptoms, such as shortness of breath, wheezing, and sinus irritation, and post-traumatic stress disorder. Of participants in the registry who completed a follow-up survey in 2006 or 2007, 10 percent reported being diagnosed with asthma since enrolling in the registry, with the highest risk being among workers involved in the rescue and recovery at ground zero.[50]

Over the next five years, the department also undertook several initiatives to prevent and respond to bioterrorist attacks. It spent $16 million to upgrade the Public Health Laboratory to biosafety level 3 (the second-highest level), enabling it to test for a wide range of highly dangerous pathogens that could be used as weapons. It began a joint inspection program with the New York Police Department to ensure that the radioactive material held at hospitals and medical research facilities was secured, and it trained medical staff on using radiation monitors.[51] It signed a joint agreement with the Police Department and the FBI establishing a protocol for investigating suspected attacks with biological weapons.[52] The Board of Health also amended the health code to give the department broadened powers to isolate and quarantine people suspected of having a contagious disease that might be linked to bioterrorism.[53] The amendment attracted little notice when it was passed in the spring of 2003. In light of the alarms that community groups and advocates had raised a decade earlier when the department had crafted new regulations for the detention of people with tuberculosis, the lack of controversy surrounding the expanded authority was a striking indication of how much the political climate had changed in the aftermath of terror.

These initiatives were part of a broader national effort to strengthen state and local health departments. The events in the fall of 2001 highlighted both the importance and the inadequacy of the nation's public health infrastructure, especially in the areas of epidemiologic surveillance and laboratory analysis. At the annual meeting of the American Public Health Association in Atlanta two months after the September 11 attacks, U.S. Secretary of Health and Human Services Tommy Thompson told the crowd, "We must take this opportunity to do everything we can to strengthen the public health system."[54] Many public health professionals hoped that their critical role in keeping the country safe would bring new resources to a field that politicians, policymakers, and the public had long taken for granted.

Federal funding to help public health agencies prepare for bioterrorism increased from $67 million in 2001 to around $1 billion in 2002.[55] Many observers questioned, however, whether the sudden infusion of money into state and local health departments was an unalloyed benefit. Public health professionals worried that once the urgency surrounding the issue faded, funds would dry up and health departments would be left scrambling to sustain programs they had painstakingly built.[56] Others feared that while energy and resources were being devoted to preparing for dire yet remote contingencies like chemical attacks, the actual causes of sickness and death would be neglected.[57] Prominent figures on the left saw bioterrorism preparedness as an attempt to co-opt public health into the agenda of the Bush administration. The Public Health Association of New York City warned in the summer of 2002 that "in a militarized political environment, we could find the anti-terrorism tail wagging the public health dog. It would be an abrogation of responsibility to permit a narrow focus on potential bioterrorism to sidetrack the city from dealing with its ongoing day-to-day health needs."[58]

For many in the field, an object lesson in the misdirection of public health energies was the federal government's hapless and ill-advised attempt to vaccinate 10 million health care workers against smallpox in the winter and spring of 2003. The plan was undertaken in spite of the fact that government officials admitted that they had no knowledge that a smallpox attack was imminent and that the vaccine could cause severe adverse reactions, including death in about one in every one million people who received it. The decision was thought to have been ordered by Vice President Dick Cheney against the advice of the CDC's immunization advisory panel, which had recommended vaccinating a much smaller pool of first responders.[59] In New York City, only a few hundred people out of a target population of thousands received the vaccine in spite of weeks of intensive effort by the Health Department's immunization staff and Mayor Michael Bloomberg's attempt to set an example by being vaccinated in a City Hall ceremony.[60]

Observers who worried that the Health Department would focus on bioterrorism at the expense of other, less sensational health issues would be surprised, however. It soon became evident that a new commissioner, appointed by incoming mayor Michael Bloomberg, would give top priority to a very different set of threats.

Chapter 8

A New Public Health Agenda

TWO MONTHS after the terrorist attacks, New Yorkers elected Michael Bloomberg, a businessman and philanthropist and the seventy-second-richest person in America, as their mayor. Bloomberg had made a fortune at the investment bank Salomon Brothers in the 1970s; in 1981 he had founded the financial news and information company that bore his name. His net worth was estimated at $4 billion. A lifelong Democrat, he switched parties to run for mayor because (as he publicly admitted) the Republican primary field was less crowded. He had never held elected office. But in the aftermath of September 11, voters seemed to want what Bloomberg offered: managerial competence, financial acumen, and pragmatism that transcended partisanship and ideology. Perhaps more to the point, he spent some $74 million of his own money on his campaign, roughly five times the amount spent by his Democratic opponent, public advocate Mark Green.[1]

Bloomberg's wealth and entrepreneurial background made him such an unusual occupant of the mayor's office that it was easy to overlook one of his most distinctive characteristics: a deep appreciation of public health. His immediate predecessors—like most politicians and policymakers—had equated health with medical care, and none had seen the Health Department as among the most valuable or consequential city agencies. The hospital sector, with its vastly greater budgets, problems, and political influence, had dominated the health arena from John Lindsay through Rudy Giuliani. Bloomberg was unique in his nuanced understanding of what the Health Department could accomplish.

Bloomberg credited his interest in public health to his friendship with Alfred Sommer, the indefatigable dean of the School of Public Health at Johns Hopkins University. Bloomberg had gotten to know Sommer while serving on the board of trustees of Hopkins, from which he had earned a degree in engineering. Sommer convinced Bloomberg of the value of preventing disease rather than curing it and the importance of interventions designed to protect entire populations. In 1995, Bloomberg made his first gift, of $20 million, to the School of Public Health at Hop-kins; in April 2001, after he had given another $15 million, the university renamed the school after him.[2]

After the election, Bloomberg turned to Sommer to lead the search for a new health commissioner. Thomas Frieden, who had won wide ac-claim among the city's health establishment for his leadership against drug-resistant tuberculosis, was an obvious choice. Frieden had served as the director of the Bureau of Tuberculosis Control until 1996, when he accepted an offer from the World Health Organization to support the fight against the disease in India. There, against even longer odds than he had faced in New York City, he marshaled a massive effort using di-rectly observed therapy and achieved similarly remarkable improve-ments in the detection and cure of patients.[3] He was in New Delhi when he got the call from Sommer asking if he wanted to come back to the city. A native New Yorker, Frieden felt a strong connection to the Health De-partment, where he had cut his professional teeth and scored his early career success. He had also been deeply affected by the attacks on the World Trade Center. He later told a reporter that the position of commis-sioner was "the only job in the United States that I would have come back for."[4]

Bloomberg quickly became known for giving his commissioners wide latitude to run their agencies as they saw fit. Over the next several years, Frieden—sometimes with the mayor's active support, always with his implicit backing—would pursue a series of innovative and controversial policies and programs. As local journalists covering the mayor and his health commissioner noted, Bloomberg and Frieden had so many affini-ties that their partnership in public health seemed almost foreordained.[5] Both were technocrats who exuded brusque efficiency. Both had a keen understanding of the political maneuvering that was often necessary to achieve health goals, yet could approach the process with an impatience that came across as arrogance. Most important, both were devoted to quantification. "In God we trust; everyone else, bring data" was one of the mayor's favorite quips. "Data analysis is religion for Mr. Bloomberg, and numbers are the lifeblood of his administration," according to an admiring profile in the *Times*. "They drive policy rather than just track progress."[6] This statement was equally true of Frieden, who had made enhanced surveillance the foundation of his fight against tuberculosis in the 1990s and had obsessively tracked statistics such as treatment com-pletion and cure rates. "If you can't measure it," he said, sounding as much like a CEO as an epidemiologist, "you can't manage it."[7]

Improving the measurement of New Yorkers' health status was one of Frieden's first priorities as commissioner. Until the 1970s, the depart-ment had conducted ongoing surveys of patterns of illness and use of health services in each borough. This surveillance was another victim of the fiscal crisis.[8] Several national surveys collected information about Americans' health risks and behaviors, but few of these had a large enough sample size to provide useful information about localities.[9] In May 2002, a few months after Frieden became commissioner, the department began conducting the first annual Community Health Survey, which asked almost ten thousand randomly selected New Yorkers in all five boroughs more than one hundred questions closely modeled on the CDC's annual health survey, the Behavioral Risk Factor Surveillance System. Questions covered a wide range of topics, including whether respondents saw a doctor, how many servings of fruits and vegetables they consumed each day, how much they exercised, whether they smoked cigarettes or drank alcohol, whether they were exposed to secondhand smoke at home or on the job, and whether they had undergone cancer screening.[10] Two years later, the department instituted a second survey, modeled on the National Health and Nutrition Examination Survey, that included a physical examination of a subset of the respondents.[11] The physical exam measured, among other things, blood pressure, cholesterol, and blood glucose levels.[12]

In addition to being a devotee of data, Frieden was a student of history, and he would self-consciously model his efforts on those of Hermann Biggs, the city's most visionary public health official at the turn of the twentieth century. Surveillance as a basis for action had been one of Biggs's trademarks; data collection, Biggs had asserted, was never conducted merely "to keep clerks or adding machines busy."[13] One hundred years later, the information gathered through community surveys would guide decisionmaking as Frieden pressed ahead with a new public health agenda.

"Epidemics of the Modern Era"

Frieden's determination to act against the conditions responsible for the greatest amount of sickness and death in the city pointed clearly to chronic diseases, or "the epidemics of the modern era," as he and several colleagues would label them in a journal article.[14] The fight against cancer, cardiovascular disease, obesity, and diabetes would be the department's signature issue during Bloomberg's first two terms. The new agenda would prove controversial because these diseases were often viewed, however erroneously, as the result of "lifestyle choices." Debates would center not only on what kinds of interventions were justified, but more fundamentally on whether chronic illnesses could properly be considered "epidemics" at all and therefore appropriate targets for government action.

Arguably the greatest failure of the American public health profession in the twentieth century was its decades-long inaction on the epidemiological transition from infectious to chronic diseases. Heart disease, cancer, and stroke had displaced contagions as the leading causes of death in the United States by the 1920s. The change had not gone unnoticed by public health and medical experts. "Measured in any terms," wrote a statistician with the U.S. Public Health Service in 1945, "the chronic diseases are a staggering national burden, a major cause of insecurity and a challenge to society for action."[15] Yet the public health rank and file, especially in state and local health departments, had failed to take up this challenge.

In spite of their economic and human costs, chronic diseases lacked the appearance of crises. They developed insidiously, sometimes over many decades, and their etiologies were complex and poorly understood. Some of their causes—especially cigarettes and diets high in fat and cholesterol—were sources of pleasure and symbols of affluence in modern American society.[16] "One is hard put to find profit or enjoyment from or a kind word to say for tuberculosis, typhoid, or streptococcal throat," CDC head William Foege had written in 1978. "However, overeating, overdrinking, smoking, and fast cars are frequently depicted as part of 'the good life.'"[17] Not incidentally, powerful commercial interests had a financial stake in perpetuating unhealthy lifestyles. "There is no pro-TB or pro-Ebola lobby," Frieden, echoing Foege, said in 2004, "but there is a pro-tobacco lobby."[18]

Even in New York City, so often the site of public health innovation, efforts to fight chronic illness in the post–World War II era had been limited and piecemeal. In the 1950s, the department established a Bureau of Nutrition to provide community-based education programs about healthy eating.[19] The bureau followed more than 1,500 participants in a fifteen-year study of the connection between dietary fat and cholesterol and heart disease. The study—called the "Anti-Coronary Club"—determined that changes in diet could lower cholesterol and the risk of heart disease.[20] In the 1960s, health commissioner George James had hired a coordinator for chronic illness, who was envisioned as having a broad mandate related to diet and lifestyle risks, although in practice the position was devoted mostly to smoking cessation clinics and education about the dangers of narcotic use.[21] Gordon Chase had promoted community-based blood pressure screening in the early 1970s, but this effort was not part of a coherent plan for reducing hypertension.

None of these efforts ever accounted for more than a tiny fraction of the department's budget and staff, and they did not survive the fiscal crisis of the 1970s. In the 1980s, commissioner David Sencer had candidly admitted to a colleague that the department devoted only "a pittance" to chronic disease because of budgetary constraints; his successor, Stephen Joseph, had told the mayor's office, "I continue to believe that this Department's lack of an organized program to address chronic diseases is a serious shortcoming in our City's public health efforts."[22] Categorical funding from the Centers for Disease Control was critical to the work of local health departments, and the CDC did not have a center devoted to chronic disease prevention until 1989.[23]

By the turn of the twenty-first century, chronic diseases were responsible for about 70 percent of deaths nationwide, yet major city and county health departments around the country spent less than 2 percent on average of their annual budgets to prevent or control these conditions; in New York City the amount was just 1 percent.[24] In a manifesto with the provocative title "Asleep at the Switch," published in the *American Journal of Public Health*, Frieden offered a harsh assessment of his profession. "Local health departments," he charged, "generally do a good job of monitoring and controlling conditions that killed people in the United States 100 years ago."[25]

In his first year as commissioner, Frieden established a new unit, the Division of Health Promotion and Disease Prevention, to house efforts against chronic diseases, primarily tobacco-related illness, cardiovascular disease, diabetes, and cancer. There were no staff members devoted to these conditions when Frieden began; within five years there would be around one hundred.[26] Funds devoted to chronic disease programs increased sharply, to about 10 percent of the department budget. The money came entirely from city taxes, since federal grant support for chronic disease prevention remained negligible. One of the unit's core philosophies was that traditional behavior-change strategies were, by themselves, insufficient to bring about significant and lasting improvements in the area of chronic illness. Mary Bassett, whom Frieden hired as the first head of the Division of Health Promotion and Disease Prevention, bluntly declared that relying on health education methods such as pamphlets, brochures, and mass media was a "failed strategy."[27] Instead, the department would seek to modify policies, laws, and regulations to alter the social and economic contexts that shaped people's choices.

Moving forcefully against smoking and high-fat diets would require Bloomberg and Frieden to confront the antipaternalistic ethos that pervaded American civic and political culture—the belief that coercive government action was acceptable only to prevent individuals from harming others. Compulsory health measures enacted for people's own good had sparked controversy in areas as diverse as fluoridation of water supplies and mandatory seat belt laws.[28] Many New Yorkers believed that whether they smoked and what they ate were freely made decisions in which city government had no claim to intervene. In a speech at a public health conference, Bloomberg acknowledged the sensitive nature of his administration's efforts. "Clearly, there are many matters of personal behavior and personal taste that we have no business regulating," the mayor said. "But just as clearly, there are also areas in which we have an obligation to act on what we know."[29]

Rebutting charges of paternalism would be a central task in Frieden's first and in many ways most successful campaign: the effort to decrease rates of smoking, the city's leading cause of preventable sickness and death. When Alfred Sommer contacted Frieden to ask if he was interested in serving as health commissioner, Frieden had said that he would take the job only if the mayor would agree to back strong antitobacco measures. When Sommer—who was making the call just weeks after the September 11 attacks—expressed surprise that Frieden did not identify bioterrorism rather than cigarettes as his top priority, Frieden replied that tobacco-related illnesses killed far more people.[30]

Frieden began his antismoking campaign as soon as he became commissioner in early 2002. By this time, the public health war on cigarettes was several decades old. None of the approaches that Frieden would eventually employ—taxation, regulation of public smoking, mass media campaigns, and cessation programs with counseling and nicotine replacement—was novel. All had been used in New York City and elsewhere at various times over the previous forty years. Frieden's innovation was to apply all these tactics far more aggressively than had been thought possible. He was able to do so because he had the support of a mayor who was willing to expend political capital to promote health and to take the heat these policies generated.

The War on Cigarettes

By the middle of the twentieth century, smoking was deeply engrained in the country's social fabric and the cigarette was a symbol of freedom, glamour, and modernity.[31] The incidence of lung cancer, coronary heart disease, emphysema, and numerous other illnesses inexorably increased in proportion to the rising prevalence of smoking, which peaked in the early 1960s at around 50 percent of men and 30 percent of women. Scientific evidence of the dangers of smoking had steadily accumulated by 1964, when the U.S. surgeon general released the landmark report *Smoking and Health*, which galvanized the modern-day antitobacco movement.[32]

The New York City Health Department moved swiftly to respond to the surgeon general's 1964 report. Within a few months, it began offering "smokers anonymous" clinics at which participants received individual and group counseling and the drug Lobeline to ease their withdrawal from nicotine.[33] The program expanded under the vigorous leadership of Donald Fredrickson, a thirty-two-year-old physician who had served in the Peace Corps and had run a clinic in Harlem before joining the department. Fredrickson was an outspoken advocate of far-reaching policy changes to reduce smoking. He called upon television networks to end the depiction of smoking by protagonists of popular shows, for example, arguing that the cultural climate needed to be altered so that smoking became unfashionable.[34] Such recommendations would become commonplace decades later.

In 1967, while still working at the Health Department, Fredrickson helped his friend John Banzhaf, a Washington, D.C.–based lawyer, found an organization they called Action on Smoking and Health (ASH), with Banzhaf as the executive director and Fredrickson as a trustee.[35] The group soon became an influential player on the national tobacco control scene; one of its first victories was a lawsuit that resulted in television networks' being required to devote time to antismoking advertisements.[36] Fredrickson's involvement with ASH was arguably as beneficial as his work with the Health Department, but his dual role of civil servant and activist proved untenable. After health commissioner Edward O'Rourke learned that Fredrickson's name was on ASH's letterhead, he consulted with the department's legal counsel, who opined that a business regulated by the department might receive a letter from ASH, see Fredrickson's name, and perceive the communication as unduly coercive. Fredrickson appealed to the city's Board of Ethics and was dismayed when he was told that "it would be in the best public interest if you did not serve as one of the three trustees" of ASH.[37] He left the department shortly thereafter to take a post with the Intersociety Commission for Heart Disease Resources, a nongovernmental organization.

After Fredrickson's departure, the department's antismoking program languished. In 1974 health commissioner Lowell Bellin undertook an ill-fated effort to amend the health code to require nonsmoking sections in restaurants. "We hope," Bellin said with characteristic bluntness, "to create a climate in which the smoker is uneasy."[38] But the measure was too radical for the times—smoking remained ubiquitous, and no other U.S. city had such a requirement—and the emerging fiscal crisis relegated the issue to the back burner. Two years later, Madison, Wisconsin, became the nation's first city to require restaurants to set aside seats for nonsmokers.[39]

Bellin's effort was an early strike in what was becoming the central battleground of tobacco control: the demarcation of public spaces where smoking would be allowed or prohibited. This fight advanced on the backs of two distinct but related claims about "sidestream smoke": that it was annoying and that it posed a health threat. Evidence for the latter claim remained fragmentary and disputed for many years, but opponents of smoking effectively elided the distinction between the unpleasant and the unhealthy.[40] Antismoking measures were often pushed forward by grassroots activists working with and through elected officials sympathetic to their cause. Organizations such as GASP (Group Against Smoking Pollution) and Americans for Nonsmokers' Rights (ANR), influenced by the mobilizations around environmental and civil rights issues and employing similar rhetoric, would prove more influential than state or local health officials.[41] This was true in New York City, which adopted two major pieces of anti-smoking legislation in the 1980s and 1990s. In neither case did the Health Department play a critical role in the passage of the law; instead, politicians and activists drove the antitobacco agenda.

New York's first major smoking control bill emerged from the City Council and the office of Mayor Ed Koch. Every year beginning in 1981, City Council member Stanley Michels of Manhattan, an ardent health advocate who had championed the cause of eliminating lead paint poisoning in children, introduced a bill to limit smoking in public, and every year it died in the council's health committee.[42] Mayor Koch was an ex-smoker and a longtime foe of cigarettes, but he consistently opposed Michels's bill, arguing that in the city's fragile postcrisis economic situation it was unwise to pass a measure that would burden businesses.[43] The furthest Koch was willing to go was asking restaurants to voluntarily set aside one-quarter of their seats for nonsmokers.[44]

A few months after beginning his third term in 1986, however, Koch reversed his position and sought significant restrictions on where smoking was allowed.[45] The city's economy had improved enough, Koch said, that concerns about hurting the business community were less acute. Moreover, increasing scientific evidence about the health risks of secondhand smoke had accumulated over the previous several years, and nationwide polls showed large increases in public support for restricting smoking in public.[46] Although health commissioner Stephen Joseph advised the mayor on the issue, the decision to make smoking curbs a priority was Koch's.[47]

The bill faced stiff opposition from the tobacco and restaurant industries and the city's chamber of commerce; African American and Latino City Council members objected that the measure would disproportionately affect the smokers and business owners in their districts.[48] After eighteen months of contentious political negotiations, the City Council overwhelmingly passed a bill that went beyond what Stanley Michels had proposed, though not as far as Koch had hoped. Smoking was banned in classrooms, public restrooms, banks, taxis, and on public transportation. Restaurants with more than fifty seats were required to set aside at least half of them for nonsmokers. (Koch had sought nonsmoking sections in all restaurants.) Large enclosed public spaces such as hotels, sports arenas, and convention halls had to designate nonsmoking areas.[49]

The city's next significant limits on tobacco came primarily through the work of community activists. The leading figure was Joseph Cherner, a millionaire bond trader who in 1987, at the age of twenty-four, quit his Wall Street job to begin a new career as an antismoking crusader. Unlike many activists, Cherner was not a reformed ex-smoker, nor had he lost a loved one to cancer; rather, he held an avowedly Manichaean view of the world in which tobacco companies were forces for evil. Over the next several years, Cherner worked on his own through a nonprofit organization he founded, Smokefree Educational Services, and as part of the Coalition for a Smoke-Free City, a network of more than one hundred health-related community organizations. Cherner and the coalition scored a series of minor victories, including the elimination of most cigarette vending machines from the city and a ban on smoking in schools and day care centers.[50]

In 1993, after the Environmental Protection Agency issued a widely cited report classifying secondhand smoke as a Class A carcinogen, Cherner and the coalition set their sights on extending the restrictions set forth in the 1988 law.[51] They found a sympathetic audience with City Council speaker Peter Vallone, a former pack-a-day smoker, who introduced a bill to eliminate smoking from almost all enclosed public spaces and many outdoor settings, including sports stadiums and playgrounds. The bill quickly attracted the support of a majority of council members, but it also provoked a torrent of opposition, led by tobacco giant Philip Morris. The company publicly threatened to move its headquarters out of New York City and end its donations to local arts and cultural organizations; it also leaned on its grantees to express their concerns to council members about the potential loss of funding.[52] The company took out full-page newspaper ads and set up front groups pretending to represent restaurant and hotel operators, which inundated council members with faxes, letters, phone calls, and personal visits. The Coalition for a Smoke-Free City had a well-planned counterattack, including mass mailings to restaurant owners and radio and print ads promoting the bill. The group also commissioned a Gallup poll to demonstrate public support for the measure.[53]

The public relations battles culminated in a series of contentious City Council hearings in 1994. Standing-room-only crowds packed three public hearings that fall, with attendees alternately cheering or booing the more than two hundred people who testified. On one side were those worried about the encroachment of "health fascists" on the right of smokers to enjoy a legal behavior; on the other were people who spoke with equal fervor about health problems they had suffered from having to breathe secondhand smoke.[54]

The bill went through several iterations on the way to passage, expanding at one point to include a ban on smoking in all restaurants. To gain the support of wavering council members, Vallone made concessions to reduce the economic hardships that the law might impose; restaurants with thirty-five or fewer seats were exempted from the ban, for example. The bill passed the City Council at the end of 1994. Mayor Giuliani, who did not take a prominent role in the debates but who in general supported smoking restrictions, signed it into law a few weeks later.[55]

The 1988 and 1995 antismoking laws were significant and hard-won victories for clean indoor air in New York City. Their effect on the city's smoking rates, however, was negligible. The prevalence of smoking barely budged during the 1990s, hovering at around 21 percent. Although this was slightly better than the national average of 23 percent, many metropolitan areas had lower rates.[56] When Frieden assumed the leadership of the Health Department with a central focus on tobacco, the goal of fewer smokers was clearly attainable, though bold measures would be needed.

Given the administration's devotion to data, it was not surprising that the first measure Bloomberg proposed was one whose efficacy was well supported by research. Econometric studies had found that cigarette buyers were price-sensitive and that increases in cost drove down consumption. The city's cigarette tax had not risen since 1976, when the tax per pack had gone from four to eight cents, even though the state sales tax had climbed steadily during those years, from fifteen cents to $1.50.[57] Although an increase seemed long overdue, the timing was politically risky. Bloomberg confronted a $4.76 billion deficit and a badly wounded local economy when he took office. Tax increases were a time-honored way of closing budget gaps, but the mayor resisted them, believing that they would put a damper on the city's recovery at a time of national recession and post-9/11 economic weakness. He was willing to make an exception for cigarette taxes, however, and he secured the state legislature's approval for a tax increase in time for the start of the new fiscal year July 1. This was a sign that Bloomberg's antismoking zeal was strong enough to trump his other principles; a more cynical interpretation offered by critics was that the New Yorkers most burdened by the tax were also the poorest and most lacking in political power.[58] Like most other health problems, smoking was disproportionately found among people of lower income and education levels.

Of all the smokers who stood to be affected by the tax increase, young people were the most influenced by cost, and when he announced the measure, Bloomberg underscored its anticipated effect on youth smoking. "The numbers," he said, "are clear: you raise cigarette taxes, the kids smoke less."[59] While the mayor's concern for the health of minors was no doubt genuine, his framing also reflected a strategic shift in rhetoric that had taken place. Activists had increasingly recast antitobacco policies as child protection measures, since most adult smokers began when they were teenagers.[60] Frieden put a fine point on it when he said of tobacco companies, "They're out for our children."[61] The protection of young people from harm could provide an ethical justification for strict antitobacco measures that might be seen as unacceptably paternalistic when applied to adults.[62]

The mayor faced criticism from bodega owners in poor neighborhoods, who warned that the tax would hurt their business by causing customers to turn to the Internet or out-of-state sales for their cigarettes. Other skeptics warned that the increase would lead to a black market. Such concerns were not new, nor were they unfounded: when the city had imposed its first sales tax on high-tar-and-nicotine cigarettes, in 1971, the measure sparked a wave of bootlegging as organized crime families brought in truckloads of contraband cigarettes from out of state.[63] In 2002 these fears were given a new spin for the post-9/11 era by a representative of the Libertarian Party, who warned that terrorists would finance their activities with cigarette smuggling.[64]

Bloomberg brushed aside such criticisms. Six months after taking office, he signed a bill at a City Hall ceremony raising the cigarette tax to $1.50 per pack. The increase gave New York City the country's highest municipal cigarette tax. Combined with the state tax, the price of a pack of cigarettes would be almost twice the national average. Although subsequent evaluations showed that the tax increase did reduce consumption, some smokers found ways to evade it. In the months after the tax took effect, a new figure, dubbed by residents "the $5 man," appeared on the streets of Harlem hawking bootleg cigarettes for well below the legal price of about $7.50 per pack. In at least one economically hard-hit neighborhood, buying cigarettes from a bootlegger, not quitting or cutting down on smoking, seemed to be the primary response to the tax hike.[65]

By the time Bloomberg signed the tax increase, Frieden had already mapped out the next phase of the city's antitobacco strategy: banning smoking in all workplaces, including restaurants and bars. To make the case for what was certain to be a controversial proposal, he assembled a briefing book for the mayor showcasing the health benefits and economic impacts in jurisdictions where comprehensive smoking bans had been implemented. Data from California, for example, where all restaurants and bars had been smoke-free since the mid-1990s, showed that the laws did not have negative economic effects but in fact were good for business. When Frieden presented the plan to Bloomberg, the mayor needed little encouragement. His top deputies, however, were dismayed, not just by the possibility that the measure would hurt the economy at a time when it remained fragile—the city had lost thousands of jobs in the period after September 11, with the hospitality sector being especially hard-hit—but by the political capital it would no doubt cost the mayor.[66] Bloomberg asked Frieden whether the law would save lives; his press secretary asked Frieden, "What were you thinking?"[67]

In preparation for the initiative, Frieden also consulted with Joseph Cherner, who shared the lessons learned during the battle over the 1994 legislation and offered advice on the political strategies that would be needed to get the measure through the City Council.[68] Cherner had laid some of the groundwork for additional restrictions during the 2001 campaign by gaining a commitment from several City Council and mayoral candidates to support comprehensive smoking bans. In preparation for moving forward, Frieden held a series of meetings with members of the City Council and representatives of community boards to allay their concerns and secure their support for the plan.[69]

In August 2002, just five weeks after signing the tax increase, Bloomberg announced that he was asking the City Council to extend the anti-smoking law to all 22,000 of the city's restaurants and bars.[70] The measure was promoted to the public with a simple and consistent message: secondhand smoke was a threat to the health of workers. This framing—like the argument that tax increases protected children—was both principled and politically advantageous. Claiming to protect vulnerable bystanders such as waiters and bartenders was a way to mitigate the charges of paternalism that had been leveled against the mayor and the Health Department since the antitobacco effort began. The department rolled out a series of radio and newspaper advertisements to drive home the message. "Bartenders who work an 8-hour shift in a smoky bar," said one of the print ads, "inhale the same amount of cancer-causing chemicals as if they'd smoked more than half a pack of cigarettes."[71] The proposal was nevertheless met with incredulity in some quarters. New Yorkers saw their city as the nation's capital of nightlife and cosmopolitanism, and many found the prospect of bars without cigarettes almost as far-fetched as the idea of bars without liquor.

City Council member Christine Quinn of Manhattan, chair of the council's health committee, introduced a bill a few days after Bloomberg's announcement. In spite of Frieden's efforts to reach out to council members, the measure faced an uncertain path to approval. Bloomberg took an unusually aggressive role in promoting the legislation, privately telling some council members that he would retaliate against them by backing their opponents in the next election if they voted against the bill.[72] City Council speaker Gifford Miller, who was thought to have mayoral aspirations, refrained from publicly backing the bill for weeks, using his support for smoking control as a bargaining chip to gain the mayor's cooperation on other issues. Meanwhile, some council members expressed resentment at what they perceived as Bloomberg's dismissive attitude toward the concerns that were being raised about the measure's potential economic impacts.[73] Restaurant and bar owners pressured council members, as did tobacco giant Philip Morris.

The City Council held more than twenty hours of public hearings at three sessions in October and November. As had been the case the last time the city sought to limit public smoking, the hearings were raucous. At the first event, a crowd of supporters and opponents—including three people dressed as grim reapers and a man outfitted in a giant cigarette costume holding a sign that said I ♥ SECONDHAND SMOKE—rallied in front of the council chambers before the start of the hearing. Inside, the testimony was repeatedly interrupted by shouts and heckling.[74] Opponents claimed that the law would harm workers more than help them because businesses would be forced to lay off staff. Owners of small bars in blue-collar neighborhoods were especially concerned about the threat to their livelihoods. In his testimony, Frieden drew on data from the Community Health Survey to argue that the measure would further social justice.[75] "African Americans, Latinos or Latinas, and those with low incomes are twice as likely to have to breathe second-hand smoke on the job," he said. "The fundamental principle of worker safety is that workers should not have to choose between their health and their jobs."[76]

As the debate raged on during the fall of 2002, the local media had a field day poking fun at Bloomberg as the city's nanny. Much of the coverage indicated that editors and reporters were unconvinced that the ban was truly about worker safety rather than Bloomberg's puritanical tendencies.[77] A full-page cartoon on the cover of the Post depicted the scowling mayor in front of the "Bloomberg Bar and Grill," in the window of which hung signs with the universal "no" slash over the words SMOKING and FUN. The headline: "Bar Humbug."[78]

Several compromises were negotiated, including an exemption for cigar bars already in business, owner-operated bars with no employees, and private membership clubs with no employees. Speaker Gifford Miller eventually came around, and the bill passed the council by a wide margin the week before Christmas 2002. The passage gave momentum to a long-running battle to enact a similar measure statewide: three months after the City Council enacted the Smoke-Free Air Act, New York governor George Pataki signed into law an amendment to the state's Clean Indoor Air Act, enacting new smoking restrictions in the entire state.[79]

Both the city and state laws drew a swift legal challenge from the group C.L.A.S.H. (Citizens Lobbying Against Smokers' Harassment), which was one of the most outspoken opponents of the mayor's public health agenda. C.L.A.S.H. predated Bloomberg's election, having formed in the summer of 2000 when New York State doubled its cigarette tax. The group was founded by Audrey Silk, a Brooklyn police officer who was Joseph Cherner's prosmoking doppelganger: Silk fought back against the steady and seemingly inexorable advance of smoking restrictions with all of the passion and determination, but none of the success, with which Cherner had advanced them in the 1990s. C.L.A.S.H. framed the battles over cigarette smoking as an issue of fundamental rights and freedoms. An intolerant majority was intent on denying the rights of smokers, the group argued, using exaggerated scientific claims about the dangers that smoke posed to others. According to the group's website, its mission was "to end the discrimination against smokers by exposing the anti-smoking lies."[80]

C.L.A.S.H.'s lawsuit sought to overturn both the city and the state laws, alleging that the restrictions on public smoking violated smokers' constitutional rights to freedom of association, assembly, speech, and equal protection. The group compared the diminishment of the freedom to smoke to the denial of the rights of disfavored minorities; smokers, they said, were being turned into "social lepers" and "second-class citizens." A federal district court judge rejected the group's claim that smokers as a class had qualities that merited the strict scrutiny of governmental actions affecting them.[81]

In spite of the controversy the smoking ban created, the law was largely well accepted once it went into effect, with New Yorkers favoring it by an almost two-to-one margin. Nor did the dire economic effects predicted by opponents come to pass: a department evaluation a year later showed that business in bars and restaurants was up almost 10 percent and the hospitality sector had added more than 10,000 jobs.[82]

Frieden's next two campaigns in the war on cigarettes sought to encourage smokers to quit using persuasive rather than coercive means. In the spring of 2003, the department launched a cessation campaign in collaboration with the state health department and Roswell Park Cancer Institute, a research center in Buffalo. Frieden secured from the pharmaceutical company Pfizer a donation of millions of dollars' worth of the firm's nicotine replacement patch kits, and the department launched a program to distribute the patches free to the first 35,000 callers to the state's stop-smoking hotline. Those reached by the program, a subsequent evaluation showed, were likely to be nonwhite, foreign-born, or poor.[83] When the program was repeated in 2005, more than 45,000 patch kits were distributed.[84]

The final element of the city's antismoking efforts was a public education campaign via television and print ads between January and October 2006. With a budget much higher than usual for a public health announcement, the ads ran in heavy rotation on broadcast networks and basic cable channels, including the Spanish-language cable networks Telemundo and Univision. The theme of the campaign was "Nothing Will Ever Be the Same"; it showcased the personal stories of several smokers whose lives were changed by the devastating effects of tobacco-related illnesses. One ad featured Ronaldo Martinez, a fifty-three-year-old Bronx resident who had had his larynx removed after years of smoking and who spoke in a synthesized voice from an artificial voice box. A subsequent evaluation suggested that the spot had reached its desired audience. Whereas the smoking rate overall had remained flat in 2005, it dipped significantly among men and Hispanics.[85]

The results of the department's four-pronged attack on tobacco between 2002 and 2006 were dramatic. During the 1990s, smoking prevalence in the city had remained stagnant, but from 2002 to 2003, during which time the tax increase and the smoking ban were implemented, it dropped by about 11 percent, representing some 140,000 fewer smokers. It dipped further, to 18.4 percent, in 2004, and in 2006 it fell to 17.5 percent. Over four years, the percentage of smokers in the city decreased by almost 20 percent.[86] The declines were greatest among women, eighteen- to twenty-four-year-olds, those in the city's highest and lowest income brackets, and heavy smokers. Although the ban on smoking in restaurants and bars had produced by far the largest amount of controversy, the department's evaluations showed that it was the tax increase that had spurred the most smokers to quit.[87]

Fighting Fat: Diabetes, Cardiovascular Disease, and Obesity

Health problems related to diet, including high cholesterol, cardiovascular disease, and diabetes, were among the most serious and seemingly intractable conditions for the department to address. Data from the department's health surveys showed that about 61 percent of New Yorkers were overweight or obese. One-quarter of city residents had high cholesterol, and around one in eight had diabetes.[88] And the picture in the city was worsening, as it was nationwide. Between 2002 and 2004, the prevalence of both obesity and diabetes in the city rose by 17 percent, representing more than 17,000 new cases of diabetes.[89] Frieden's preferred sound bite in his public statements was that obesity and diabetes were the only health problems in the city that were getting worse, and getting worse rapidly.

Diabetes extracted a particularly devastating toll in health care expenses and human suffering. When not properly controlled through diet or medication, it could lead to a host of debilitating complications, including kidney disease, blindness, and leg, foot, and toe amputations. The prevalence of diabetes in the city had more than doubled since the 1990s. The increase was almost entirely in type 2 diabetes, which was the result of obesity; it had been known as "adult-onset diabetes" but was increasingly developing in children. As with so many of the city's health problems, diabetes disproportionately burdened poor people of color. It was twice as prevalent among blacks and Hispanics as among whites; the South Bronx, Harlem, Washington Heights, and north-central Brooklyn were the hardest-hit areas.[90]

In the summer of 2005, the department unveiled a new proposal designed to improve the clinical management of diabetes. Under an amendment to the health code, laboratories would be required to report patients' levels of hemoglobin A1C, a marker of blood glucose, to a registry at the Health Department. Each lab report would include the patient's name, date of birth, and address. The registry would enable the department to track the epidemiology of the condition, plan services, and target interventions to both clinicians and patients that would improve care and prevent complications. The program was modeled on a successful system in Vermont made up of more than one hundred private managed care practices.[91]

As the first population-based registry in the country to conduct ongoing monitoring of diabetics' blood sugar levels, it was an innovative program but not an entirely unprecedented one. Although surveillance had originally and most frequently been used to track infectious conditions, registries of noncontagious or chronic health problems such as cancer, blood lead levels, and birth defects had existed for decades. All of these systems had sparked debates about the right and the duty of government to collect personally identifiable medical information. What made the diabetes registry potentially more controversial was its explicit aim of improving medical care. The Community Health Survey had shown that while most of the city's diagnosed diabetics had had an A1C test, only a small percentage of them knew their result—a sign that many doctors were either not sharing the results or were not adequately explaining them.[92] Beginning with a pilot program in the South Bronx, the registry would generate quarterly listings sent to physicians of their diabetic patients' most recent A1C levels, ranked in descending order so that doctors could quickly see which patients needed the most attention. The system would also generate letters printed in English and Spanish to patients who had elevated A1C levels, explaining the result and its medical implications.[93] Patients could opt out of receiving the letter, but not out of having their A1C levels reported.

As an effort to improve clinical practice, the initiative recalled Lowell Bellin's program of Medicaid auditing and standard-setting in the 1960s, which had sought to use the department's regulatory powers to monitor medical care it did not directly provide. Physicians had bitterly resisted Bellin's efforts, but the announcement of the diabetes registry in 2005 drew no formal opposition from the medical community. Neither the state nor the county medical society took a formal stance on the health code amendment. Since the 1960s, the health care landscape had changed dramatically, and physicians had lost the self-policing autonomy they once had. The rising influence of third-party insurance and managed care plans had made it routine for outsiders to review and evaluate doctors' treatment decisions under the mantle of "quality assurance."[94] Frieden repeatedly stressed, moreover, that the registry was designed to help doctors improve diabetes care, not to punish them or impugn their competence.

It was not just physician groups that were silent on the proposal; only thirty-one comments were received during the public comment period, and only ten people testified at the hearing in the summer of 2005. Once the measure had been approved, however, the program drew concerns from some scholars of public health law and bioethics, who worried that a government agency's sending letters to patients telling them that their disease was poorly controlled smacked of victim-blaming and might inadvertently drive patients away from care. They also warned that the unintentional disclosure of information in the registry might endanger patients' ability to obtain life, health, or disability insurance or lead to job discrimination.[95] Some critics raised more fundamental questions about the legitimacy of a public health agency having access to private medical information in the absence of a compelling societal threat. "The general goal of improving public health is too vague and malleable a concept to justify depriving individuals of their personal privacy," wrote Boston University law professor Wendy Mariner. "The limitless nature of the apparent principle underlying the A1C Registry transforms a well-intentioned program to improve health into a threat to personal liberty."[96]

Privacy concerns were also raised by the American Diabetes Association, which had supported the initiative but recommended that patients' consent be required before their A1C levels could be reported.[97] Those in charge of the registry insisted that obtaining the consent of every patient would be unworkable and would lead to incomplete ascertainment that would compromise the registry's ability to give an accurate picture of the problem.[98] They assured skeptics that the system would have strict privacy protections—as did all the department's surveillance activities—to prevent disclosure of the A1C results to anyone other than the patient and the physician who ordered the test.

In response to those who questioned the appropriateness of the department using its surveillance capacity to intervene in the care of a chronic illness, Frieden and the staff of the diabetes program insisted that the registry fulfilled a moral duty to act in the face of human suffering. That diabetes was not contagious and did not threaten others, they held, did not lessen the urgency of addressing it. Nevertheless, the A1C reporting system, like directly observed therapy for tuberculosis, revealed the protean nature of public health intervention. Was tracking the health status of diabetes patients a helpful service or a burdensome invasion of privacy? Would the physicians and patients affected by the registry see the Health Department as a beneficent "protector" or a threatening "enforcer"?

The Board of Health approved the new requirement in late 2006, and the following summer the department began conducting outreach to around seventy medical practices in the South Bronx, seeking their participation in the pilot system of doctor and patient notification. The response was largely favorable: health care providers for more than 80 percent of patients with high A1C levels signed up to have their patients receive letters. The program was complemented by efforts to help patients manage their condition, including distribution of blood pressure monitoring cuffs, blood glucose measurement strips, and free memberships to city recreation centers. By 2009, more than four million test results had been submitted.[99]

The problem of rising obesity rates had complex and far-reaching causes, including broad economic and societal factors that made high-fat, high-calorie food cheap and abundant.[100] Determining how to prevent obesity-related illnesses—especially cardiovascular disease, the city's leading cause of death—was therefore difficult. In mapping out a strategy, the staff of the Division of Health Promotion and Disease Prevention consulted with several experts in food policy, including Michael Jacobson, founder and director of the Center for Science in the Public Interest, a Washington, D.C.–based advocacy group that had been working on nutrition issues since the 1970s; Kelly Brownell, founder of the Rudd Center for Food Policy and Obesity at Yale University; and Walter Willett, the chair of the department of nutrition at the Harvard School of Public Health.[101]

One factor that many researchers believed was contributing to obesity rates was the consumption of meals prepared outside of the home, which had risen sharply since the 1970s. Food from restaurants, especially from fast-food outlets, was generally higher in calories, cholesterol, and saturated fats than food prepared in the home.[102] Using its regulatory authority over the city's restaurants seemed a promising point at which the Health Department might intervene. Because such efforts would affect a much greater number of New Yorkers than the diabetes registry and would necessarily have an impact on commercial interests, they had the potential to provoke wide public controversy.

Both Walter Willett and the Center for Science in the Public Interest had warned for many years about the adverse effects on cholesterol and cardiovascular health of artificial trans fats. Although they occurred naturally in some foods, the majority of trans fats in Americans' diets were artificially produced, contained in the partially hydrogenated oils used in processed foods. Many cooks liked artificial trans fats because they enhanced the taste and texture of foods—they made pastries flakier and French fries crisper, for example—and because they had a longer shelf life than natural alternatives such as butter or olive oil. But several scientific bodies, including the Institute of Medicine and the American Heart Association, had raised concerns about the negative health effects of artificial trans fats. After the Food and Drug Administration enacted a regulation in 2003 requiring packaged foods to display trans fat content, several corporate food manufacturers and restaurant chains began to reduce or eliminate their use.[103]

Many people in the food and restaurant industries were reluctant to stop using trans fats and feared that the change would make their products less enjoyable for customers. Some nutrition experts questioned whether it was appropriate to single out trans fats as a problem, arguing that they accounted for only a small amount of the average person's daily caloric intake and that most of the likely substitutes were only slightly less unhealthy. But research indicated that artificial trans fats were uniquely harmful. Like saturated fats, they raised "bad" cholesterol; unlike saturated fats, however, they also lowered "good" cholesterol.[104] "Even if you switch to suet," Frieden said, "you do better."[105]

In the summer of 2005, Frieden sent a letter to the city's thirty thousand food establishments encouraging them to phase out trans fats from their ingredients. ("Grease and desist," quipped the *Post*.[106]) At the same time, the department sent out a mass mailing urging consumers to ask restaurants about the cooking oils they used. Over the next several months, Health Department staff members went on site to train almost eight thousand restaurant owners about using healthier oils. Nine months later, when inspectors returned for follow-up visits, the results were disappointing but hardly surprising: the use of trans fats had not changed.[107] In September 2006, Frieden turned to regulation to achieve what he had been unable to win through persuasion. He introduced an amendment to the city health code requiring the city's restaurants to eliminate all but minute amounts of trans fats from their food within eighteen months.

The trans fat measure was paired with another initiative aimed at meals prepared outside the home: a requirement that certain chain restaurants post on their menu boards the caloric content of their meals. The measure was intended to help guide consumers toward lower-calorie foods and to encourage restaurants to offer a wider range of low-calorie items.[108] The requirement was needed because of what the department called a "calorie information gap" (a version of information asymmetry, which in economic theory could justify government regulation). People had no idea, for example, that a McDonald's "deluxe breakfast"—pancakes with syrup and butter, bacon, sausage, hash browns, biscuit, and scrambled eggs—had more than 1,600 calories, almost an entire day's recommended caloric intake for many people.[109]

Although calorie posting would in theory be beneficial in all restaurants, the department determined that the requirement would be most feasible and effective in fast-food chain establishments, which had standardized menus and ingredients. These businesses accounted for 10 percent of the city's restaurants but 30 percent of the restaurant traffic. The measure would apply to chains that already made calorie information available but typically did so in places (such as on websites, napkins, or tray liners) that were not easily accessible to consumers when they ordered.[110]

Bloomberg did not take an active role in promoting the measures, as he had done with the antismoking efforts, but he continued to lend his strong support to Frieden in his public statements. In some respects, the mayor was in a much better position to support the restaurant proposals than he had been to attack smoking. The city's economy had rebounded since 2002. Bloomberg had won reelection by a record margin in November 2005, and he continued to enjoy high favorability ratings in mid-2006 when the regulations were proposed.[111] That the ban on smoking in bars, one of the most contentious initiatives of the mayor's first term, had not affected his popularity vindicated the claim by Frieden and other tobacco control advocates that strict antismoking measures, for all the rancor they might stir when they were proposed, were appreciated by voters once they were implemented.

Pushing the trans fat regulation and menu requirement clearly carried a political risk for the mayor, however. Far more New Yorkers patronized chain restaurants than smoked, so the measures had the potential to alienate a larger proportion of the electorate. Bloomberg did not need to pick a fight with the city's restaurants, which had already (successfully) sued the Health Department over a new sanitary inspection system instituted in 2003 that made it easier for establishments to fail and sharply increased fines.[112] Bloomberg had an ambitious second-term agenda with many thorny issues, including reforming the city's perpetually troubled public school system and enacting bridge tolls and congestion pricing to deal with auto traffic in Manhattan. These initiatives would require all the administration's attention and resources, and a crusade to reform fast food could turn into a distraction.[113]

Of the two proposals, the trans fat ban attracted more attention by far. It drew media coverage not just locally but nationally and even internationally, with journalists noting that New York City was a bellwether for public health action in other jurisdictions.[114] Overall the reaction was cautiously supportive: many observers were willing to countenance government intervention in the case of a uniquely unhealthy product like trans fats, but wary of regulating other common food ingredients that might have long-term detrimental effects. Much of the commentary was skeptical or negative, however, attacking both the particular case and the general principle it illustrated. The trans fat ban was odious to free-market conservatives, who were reflexively hostile to any interference by the government in transactions between a business and its customers. A prohibition on an ingredient associated with indulgences such as snack foods and desserts, coming on the heels of the city's banishment of cigarettes from bars, reinforced the perception that Bloomberg and Frieden were attempting to impose a Spartan, abstemious version of good health that denied any role for pleasure. Critics asked whether the mayor would next seek to ban butter or mandate calisthenics.[115]

The department received more than 2,200 written comments on the two amendments during the one-month public comment period, and forty-five people testified about the proposals at a five-hour public hearing in October 2006. Most of those who spoke at the hearing focused on the trans fats ban, and most were in favor. Frieden had made sure that there would be representation not just from health and nutrition experts but also from restaurateurs who could affirm that removing trans fats did not affect their bottom line or their customer satisfaction. The owner of a popular Chicago restaurant that had voluntarily switched to healthier oils bragged that it had gone on to win that city's "best fried chicken" award.[116]

Opponents of the measure sounded familiar themes of individual choice and the right of businesses to be free from regulation. The testimony of Audrey Silk of the smokers' rights group C.L.A.S.H., who had warned about the slippery slope of health paternalism, had an air of I-told-you-so. "When the smoking bans were accepted," she said, "that was the green light to the health police that the public would offer little resistance to their controlling other areas of our lives for our own good."[117] The New York State Restaurant Association called the proposals "a recipe for disaster that could be devastating for New York City's restaurants."[118]

In December 2006, the Board of Health unanimously approved the two health code amendments, largely as they had been proposed; the deadline for complying with the ban on trans fats was extended, and restaurants were given slightly more flexibility in where they could post their calorie information.[119]

Although the trans fats ban had stirred more controversy, it was the menu labeling requirement that ended up in court. The New York State Restaurant Association, which had attacked the measure as expensive and unworkable, brought the suit. The legal challenge rested on two claims: first, that the federal Nutrition Labeling and Education Act, which required that packaged foods carry a listing of their ingredients, preempted the city's regulation; and second, that the rule violated the First Amendment's free speech protections, which forbade government from forcing people to express opinions against their will. Lawyers for the restaurant association pursued the case aggressively. They used Freedom of Information Act requests to obtain email communications between Health Department employees and the nutrition policy experts they had consulted, and they filed complaints with the court arguing that the exchanges had been inappropriate.[120]

A district court judge ultimately affirmed the city's authority to mandate the disclosure of nutrition information, but the decision held that the measure could not apply only to restaurants that already offered such information voluntarily.[121] The measure was rewritten so that it applied instead to all restaurants that were part of chains with fifteen or more outlets, and after a second challenge from the restaurant association a court upheld the requirement.[122]

Within a few years after the regulations took effect, it was difficult to find anyone seriously arguing that the city's fast food had become less delicious or that displaying calorie information was an unmanageable burden. Like the ban on smoking in bars, the two measures were well accepted once they were implemented. As proponents had hoped and critics had feared, New York was a harbinger of a new public health agenda: within a few years numerous local and state governments considered or adopted similar laws.[123]

The debates over removing trans fats and posting calorie counts revealed the conflicted public attitudes about government intervention in problems related to diet and obesity. On the one hand, there was a clear sense of crisis at the time of the Health Department's actions. References to an "obesity epidemic" in the United States had become commonplace in the popular media in the 1990s, and by the early 2000s there was widespread recognition that the increase in Americans' average weight had serious medical and economic repercussions not just for individuals but for society as a whole.[124] At the same time, however, the rhetoric of "personal choice" remained powerful. According to this belief, government could educate and cajole, but it could not legitimately invoke its regulatory authority to prevent people from harming themselves. If people wanted to eat high-fat, high-calorie meals—so said the antipaternalists—the choice should be theirs, not the state's.

To counter charges that the department was overreaching, Frieden portrayed these initiatives as continuing a time-honored, well-accepted mission to safeguard the public from harmful substances. In making the case for removing artificial trans fats from food, Frieden compared trans fats to the lead in lead-based paint: "It is invisible and dangerous, and it can be replaced."[125] In a similar vein, Mary Bassett and Lynn Silver, staff members with the Division of Health Promotion and Disease Prevention who had spearheaded the trans fat and menu proposals, analogized their efforts to past consumer protection measures. "The modern food supply is tainted—it is too salty, too fatty, too sugary, and too rich in calories, and there is simply too much of such food easily available," they wrote in an editorial in the *Journal of the American Medical Association*. "Just as society protected the public from microbes, adulterants, and additives in food during the 20th century, public health systems must reduce the contribution of food to the epidemics of obesity and chronic disease that characterize the current era."[126]

Nevertheless, it was clear that many New Yorkers were devoted to the habits of consumption that the Health Department was attempting to alter. Whether they could be persuaded to equate Big Macs with asbestos remained to be seen. Even more challenging would be the opposition of the corporate interests with political power extending far beyond any one municipality; they were clearly prepared to fight efforts to recast their products as unhealthy. How much legitimacy public health professionals could claim as they sought to adapt their traditional functions to a new epidemiological context continued to be contested.

"Lightning Does the Work"

In May 2009, four months after his inauguration, President Barack Obama announced that he had selected Thomas Frieden to serve as the head of the Centers for Disease Control.[127] The appointment was no surprise, since Frieden was arguably the highest-profile public health official in the country. He had served as the commissioner in New York City for more than seven years, the longest tenure since the legendary Leona Baumgartner from 1954 though 1962. His initiatives on smoking, obesity-related illnesses, and a host of other health issues had seized the attention of both admirers and critics. He owed his success—as he readily acknowledged—to the consistent backing of the mayor he served. Together, Frieden and Bloomberg had achieved much more than either one would have been able to accomplish separately—whether Frieden under a less committed executive or Bloomberg with a less visionary commissioner.

The partnership of the two men was notable not just for their efforts to extend the public health mandate into new realms but for their use of far-reaching policy changes to achieve this goal. To be sure, the Health Department mounted traditional education campaigns that exhorted individuals to take steps to improve their health. The splashiest of these was "Take Care New York," which urged people to adopt an array of preventive health behaviors: see a doctor regularly; get screened for cancer, HIV, and depression; improve diet and stop smoking; get immunized. The message was spread through a media blitz that included 400,000 pocket-sized brochures in English and Spanish, subway posters, and outreach through community groups.[128] But such efforts were adjuncts to the more powerful tool of law.

Bloomberg made his administration's focus explicit in a keynote address he delivered at a CDC conference in June 2006. "We rely on the forceful application of the law—democratically debated and approved—as the principal instrument of our public health policy," Bloomberg told the audience. "Certainly, public information campaigns about health issues are indispensable—and we use them. But we must also recognize that, alone, public information campaigns are insufficient to the enormous tasks at hand. It's like the way Mark Twain once described his appreciation for the nature of thunderstorms. 'Thunder,' Twain said, 'is good. Thunder is impressive. But lightning does the work.' In the realm of public health, law really does the work."[129] Beyond the efforts on smoking and diet, the Health Department invoked its regulatory authority in a variety of ways, including broadening powers to quarantine people in the event of bioterrorism, making sanitary inspection of restaurants more rigorous, mandating the reporting of adolescent immunizations, and requiring licensed day care facilities to eliminate sugar-sweetened beverages, provide more exercise time, and limit the amount of television-watching by children.

In wielding the stick of regulation, the Health Department was returning to its nineteenth-century roots. During the sanitary revolution, states and localities enacted a robust network of laws aimed at making workplaces, tenements, and public spaces healthier by abating or removing the hazardous conditions that were by-products of urbanization and industrialization. Public health pioneers in this era incurred the wrath of their fellow citizens, who were often reluctant to subordinate private interests to the common welfare, and as a result these laws were subject to constant contestation and legal challenge.[130] Frieden saw himself as continuing within the venerable tradition of reformers like his idol Hermann Biggs. He was fond of quoting Biggs's maxim: "Public health is purchasable." But he was clearly guided by another, lesser known of Biggs's beliefs: that "the sanitary measures adopted are sometimes autocratic, and the functions performed by sanitary authorities paternal in character."

The proposition that public health is, at least sometimes, an autocratic or paternalistic enterprise cuts against the grain of political and cultural beliefs central to American society. The model of muscular public health that Bloomberg and Frieden advanced has skeptics across the political spectrum: from civil libertarians on the left, fiercely protective of the rights of individual privacy and autonomy, to free-market conservatives on the right, hostile to infringements on commercial and property interests.

The assertive use of law, regulation, and policy change raised questions about how the public should be involved in public health decision-making. "Health never improves without the engagement of the community," was the assessment of Mary Bassett, who led the department's efforts against chronic illness under Frieden. "You have to change the policy environment, but health never improves through engineering alone."[131] Yet there may be tension between community input and the forceful action of health officials. Bloomberg and Frieden conceded the value—or at least the necessity—of democratic processes, whether City Council deliberations or the public comment and hearings required for amendments to the health code. Yet they were also driven by the conviction that they knew what was best for the city's health, and they were prepared to push ahead with their vision even in the face of clamorous opposition.

Bloomberg's readiness to put his popularity on the line to back potentially unpopular health initiatives enhanced the influence of the Health Department as much as increasing its size and fiscal resources would have done. The department's budget and staff did not increase substantially during the eight years of Bloomberg's first two terms, remaining relatively constant at $1.3 billion to $1.5 billion annually and between 5,500 and 6,000 employees.[132] More important to its success was that Bloomberg explicitly and repeatedly articulated the health of the public as a goal worth prioritizing over competing demands.

Conclusion

The Politics of Public Health

THE COMPLICATED relationship between public health initiative and the conditions of democracy is a theme running through the history of the New York City Department of Health in the decades around the turn of the twenty-first century. The technical tools of public health—data gathering and analysis, health education and promotion, sanitary inspection and regulations, community-based screening and prevention, among many others—have continuously been mediated through politics, not in the narrow sense of partisanship but in the more general meaning of struggles between interest groups over collective decisionmaking in society. "Public health is inherently a political process," observed Stephen Joseph, who as commissioner in the 1980s was at the center of some of the era's most pitched battles over how to protect the city from disease, "and if you're true to the profession and you're lucky you can work your way to and through the issues that protect the public's health. But you have to do it within the political arena. Anybody who thinks that they can stay aside from that, whether it's in a small rural county in Kansas or in New York City, is either ignorant or fooling themselves."[1]

But what does it mean to "do public health" in the political arena? From the 1960s through the early 2000s, the Health Department sought to negotiate complex legislative, legal, and bureaucratic terrains; to balance and respond to the needs and demands of a broad range of individuals and interest groups; to implement programs amid fiscal instability; and to address health problems that were rooted in racial, ethnic, and economic inequities. Political circumstances shaped and constrained the department's responses to issues as diverse as they were challenging, including outpatient care for the poor, heroin addiction, lead paint poisoning, abortion, childhood immunization, infant mortality, AIDS, homelessness, tuberculosis, West Nile virus, bioterrorism, tobacco-related illnesses, diabetes, and cardiovascular disease.

The health concerns that this book has highlighted demonstrate the

257

varied ways in which an issue may become prominent on the public health agenda. Besides initiative from within the department, numerous other forces played a role in giving these issues urgency, including broad-based changes in societal attitudes (heroin addiction, abortion, tobacco), pressure by activists or politicians (lead paint, abortion, AIDS, homelessness, immunization), popular fears that a disease would spread from a feared or despised minority group into the "general population" (heroin addiction, AIDS, tuberculosis), concern about a group perceived as vulnerable or sympathetic (lead paint, immunization, infant mortality), or some combination of these factors.

The diseases that generated the most public controversy and attention in the media were not the ones responsible for the greatest morbidity and mortality. Diseases that accounted for only a handful of illnesses and deaths, such as West Nile virus and anthrax poisoning, provoked enormous public alarm because of their exotic and unprecedented nature. In contrast, the city's leading causes of death throughout this forty-year period, cardiovascular disease and cancer, received attention only in the early 2000s, largely as a result of the initiative of Thomas Frieden, who was aided in his efforts by increasing public concern about the economic costs of obesity-related illnesses and decreasing societal tolerance for smoking.

From the standpoint of public perception, the department's task in pursuing an attack on chronic illnesses was the reverse of the situation during the bioterrorism episode a few years earlier. Instead of reassuring the city that there was relatively little risk from rare pathogens, the department had to convince people that something ordinary and seemingly benign—cheap, abundant, delicious food—in fact posed a grave threat to their health. It was also necessary to counter the widespread perception that chronic diseases were problems of individuals' own making—that people developed obesity-related illness because they were too gluttonous and too slothful, because they lacked willpower and made poor choices. These attitudes reflected strongly moralistic beliefs—rooted in ancient notions of disease as divine punishment—equating good health with upright character.

Even labeling noncontagious conditions such as cardiovascular disease and diabetes as "epidemic" was contested. The libertarian legal scholar Richard Epstein sought to buttress an ideological argument that government may not legitimately intervene in the behaviors of competent adults when he declared in 2003, "There are no non-communicable epidemics."[2] This claim was scientifically erroneous—standard epidemiology textbooks define an epidemic as incidence of any disease above the normal or expected amount—but politically powerful.[3] It underscored how greatly the meanings assigned to an illness can shape views of the appropriate response.

Influencing popular perceptions of what constitutes a crisis and what should be done about it is therefore a critical task for public health professionals. Health departments have several tools at their disposal: mass communication via posters, pamphlets, and the Internet; interactions with the press; and meetings and consultations with community organizations and key opinion leaders. Their work is complicated, however, by the fact that many groups and individuals may also be attempting to magnify or downplay a given problem. The support of these figures—or, at minimum, their lack of active opposition—is essential.

Mark Barnes, who as associate commissioner for policy marshaled the support of the city's medical community to gain passage of the new tuberculosis detention regulations in 1992, later reflected on the need to engage diverse constituencies, especially those who might otherwise be excluded or overshadowed, in advancing a public health agenda. "The main problem with interest-group liberalism in our postmodern society is that the ability to articulate positions has no necessary relationship to the legitimacy of those positions," he recalled. "The task, therefore, of savvy public officials is to try to make sure that voices are heard that have a legitimate argument to make."[4] Thomas Frieden clearly followed this advice in 2006 when he lined up support from a vast array of local and national health experts, academics, businesses, and elected officials behind the proposed ban on trans fats, to the extent that favorable public comments outnumbered opposing ones by a ratio of thirty-one to one.[5]

The increasing influence of citizen activists who mobilized around health issues, a phenomenon that had emerged in the civil rights era, was one of the most salient shifts over the forty years covered by this narrative. On many issues, the advocacy of health-related organizations was a critical adjunct to the Health Department's efforts, bringing much needed public attention and fiscal resources to the work of the department. At times, the department encouraged and even orchestrated activist pressure on city government, and the involvement of these groups and individuals enabled successes that would have been impossible without their efforts.[6] Community-based organizations and advocates were critical forces in bringing attention to the issues of lead paint poisoning, homelessness, and infant mortality, for example. Yet activists often had a complicated and ambivalent relationship with the Health Department, differing with the department leadership on goals and strategies and sometimes perceiving health officials as complacent or insufficiently willing to press the mayor's office for resources. (The categories of Health Department employee and activist were not mutually exclusive, of course; numerous staff members pursued political activism before, during, and after their employment by the city.)

Communities are not monolithic in their views about health issues, moreover, and do not speak with one voice. During the early days of the

AIDS epidemic, for example, the gay community was fractious and sharply divided. Diseases often affect multiple communities whose priorities and values differ, as was evident in the varied public reactions to the prospect of detaining non-adherent tuberculosis patients or supplying clean needles to injection drug users.

One important way in which activists concerned with health issues framed and advanced their claims was to use what political scientists refer to (sometimes skeptically) as "rights talk"—attempting to add moral weight to a demand by framing it in terms of a fundamental right.[7] Several issues addressed by the Health Department after the 1960s were couched in rights talk: the right of children to homes untainted by lead paint; the right of people with AIDS to be free from discrimination; the right of women to abortion; the right of the homeless to decent housing. This discourse served to raise the stakes—failure to advance a public health program becoming not just a professional shortcoming but a moral affront—and although it was often effective, it also polarized issues and strained relations among those involved in addressing the problem.

The language of rights, though often associated with the struggles of disenfranchised communities, is available to the powerful as well as the downtrodden: corporate interests co-opt it in resisting government regulation. The tobacco industry fought restrictions on public smoking by setting up "smokers' rights" groups ("Astroturf," as opposed to grassroots, organizations); one of the most outspoken critics of New York's trans fat ban and menu labeling requirements was a restaurant industry–supported lobbying group that named itself the Center for Consumer Freedom.[8]

Public health, some analysts have argued, is at a disadvantage in the political arena because it typically speaks in terms of collective responsibilities—an idiom different from the country's dominant language of individual rights.[9] As an essentially community-focused, collective enterprise, public health depends to at least some extent on the conception of the government as an appropriate guardian of the common welfare. Yet one of the most defining features of American civic culture is its preference for private, voluntary initiatives over state-centered action.[10] Public health officials often seek to articulate in a compelling fashion the essential interrelatedness that justifies their programs. "We are all connected by the air we breathe," Thomas Frieden was fond of saying when discussing tuberculosis.

More than persuasive rhetoric is needed, however, for municipal public health officials to be able to advance a robust or innovative agenda. They require the backing of elected leaders (not only the mayor but City Council members, state senators and assembly members, and U.S. Congress members), who in turn must have the support of their constituents or risk the consequences of defying the will of the electorate. The successes under Mayor Michael Bloomberg threw into relief the extent to which support from a chief executive can be a critical determinant of success—especially on highly contentious issues or ones that depart from the traditional public health mission. New York City's mayors from the 1960s through the 1990s only occasionally risked voters' anger by supporting a controversial public health program. John Lindsay backed Gordon Chase's expansion of methadone maintenance for heroin addicts in 1970, but only after he had been elected to a second term. Ed Koch took on public smoking and defended Stephen Joseph's needle exchange trial as it was being pummeled by critics. ("Keep it up!" Koch wrote to Joseph during the uproar. "If they hit you, hit back."[11]) But Koch backed down in the face of opposition when Joseph tried to require named reporting of HIV cases. David Dinkins, at Margaret Hamburg's urging, reversed his earlier opposition and approved the establishment of city-funded needle exchange.

Health officials may have difficulty advancing any proactive agenda, controversial or not, because so much of public health work is driven by crises, whether they emerge "naturally" (as in the appearance of a new pathogen) or are constructed by interest groups. Unforeseen events have often put the department in a defensive posture. Woodrow Myers, whose brief tenure as health commissioner in 1990 and 1991 gave him ample opportunity to manage crises, later reflected on the inevitably reactive nature of much of the work. "I've always described the job of the health commissioner as one of putting your fingers in the holes in the dyke," he said, "and when the dyke springs a new hole, your job is to figure out a way to grow a new finger."[12]

The ability to manage crises in the political arena is a critical skill for public health professionals. Thomas Frieden described effective management of an epidemic as "the art of controlled hysteria. You want people to be worried enough to give you more resources, but not so worried they make you do all sorts of stupid things."[13] Margaret Hamburg skillfully exploited the public fear, verging on hysteria, about the spread of drug-resistant tuberculosis to bring desperately needed federal resources into the city. She managed to strike the right balance between concern and alarm. Given the sensationalist media coverage portraying people with tuberculosis as dangerous and irresponsible vectors of illness, however, it is easy to imagine a counterfactual scenario in which the tubercular poor would be subject to draconian measures; history provides many examples of vulnerable populations suffering rights violations in the name of protecting the public health.[14] The complexity of managing crises was acutely apparent in the early days of AIDS in the 1980s. David Sencer's low-profile approach to the disease proved doubly unsuccessful: he was unable to tamp down the hysteria among people prone to irrational fears of contagion, and for his efforts he was accused by activists of indifference and neglect.

Aggressive measures to control disease, whether proposed by health officials or by members of the public, reveal the Janus-faced nature of public health. It is alternately protector and intruder; at various moments health departments may be providers of services or enforcers of regulations (or both simultaneously, as in the case of mandatory directly observed therapy for tuberculosis). Citizens at times pressed the department to fulfill its role as protector, as when the Committee to End Lead Poisoning demanded more testing of children in slums, the Committee for Sexual Responsibility called on the department to regulate conduct in gay bathhouses, and the Coalition for the Homeless sought preventive services for shelter residents. At other times, in contrast, activists sought protection *from* the department, as when ACT UP resisted named reporting of HIV cases, civil liberties groups fought the department's powers to detain non-adherent patients with tuberculosis, C.L.A.S.H. declared that smokers were being persecuted by restrictions on public smoking, and environmental groups objected to pesticide spraying to combat West Nile virus.

An additional factor complicating public health action is the lack of clearly defined boundaries between the field and other, related professions. In the case of outpatient clinics, lead paint poisoning, homeless health, and methadone, action was impeded by the lack of consensus about whether the problem should be addressed by public health or by (respectively) the hospital system, the city housing authority, the social welfare system, or drug treatment professionals. In the aftermath of the terrorist attack of 2001, difficulties in coordinating efforts with law enforcement and environmental protection officials complicated the response to the threat of anthrax and questions about air quality. All these issues revealed, once again, that the question of whether a given public problem constitutes a public *health* problem is by no means straightforward.

"It is inconceivable," Myron Wegman, a prominent public health scholar, wrote in 1977, "that modern society, regardless of its form of government, should not have a government agency whose primary concern is with the health of the populace."[15] Yet even as these words were being written, the view that public-sector agencies such as health departments were the best form for advancing the common welfare was beginning to be eclipsed by antigovernment, proprivatization ideologies. Turning what were traditionally considered public services—transportation, fire, and sanitation, for example—over to for-profit managers as a way to reduce the size of government and improve efficiency was one of the cornerstones of a political philosophy that became hegemonic in the 1980s, most notably under Ronald Reagan in the United States and Margaret Thatcher in England.[16] "Government is not the solution to our problem," Reagan famously declared in his 1981 inaugural address. "Government is the problem."[17] The effects of the limited-government philosophy on public health outcomes was apparent in New York City in the 1980s, when the severity of AIDS, tuberculosis, homelessness, and infant mortality was exacerbated by cuts to federal safety net programs.

New York has long stood out among the nation's largest cities for the strength of labor and union activists and its commitment to generous and humane social welfare provisions. The fiscal travails of the 1970s through the 1990s, however, sorely tested the city's commitment to those ideals.[18] Thanks to Margaret Hamburg's political skills, the department managed to come through the Giuliani administration relatively unscathed, surviving the mayor's attacks on public agencies as havens of bureaucratic mediocrity (an ironic charge given that his administration was notorious for using city agencies, especially the public hospitals, as dumping grounds for patronage jobs[19]). Although Mayor Michael Bloomberg has also pursued neoliberal policies (the most high-profile battle of his tenure was taking on the powerful teachers' union), his support for public health as a core function of government has been a hallmark of his administration.

Public health is a kind of public good, in the economic sense of the term: it benefits all members of society, it is available to everyone, and it is not diminished by common usage. The protection and promotion of public goods are traditionally considered to be among the principal roles of government. Although many public health functions, such as the maintenance of clean water supplies, are widely recognized as public goods, the abstract and vaguely defined nature of the field impedes widespread appreciation of its value and the necessity of government support. It is difficult to rally popular enthusiasm around the routine work of a municipal health department because the benefits it produces are mostly negative ones—the absence of illness and death—whose direct impact on any individual in the community may be remote or imperceptible. In the words of Alfred Sommer, the Johns Hopkins dean who recommended Thomas Frieden as health commissioner, public health is "an invisible health system that promises, as an outcome, abstract non-events."[20] In a contest for public recognition, those who seek to prevent illness are inevitably disadvantaged compared to those who cure it. This ironic paradox helps to explain the gross imbalance in the country's spending: as much as 95 percent of health dollars in the United States are directed toward medicine or medical care and less than 3 percent toward prevention.[21]

Yet neither medical care nor public health intervention is the most significant factor influencing the health of populations. The fundamental structures of society—the distribution of wealth, power, and resources—lie at the root of the challenges confronting public health. A robust body of empirical research, drawing on data from both industrialized and economically developing countries around the world, has shown the powerful effects on physical and mental health of one's position in the social and economic hierarchy. Health improves at every point along this gradient, from bottom to top.[22]

The effects of social and economic determinants have been significant throughout New York City's history and were as pronounced as ever at the turn of the twenty-first century. The gradient in health is made visible on the map of the city's thirty health districts. For virtually every major health indicator, a handful of districts—Harlem, Washington Heights, and the Lower East Side in Manhattan, Bedford-Stuyvesant and Brownsville in Brooklyn, Mott Haven and Morrisania in the Bronx— consistently had the worst statistics during these four decades. Perhaps the starkest documentation of this phenomenon was the widely cited 1990 report in the *New England Journal of Medicine* by two Harlem-based physicians, Colin McCord and Harold Freeman, showing that residents of that neighborhood had a mortality rate more than double that of whites in the United States and more than 50 percent higher than for blacks in the United States.[23] Some of the gaps in the city's health outcomes narrowed over the past two decades, such as the differential life expectancy between blacks and whites, but disparities along lines of income and race remained in many causes of illness and death (notably AIDS, diabetes, and homicide).[24]

The most durable and effective improvement in health entails intervening in income, education, and the basic material conditions of people's lives. Nevertheless, even if a kind of radical egalitarianism would be the most effective and durable path to improving the well-being of populations, the field of public health lacks the mandate, much less the ability, to redistribute income or societal resources. There remain, moreover, deep divides within the profession about the extent to which it should seek to alter fundamental structures and attack racism, sexism, homophobia, and other varieties of bigotry and discrimination that reinforce inequity. Political liberals and progressives in the profession have been vocal in urging more forthright engagement with these determinants of health, but the belief that the field should pursue a social justice agenda is by no means universal.[25]

The work of municipal public health—reducing preventable sickness and death and improving quality of life—seems in some respects straightforward and self-evidently beneficial. Yet the experience of New York City reveals that public health is a field rife with ambiguities and contradictions. Its mission is potentially expansive yet vaguely defined; it is powerful in theory, yet often weak in practice. The social determinants of health are so varied as to constitute an almost limitless range of possible interventions. The police powers wielded by municipal and state governments provide a basis for forceful action, yet this authority has often gone unexercised because of a lack of societal consensus about the appropriate scope and mandate of public health.

The creation of local departments of health stands among the great achievements of the sanitarian movement of the nineteenth century. But what will be the fate of urban public health in the twenty-first century? Given the enormous political challenges that innovation in public health will face—attacks by commercial and antiregulatory interests, conflicting or contradictory demands from elected leaders and activists, ignorance or apathy among much of the public—what are the prospects for health departments to establish a coherent mission and agenda and to secure the necessary support to advance it?

The implications of history for future policy are rarely straightforward, and the events of this book reveal no simple or obvious "formula" for effective public health action. Arthur Schlesinger Jr. aptly warned about "the inscrutability of history."[26] It is clear, however, that initiative from within the New York City Health Department has been a necessary but insufficient condition for public health success in the city. One of the department's central tasks since 1965 has been to reconcile or align the disparate and often conflicting interests of the many constituencies affected by public health policies. The events related in this volume suggest that the ability to engage with and persuade opinion leaders in government and civil society, maneuver within legislative and regulatory arenas, and communicate in a clear and compelling manner to diverse segments of the public are as essential as expertise in epidemiology, statistics, and medicine. Effectively advancing the common welfare demands all these skills.

Notes

Introduction

1. The agency's full name is the Department of Health and Mental Hygiene, following a 2001 merger with the Department of Mental Health, Mental Retardation, and Alcoholism Services (see chapter 8). The Department of Sanitation and the Health and Hospitals Corporation, the quasi-public entity that operates the city's public hospitals, are also headquartered at 125 Worth.
2. See, for example, Gusfield (1981).
3. See, for example, Kahneman, Slovic, and Tversky (1982).
4. Oliver (2006); Kingdon (1984).
5. Oppenheimer, Bayer, and Colgrove (2002).
6. See, for example, the American Public Health Association survey results (Wooley and Benjamin 2004); Public Health Association of New York City (2001).
7. Institute of Medicine (2003).
8. Colgrove, Markowitz, and Rosner (2008).
9. Mann (1999), 443.
10. On the growth in the authority of health departments and scientific medicine during this period, see, for example, Rosenkrantz (1972); Leavitt (1982); Galishoff (1975); Craddock (2000); Fee and Hammonds (1995); Schultz and McShane (1978).
11. Novak (1996).
12. Duffy (1979); Starr (1982), 180–97.
13. Starr (1982), 180–97.
14. Rosen (1971).
15. Brandt and Gardner (2000).
16. Melosi (2000); Fox (1995).
17. Emerson and Luginbuhl (1945); Smillie (1947).
18. MacLeod (1967).
19. Miller and Moos (1981).
20. Emerson and Luginbuhl (1945).
21. Duffy (1990), 163.
22. Waserman (1975).
23. Miles (1974).
24. Etheridge (1992).

25. Rosenberg (1962).
26. Kaufman (1959).
27. Duffy (1968); Baumgartner (1969); Jones (2005).
28. Hammonds (1999).
29. Biggs (1897), 28.
30. Opdycke (2000), 54–55.
31. Garrett (1961), 196–99.
32. Duffy (1968), 343–74; Baumgartner (1969).
33. Kaufman (1959).
34. Mazur (1977).
35. Pierson and Skocpol (2007).
36. Miller et al. (1977).
37. Institute of Medicine (1988), 32.
38. Sugrue (1996).
39. Cannato (2004).

Chapter 1

1. "Statement of the Department of Health on Its Proposed 1966–67 Capital Budget Request," typescript, October 22, 1965, New York City Department of Health Papers (hereafter NYCDOH), box 141979, folder: "Budget—Capital."
2. Martin Tolchin, "The Changing City: A Medical Challenge," *New York Times*, June 2, 1969, 1.
3. Terry (1964), 1799.
4. Terry (1964), 1799.
5. Roemer (1973).
6. Renthal (1971); Shonick and Price (1977).
7. Fee (1988), 231.
8. The Hill-Burton Act (formally the Hospital Survey and Construction Act) created a program of federal grants to states to fund hospital construction. By 1971 the program had distributed some $3.7 billion. See Starr (1982), 348–351.
9. Poen (1979).
10. Starr (1982), 280–86.
11. Lander (1971); Brauer (1982).
12. Stevens and Stevens (1974), 45.
13. Davis and Schoen (1978), 161–73; Lefkowitz (2007).
14. Hollister, Kramer, and Bellin (1974).
15. Shonick and Price (1977).
16. Levitan (1974).
17. Roemer (1973); Sardell (1988), 60, 64–66.
18. Roemer (1973); Fox (1995).
19. Rogers (2001).
20. Burlage (1968), 172.
21. Starin, Kuo, and McLaughlin (1962); Starin and Kuo (1966); David Sencer to Stanley Brezenoff, June 3, 1983, NYCDOH, box K-237, folder: "June."
22. Jacobziner (1965); Charles G. Bennett, "Brooklyn Clinic to Aid Children," *New York Times*, October 31, 1962, 24.

23. Mustalish, Eidsvold, and Novick (1976).
24. Mary C. McLaughlin, "Public Health and Medical Aspects of Neighborhood Ambulatory Health Services," typescript, April 24, 1967, NYCDOH, box 142013, folder: "Ambulatory Care."
25. McLaughlin (1968a), 1182.
26. "Statement of the Department of Health on Its Proposed 1966–67 Capital Budget Request," typescript, October 22, 1965, NYCDOH, box 141979, folder: "Budget—Capital."
27. "Statement of the Department of Health on Its Proposed 1966–67 Capital Budget Request," typescript, October 22, 1965, NYCDOH, box 141979, folder: "Budget—Capital." On the rise of the idea that patients are "consumers" of health care, see Tomes (2006). On the consumer movement more generally in the years following World War II, see Cohen (2004).
28. "Statement of the Department of Health on Its Proposed 1966–67 Capital Budget Request," typescript, October 22, 1965, NYCDOH, box 141979, folder: "Budget—Capital," 2.
29. Mary McLaughlin interview.
30. Mustalish, Eidsvold, and Novick (1976).
31. Cannato (2004).
32. Cannato (2004), 108–18.
33. "Report of the Mayor's Advisory Task Force on Medical Economics," typescript, February 14, 1966, NYCDOH, box 141998, folder: "Mayor."
34. Howard Brown to Louis Craco, June 7, 1966, NYCDOH, box 142007, folder: "Mayor; HSA annual report for 1966."
35. Opdycke (2000), 133–36.
36. Piore, Lieberman, and Linnane (1977).
37. Rappleye (1961); Brown (1967).
38. "Report of the Mayor's Advisory Task Force on Medical Economics," typescript, February 14, 1966, NYCDOH, box 141998, folder: "Mayor."
39. Ginzberg (1971).
40. Commission on the Delivery of Personal Health Services (1968).
41. Nora Piore to Joan Leiman, October 25, 1966, NYCDOH, box 142000, folder: "Budget—General."
42. Nat Hentoff, "The Mayor," *The New Yorker*, October 14, 1967, 120–48, 128.
43. Shonick and Price (1977).
44. "Statement of Howard J. Brown to the Council of the City of New York," September 13, 1967, NYCDOH, box 142017, folder: "HSA Reorganization."
45. Yerby (1967), 72.
46. Martin Tolchin, "Merger Put Off for Two City Units," *New York Times*, March 18, 1966, 41.
47. Arthur Bushel to Timothy Costello, February 15, 1966, NYCDOH, box 141988, folder: "City Administrator."
48. Donald C. Meyer to Leona Baumgartner, August 8, 1966, NYCDOH, box 142008, folder: "Baumgartner." See also Martin Tolchin, "City Health Aides Fear for Agency," *New York Times*, October 25, 1966, 33.
49. Louis Loeb to John Lindsay, August 8, 1967, NYCDOH, box 142017, folder: "HSA Reorganization."
50. John Lindsay to Louis Loeb, August 21, 1967, NYCDOH, box 142017, folder: "HSA Reorganization."

51. Bernard Bucove to Edward O'Rourke, February 15, 1968, NYCDOH, box 142238, folder: "Health Services Administration."

52. Howard J. Brown to Timothy Costello, September 23, 1966, NYCDOH, box 142000, folder: "Budget General."

53. Drusin et al. (1977).

54. Martin Tolchin, "Health Department Fights for Its Life," *New York Times*, May 22, 1967, 1.

55. Bernard Bucove to Edward O'Rourke, February 15, 1968, NYCDOH, box 142238, folder: "Health Services Administration." The *New York Herald-Tribune* columnist Dick Schaap dubbed New York "fun city" soon after Lindsay was elected. Cannato (2004), 108.

56. Martin Tolchin, "Health Department Fights for Its Life," *New York Times*, May 22, 1967, 1.

57. Arthur Bushel to Timothy Costello, February 15, 1966, NYCDOH, box 141988, folder: "City Administrator"; Arthur Bushel to John Lindsay, January 21, 1966, NYCDOH, box 141988, folder: "Mayor."

58. Martin Tolchin, "Health Unit Told to Begin Hiring," *New York Times*, March 29, 1966, 43; Martin Tolchin, "New Nurse Crisis May Face the City," *New York Times*, May 20, 1966, 33; "Nurses Back," *New York Times*, May 29, 1966, E2.

59. Horton (1971).

60. Paul Densen to Edward O'Rourke, October 31, 1967, NYCDOH, box 142022, folder: "Budget."

61. Hanson Blatz to Howard Brown, March 31, 1967, NYCDOH, box 142061, folder: "Tuberculosis."

62. Arthur Bushel to Frederick Hayes, December 29, 1966, NYCDOH, box 141988, folder: "Bureau of Budget."

63. Arthur Bushel to Frederick Hayes, December 29, 1966, NYCDOH, box 141988, folder: "Bureau of Budget."

64. Ginzberg (1971); Brown (1976).

65. Howard Brown to Louis Craco, June 7, 1966, NYCDOH, box 142007, folder: "Mayor."

66. Howard J. Brown to Murray Drabkin, August 10, 1966, NYCDOH, box 142002, folder: "Mayor."

67. Howard J. Brown to Sol Levine, November 20, 1967, NYCDOH, box 142273, folder: "10 Year Plan."

68. Howard J. Brown to Sol Levine, November 20, 1967, NYCDOH, box 142273, folder: "10 Year Plan."

69. Martin Tolchin, "U.S. Expert Takes Health Post Here," *New York Times*, February 18, 1967, 16.

70. Morris Kaplan, "City Plans Clinics in Neighborhoods," *New York Times*, May 19, 1967, 42.

71. On this point, see Alford (1975).

72. Martin Tolchin, "Power of Health Administrator Is Said to Upset Two Officials," *New York Times*, July 15, 1967, 14.

73. See, for example, the correspondence between Mayor Lindsay, health services administrator Howard Brown, and Marvin Perkins, head of the Community Mental Health Board, August 1966, NYCDOH, box 142000, folder: "Mental Health Board."

74. Mary McLaughlin to Howard Brown, November 29, 1967, NYCDOH, box 142013, folder: "Ambulatory Care."

75. Martin Tolchin, "Dr. Brown Quits Post as City Health Chief," *New York Times*, December 6, 1967, 1.

76. Klein (1970), 295.

77. Six years later, Brown publicly came out and called on the City Council to pass antidiscrimination legislation covering sexual orientation (Brown 1976, 15–18).

78. Martin Tolchin, "Westerner Gets City Health Post," *New York Times*, February 2, 1968, 1.

79. John Sibley, "Bucove Explains Decision to Quit," *New York Times*, November 29, 1969, 46.

80. Alford (1975).

81. Matusow (1984), 251.

82. Arthur Bushel to Frederick O'R. Hayes, December 29, 1966, NYCDOH, box 141988, folder: "Bureau of Budget"; Ginzberg (1971), 155.

83. O'Rourke (1969).

84. "Position Paper; Medicaid Program; New York City," typescript, August 21, 1968, NYCDOH, box 142239, folder: "Medicaid."

85. "Position Paper; Medicaid Program; New York City," typescript, August 21, 1968, NYCDOH, box 142239, folder: "Medicaid."

86. McLaughlin (1968b).

87. U.S. Senate (1970), 249.

88. Bellin (1969).

89. Bellin (1969); Bellin and Kavaler (1971).

90. Murray Elkins to James Haughton, April 28, 1967, NYCDOH, box 142014.

91. Cherkasky (1967).

92. Peter Levin interview.

93. Bellin (1977).

94. Bellin and Kavaler (1970).

95. Jonas (1977b); McLaughlin, Kavaler, and Stiles (1971).

96. Bernstein (1971); Parker (1973).

97. Parker (1973).

98. Bernstein (1971).

99. McLaughlin (1971).

100. Bellin, Kavaler, and Schwarz (1972).

101. Jonas (1977a).

102. Bellin, Kavaler, and Schwarz (1972); Jonas (1977a).

103. Hyman (1973); Jonas (1977b).

104. McLaughlin, Kavaler, and Stiles (1971), 2323.

105. Chowkwanyun (2010); Rogers (2001); John Sibley, "Lincoln Hospital Occupied for Two Hours in Protest," *New York Times*, February 3, 1970, 28; John Sibley, "Service Reduced in Health Center," *New York Times*, January 28, 1970, 28; Michael T. Kaufman, "Lincoln Hospital: Case History of Dissension That Split Staff," *New York Times*, December 21, 1970, 1.

106. Rodriguez (1972), 4.

107. Rodriguez (1972), 4.

108. Alford (1975), 153–57; "The Health Department, 1966–1969," typescript (n.d.), NYCDOH, box 142259, folder: "Reorganization"; McLaughlin, Ka-

valer, and Stiles (1971); "NYC Health Department Signs St. John's Contract," *New York Amsterdam News*, August 17, 1968, 20.
109. Bellin, Kavaler, and Schwarz (1972).
110. McLaughlin (1971).

Chapter 2

1. "An Action Analysis of Hippie Health," typescript, November 1967, NYC-DOH, box 142026, folder: "Reports—Misc."
2. Nutt (1976).
3. Riessman (1964); Pearl and Riessman (1965). On the use of indigenous nonprofessionals in public health, see, for example, Domke and Coffey (1966); Luckham and Swift (1969); Stewart and Hood (1970); Colombo et al. (1979).
4. *Inside Health*, December 25, 1970, NYCDOH, box 142268, folder: "Inside Health."
5. Joseph Cimino to Samuel Polatnick, December 14, 1973, NYCDOH, box 142283, folder: "School Health."
6. Olive Pitkin to Bob Trole, November 28, 1973, NYCDOH, box 142283, folder: "School Health."
7. Peter Kihss, "City Is Sued to Stop Giving Unpaid Work-Relief Jobs," *New York Times*, August 31, 1972, 1.
8. Abe Brown to Mary McLaughlin, December 13, 1967, NYCDOH, box 142273, folder: "10-Year Plan."
9. Tomes (2008).
10. Robert Carr to Howard Brown, July 5, 1966, NYCDOH, box 142000, folder: "HSA Asst."
11. Mary McLaughlin interview.
12. Citizens' Committee for Children, Lower East Side Neighborhood Association, and North East Neighborhood Association to John Lindsay, February 6, 1968, NYCDOH, box 142240, folder: "Ambulatory Care."
13. A. Ruben Mora to the mayor, members of the City Council, and the Board of Estimate, August 21, 1968, NYCDOH, box 142030, folder: "Legislation."
14. Mary McLaughlin interview.
15. Kaufman (1969).
16. Markowitz and Rosner (1996), 56–58.
17. Andrews and Edwards (2004); Bornfriend (1969).
18. Gordon (1969), 422.
19. "10-Point Health Program," flyer, NYCDOH, box 142260, folder: "Bureau of Chronic Disease."
20. Thomas W. Jones to J. Warren Toff, June 19, 1970, NYCDOH, box 142271, folder: "Tuberculosis"; Alfonso Narvaez, "The Young Lords Seize X-Ray Unit," *New York Times*, June 18, 1970, 17.
21. "Agreement Between the Young Lords Party and the City Department of Health," June 17, 1970, NYCDOH, box 142271, folder: "Tuberculosis."
22. Cannato (2001).
23. Ravitch (2000); Cannato (2001), 301–53.

24. John Maher to Warren Toff, June 29, 1970, NYCDOH, box 142262, folder: "Community Health Services."
25. Brown (1968), 2363.
26. Fairchild et al. (2010).
27. Johnson (1952).
28. Nancy Hicks, "Drive to Stop Lead Poisoning Begins," *New York Times*, October 10, 1970, 9.
29. Markowitz and Rosner (2002).
30. Kaplan and Shaull (1961); Christian, Celewycz, and Andelman (1964).
31. Greenberg et al. (1958); Jacobziner and Raybin (1958).
32. Rowland Midland to Arthur Bushel, February 28, 1966, NYCDOH, box 142007, folder: "Preventable Diseases."
33. Thomas (1983), 142.
34. Gordon (1973), 33; Jacobziner (1966).
35. See, for example, Arnold Einhorn to Harold Fuerst, January 25, 1966, NYCDOH, box 142007, folder: "Preventable Diseases."
36. "Cases of Childhood Lead Poisoning, Encephalopathy, and Deaths, NYC, 1962–1965," typescript (n.d.), NYCDOH, box 142007, folder: "Preventable Disease."
37. Blanksma et al. (1969).
38. Gordon (1973).
39. Sandra Blakeslee, "Experts Recommend Measures to Cut Lead Poisoning in Young," *New York Times*, March 27, 1969, 25.
40. Gordon (1973), 41–42.
41. Gordon (1973), 28–29.
42. Charlayne Hunter, "Panthers Indoctrinate the Young," *New York Times*, August 18, 1969, 31. See also Caron (1998).
43. Jack Newfield, "Fighting an Epidemic of the Environment," *Village Voice*, December 18, 1969, 12.
44. Jack Newfield, "My Back Pages," *Village Voice*, December 25, 1969, 24.
45. Eidsvold, Mustalish, and Novick (1974).
46. Lloyd Novick interview.
47. Young Lords Party (1971). See also Nelson (2001).
48. David Harris to Thomas Morgan, December 10, 1969, NYCDOH, box 142276, folder: "Dr. Harris."
49. Specter, Guinee, and Davidow (1971).
50. John Sibley, "Criticism Rising over Lead Poison," *New York Times*, December 26, 1969, 19.
51. Colgrove (2006).
52. Eidsvold, Mustalish, and Novick (1974).
53. Minutes, commissioner's staff meeting, February 20, 1970, NYCDOH, box 142262, folder: "Commissioner's Staff Meeting"; "New City Unit Moving Against Landlords Who Allow Poisonous Paint in Their Buildings," *New York Times*, March 18, 1970, 31.
54. Gordon (1973), 55–57.
55. Eidsvold, Mustalish, and Novick (1974), 961.
56. Bergner, Mayer, and Harris (1971); Sieben, Leavitt, and French (1971).
57. Sieben, Leavitt, and French (1971).

58. Spiegel and Lindaman (1977).

59. Musto (1999), 85.

60. *Robinson v. California*, 370 U.S. 660 (1962).

61. Chartock (1974).

62. "Activities of the Addictive Disease Control Service," typescript, March 23, 1966, NYCDOH, box 142010, folder: "Narcotics."

63. Arthur Bushel to Frederick Hayes, December 29, 1966, NYCDOH, box 141988, folder: "Bureau of Budget."

64. Samuel Oast to Alonzo Yerby, April 2, 1966, NYCDOH, box 142010, folder: "Narcotics."

65. Duffy (1990), 605; "Activities of the Addictive Disease Control Service," typescript, March 23, 1966, NYCDOH, box 142010, folder: "Narcotics"; Newman and Cates (1974).

66. Fairchild, Bayer, and Colgrove (2007).

67. Holden Johnson to Mary McLaughlin, March 20, 1970, NYCDOH, box 142275, folder: "Narcotics."

68. Samuel P. Oast to Alonzo Yerby, April 2, 1966, NYCDOH, box 142010, folder: "Narcotics."

69. "Proposal for Bureau of Drug Addiction," typescript, March 24, 1966, NYC-DOH, box 142010, folder: "Narcotics."

70. Samuel P. Oast to Alonzo Yerby, April 2, 1966, NYCDOH, box 142010, folder: "Narcotics."

71. Gordon (1973).

72. Steven Jonas to Edward O'Rourke, January 16, 1968, NYCDOH, box 142031, folder: "Narcotics"; Gordon (1973).

73. Charles G. Bennett, "Addiction Agency Called a 'Fraud,'" *New York Times*, December 11, 1968, 43.

74. Musto (1999).

75. See, for example, "Narcotics a Growing Problem of Affluent Youth," *New York Times*, January 4, 1965, 1.

76. Musto (1999), 252–53.

77. Payte (1997).

78. Dole and Nyswander (1965, 1967a, 1967b); Dole, Nyswander, and Kreek (1966); Nyswander and Dole (1967); Dole, Nyswander, and Warner (1968).

79. Gordon (1973).

80. Jane Brody, "Two Doctors Clash over Methadone," *New York Times*, February 16, 1966, L88.

81. Lewis Yablonsky, "Stoned on Methadone," *The New Republic* 155 (August 13, 1966): 14.

82. Arthur Bushel to Bernard Bucove and Edward O'Rourke, August 26, 1968, NYCDOH, box 142031, folder: "Narcotics."

83. Newman (1977).

84. Michael Dontzin to John Lindsay, August 16, 1968, NYCDOH, box 142031, folder: "Narcotics."

85. Mary McLaughlin to Edward O'Rourke, August 23, 1968, NYCDOH, box 142031, folder: "Narcotics."

86. Gordon (1973).

87. Richard J. H. Johnston, "City Plans Clinics to Treat Addicts," *New York Times*, May 30, 1969, 1.
88. Gordon (1973).
89. John Sibley, "New Health Aide Is Under Attack," *New York Times*, December 10, 1969, 30.
90. Newman (1977).
91. Newman (1977).
92. Gordon (1973); Peter Levin interview.
93. Robert Newman interview.
94. Newman (1977).
95. Gordon (1973), 99.
96. *Inside Health*, November 17, 1970, NYCDOH, box 142268, folder: "Inside Health."
97. Bayer (1978).
98. Bayer (1978).
99. Institute of Medicine (1995); des Jarlais, Paone, and Friedman (1995).
100. Newman and Peyser (1991); Rosenbaum (1995).
101. Mary McLaughlin to John Lindsay, September 30, 1970, NYCDOH, box 142275, folder: "Narcotics."
102. Musto (1999), 273.
103. Chartock (1974).
104. Des Jarlais, Paone, and Friedman (1995).
105. Jean Pakter interview.
106. Meckel (1998); Skocpol (1992).
107. Jean Pakter interview.
108. "City Aide Scored on Birth Control," *New York Times*, November 2, 1957; Edith Evans Asbury, "Birth Control Issue Again Stirs Debate," *New York Times*, August 24, 1958, E6; Edith Evans Asbury, "Birth Control Ban Ended by City's Hospital Board," *New York Times*, September 18, 1958, 1.
109. James (1966).
110. Interview with J. Joseph Speidel, Population and Reproductive Health Oral History Project, Sophia Smith Collection, Smith College.
111. "Remarks Made by Dr. David Harris at the Regional OEO Meeting on Family Planning, February 26, 1968," typescript, NYCDOH, box 142240, folder: "Maternity Service and Family Planning."
112. Reagan (1997); Nossiff (2001).
113. *Griswold v. Connecticut*, 381 U.S. 479 (1965).
114. Nossiff (2001).
115. Howard Brown, "Statement Before the Committee on Health, New York State Assembly," typescript, February 2, 1967, NYCDOH, box 142023, folder: "Legislation Abortion."
116. Sydney H. Schanberg, "Abortion Hearing Is Marked by Bitter Clashes," *New York Times*, February 9, 1967, 24; "City's Own Hospitals Perform Abortions, NY Hearing Told," *Washington Post*, February 11, 1967, E13.
117. Edith Evans Asbury, "Women Break Up Abortion Hearing," *New York Times*, February 14, 1969, 42; "Hearing," *The New Yorker*, February 22, 1969, 28–29.
118. Nossiff (2001).

119. Nossiff (2001).

120. Shirley Mayer to David Harris, July 6, 1970, NYCDOH, box 142278.

121. Jean Pakter interview.

122. Shirley Mayer to David Harris, July 6, 1970, NYCDOH, box 142278.

123. Franz Leichter to Mary McLaughlin, June 8, 1970, NYCDOH, box 142278.

124. "Aborting Abortion Reform," *New York Times*, June 3, 1970, 44.

125. Jane E. Brody, "Doctors Here Get Abortion Lesson," *New York Times*, July 2, 1970, 43.

126. Jean Pakter interview.

127. Lacey Fosburg, "Abortion Measure Stirs Alarm," *New York Times*, July 16, 1970, 24.

128. Lawrence Lader, "Undoing the Abortion Law," *New York Times*, January 4, 1971, 31.

129. "Status Report on Abortions," typescript, September 11, 1970, NYCDOH, box 142278.

130. "Progress Report: How Are We Doing on the Abortion Program?" *Inside Health*, November 27, 1970, NYCDOH, box 142268, folder: "Inside Health."

131. "Abortion Program, Bureau of Maternity Services and Family Planning—Budget Submission FY 1970–1971," typescript, NYCDOH, box 142278.

132. Harris et al. (1973).

133. Lerner et al. (1974).

134. *Roe v. Wade*, 410 U.S. 113 (1973).

135. Gordon (1973), 27.

Chapter 3

1. Thomas (1983), 137.

2. Kotchian (1997). In New York City, Lindsay's superagencies had reinforced this separation: the city's Environmental Protection Administration included the Department of Sanitation, which collected and disposed of garbage; the Department of Air Resources, which monitored airborne pollutants from light industry and transportation: and the Department of Water Supply, Gas, and Electricity.

3. Roemer (1973); Bernstein (1970).

4. Cornely (1971).

5. Starr (1982), 379–83.

6. Fuchs (1983); Illich (1976); Cochrane (1972); McKeown (1979); Knowles (1977a).

7. See, for example, Lalonde (1974); Knowles (1977b).

8. Hanlon (1973), 898.

9. Miller et al. (1977).

10. Morris (1980), 46–55.

11. Commissioner's staff meeting minutes, May 1, 1970, NYCDOH, box 142262, folder: "Commissioner's Staff Meeting."

12. Peter Levin interview; John Sibley, "Chase Builds Up Health Services," *New York Times*, April 5, 1970, 91.

13. Margaret Grossi interview.

14. Mindlin and Densen (1969).

15. Novick, Mustalish, and Eidsvold (1975).
16. Denerstein et al. (1976).
17. Kilcoyne (1973, 1976); Wassertheil-Smoller, Bijur, and Blaufox (1978); Bluestone (1976).
18. Imperato (1983).
19. Levenson and Weiss (1976), 25.
20. Mustalish, Eidsvold, and Novick (1976).
21. John Sibley, "Chase Is Leaving Health Services," *New York Times*, July 28, 1973, 21.
22. Morris (1980), 215.
23. Francis K. Clines, "Beame Urges Cut in Mayor's Power," *New York Times*, October 26, 1972, 47.
24. Imperato (1979).
25. Imperato (1983).
26. Lloyd Novick interview.
27. Lloyd Novick interview.
28. Lowell Bellin, "The Fall and Rise of the New York City Department of Health," typescript, May 24, 1974, NYCDOH, box 142291, folder: "Public Health Association of New York City Annual Meeting."
29. Pascal Imperato interview.
30. Brown (1998).
31. Blum (1991).
32. "Maternity and Infant Care Family Planning Projects," *Progress Report 1972*, NYCDOH, box 142284, folder: "Maternity and Infant Care."
33. The literature on the causes and consequences of New York City's fiscal crisis is voluminous. The account here is drawn from Shefter (1992); Morris (1980); Shalala and Bellamy (1976); Steven R. Weisman, "How New York Became a Fiscal Junkie," *New York Times Sunday Magazine*, August 17, 1975, 8–34; Tabb (1982); Brash (2003); Newfield and DuBrul (1977); and MacMahon and Siegel (2005).
34. Katz (1986).
35. Shefter (1992).
36. Morris (1980), 157.
37. Morris (1980); Glaser and Kahn (1999).
38. Donovan (1990), 13–15.
39. Jackson (1985).
40. Sayre and Kaufman (1960).
41. Morris (1980), 225; Shefter (1992), 131–32.
42. Andy Logan, "Around City Hall," *The New Yorker*, August 4, 1975, 78–88.
43. Russell Baker, "Monty Python's Flying City," *New York Times*, November 1, 1975, 29.
44. Peter Levin interview.
45. John Marr interview.
46. Peter Levin interview.
47. Nestlebaum (1979).
48. Imperato (1978).
49. Imperato (1983), 99.
50. Pascal Imperato interview.

51. Brill (1966); Baumgartner (1969).

52. City of New York (1977a, 1977b).

53. Imperato (1978).

54. Peter Levin interview.

55. Jill Gerston, "Twelve Nutritionists Get Layoff Notice," *New York Times*, January 18, 1875, 32.

56. Imperato (1979); Feygele Jacobs to Ellen Rautenberg, October 27, 1983, NYCDOH, box K-252, folder: "Medical and Health Research Association."

57. *Sorbonne Apartments Co. v. Board of Health of the City of New York*, 390 N.Y.S.2d 358 (1976).

58. Frank J. Prial, "Landlords Resisting City Mandate for Window Guards for Children," *New York Times*, March 14, 1978, 1.

59. Joseph P. Fried, "Window Guard Provision Postponed Until the Fall," *New York Times*, April 30, 1976, 34; Michael Goodwin, "For Window Guards, Resistance and Uncertainty," *New York Times*, April 16, 1978, 275.

60. Pascal Imperato interview.

61. City of New York (1978).

62. M. Spar to Melvyn Matlins, June 6, 1980, NYCDOH, box 142304, folder: "Ferrer's Personal File."

63. Ellen Rautenberg interview.

64. Peter Levin interview.

65. John Marr interview.

66. Opdycke (2000).

67. Max H. Seigel, "City Weighs Closing of Eight Municipal Hospitals," *New York Times*, February 16, 1975, 40.

68. Starr (1982).

69. See, for example, Lowell Eliezer Bellin, "Disjointed Notes on Favorite Health Administration Chestnuts," typescript, NYCDOH, box 142291, folder: "American Association for the Advancement of Science."

70. Opdycke (2000).

71. David Bird, "City Hospitals' Role a Fiscal Crisis Issue," *New York Times*, October 22, 1975, 93.

72. David Bird, "Hospitals Chief Quashed Studies Urging Cutbacks," *New York Times*, August 17, 1975, 1.

73. Max H. Seigel, "Holloman, a Black, to Head City Hospitals," *New York Times*, March 15, 1974, 69.

74. David Bird, "Bellin Charges Hospital Corporation Is 'Bereft' of Experienced Managers," *New York Times*, August 29, 1975, 55.

75. David Bird, "Protestors Mob the City Hospitals' Office," *New York Times*, May 16, 1975, 18.

76. Peter Levin interview.

77. Pascal Imperato interview.

78. Ralph Santiago to Lowell Bellin, February 7, 1975, NYCDOH, box 142291, folder: "Dr. Bellin."

79. J. Zamgba Browne, "Ministers Take Over Mayor Beame's Office," *Amsterdam News*, October 1, 1975, 1; "Metropolitan Briefs," *New York Times*, September 24, 1975, 49.

80. "Gotbaum Union Asks Ouster of Bellin as Health Chief," *New York Times*, September 7, 1975, 103.

81. "Union Leaders Want Dr. Bellin Fired," *Amsterdam News*, September 17, 1975, A1.

82. Nathaniel Sheppard Jr., "Health Agency Chief for New York Quits," *New York Times*, October 7, 1976, 23.

83. Ronald Sullivan, "Hospital Corporation Votes Nine to Seven to Remove Holloman as President," *New York Times*, January 27, 1977, 1.

84. Interview with Robert F. Wagner Jr., Koch Administration Oral History Project, Columbia University Oral History Research Office.

85. Ronald Sullivan, "Koch's Plan to Close Four Hospitals Voted Amid Protestors' Shouts," *New York Times*, June 29, 1979, B1; Jill Smolowe, "Hospital Hearing Brings Criticism of Koch's Policy," *New York Times*, February 20, 1980, B3.

86. Opdycke (2000).

87. Olive Pitkin to Lowell Bellin, August 6, 1976, NYCDOH, box 142299, folder: "School Health."

88. "School Health Expansion—Briefing Paper," typescript (n.d.), NYCDOH, box K-201, folder: "School Children's Health Program"; Irene Clark to Reinaldo Ferrer (n.d.), NYCDOH, box 142361, folder: "School Health"; Heyward Davenport, "Summary Anecdotal Opinion Survey of School Officials Involved in 1981 Immunization Campaign in the Public Schools of New York City," typescript (n.d.), NYCDOH, box K-225, folder: "Immunization."

89. New York City Department of Health (1981).

90. Eric Broder to Margaret Grossi, September 18, 1980, NYCDOH, box K-234, folder: "Mayor's Office of Management and Budget."

91. Eric Broder to Margaret Grossi, September 18, 1980, NYCDOH, box K-234, folder: "Mayor's Office of Management and Budget."

92. Colgrove (2006).

93. Heyward Davenport, "Summary Anecdotal Opinion Survey of School Officials Involved in 1981 Immunization Campaign in the Public Schools of New York City," typescript (n.d.), NYCDOH, box K-225, folder: "Immunization."

94. Colgrove (2006).

95. Ensminger (1980); Joseph B. Treaster, "School Inoculation Data Missing; Director of City Program Ousted," *New York Times*, November 19, 1978, 47.

96. William G. Blair, "Eleven School Principals Accused of Violating Immunization Statute," *New York Times*, June 2, 1981, B2.

97. Pascal James Imperato, "The High Cost of Attempting to Rid America of Measles," *New York Times*, October 28, 1981, A26.

98. Ronald Sullivan, "Diseases Cut by Policy of No Shots, No School," *New York Times*, May 22, 1982, 31; David Sencer to Maria Mitchell, August 5, 1985, NYCDOH, box K-149, folder: "NYC Dept. Health."

99. Michael Arena, "Childhood Diseases Down in City," *Newsday*, May 22, 1982, 5.

100. City of New York (1979).

101. City of New York (1980), 177–78; Reinaldo Ferrer to Nathan Leventhal, October 1, 1980, NYCDOH, box 142304, folder: "Ferrer's Personal Folder."
102. "Bureau of Venereal Disease Control, Summary of Bureau Activities, 1976–1981," typescript (n.d. [1981]), NYCDOH, box 232.
103. See, for example, Reinaldo Ferrer to Nathan Leventhal, October 1, 1980, NYCDOH, box 142304, folder: "Ferrer's Personal Folder."
104. See, for example, Imperato (1979); A. O. Sulzberger, "City Health Department Aims to Reverse Decline," *New York Times*, October 22, 1981, B1.
105. Pascal Imperato to Edward Koch, February 24, 1978, NYCDOH, box 142298, folder: "Vital Records."
106. Imperato (1983); City of New York (1977b).
107. Pascal James Imperato to Edward Koch, February 24, 1978, NYCDOH, box 142298, folder: "Vital Records"; Reinaldo Ferrer to Nathan Leventhal, August 28, 1981, NYCDOH, box 142359, folder: "Monthly Reports 1981."
108. See, for example, Jonas (1977a); Imperato (1979).
109. Committee on Public Health (1985).
110. Lawrence K. Altman, "Dispute on Death Ruling Called Key Factor in Baden Case," *New York Times*, August 3, 1979, B6; *Baden v. Koch*, 799 F.2d 825 (1986).
111. "Chief Will Quit City Health Post," *New York Times*, April 7, 1981, B4; Clyde Haberman, "Tough, Yet Benign Mayor," *New York Times*, November 24, 1981, B3.
112. Anna Mayo, "A Sick Joke: The Collapse of the City Health Department," *Village Voice*, April 28, 1980, 1, 13–16.
113. Traub (2004).
114. Mahler (2005).
115. Shefter (1992).
116. Austin (2001).
117. Traub (2004), 113–27.
118. Leonard Buder, "Murders at Record During 1979 in City," *New York Times*, March 2, 1980, 47.
119. Brecher and Horton (1993), 6.

Chapter 4

1. "Outline of Protocol for Pathologic Record Review for Secular Trend Assessment of Lymphadenopathy Syndrome," typescript (n.d. [May 1982]), NYCDOH, box K-231, folder: "May."
2. Bayer and Oppenheimer (2000).
3. Shilts (1987).
4. Masur et al. (1981).
5. Centers for Disease Control and Prevention (1981).
6. Pauline Thomas interview.
7. Pauline Thomas interview; Chamberland et al. (1985); New York City Department of Health (1986).
8. Stephen Friedman interview.
9. Jaffe et al. (1983).
10. Epstein (1996); Shilts (1987).

11. Centers for Disease Control and Prevention (1982a); David Sencer to Nathan Leventhal, February 3, 1982, NYCDOH, box K-231, folder: "February"; James Monroe to David Sencer, May 17, 1982, NYCDOH, box K-231, folder: "May"; Miller et al. (1984).

12. William Darrow to the coordinator of the Task Force on the Acquired Immune Deficiency Syndrome, September 3, 1982, NYCDOH, box K-228, folder: "Preventable IV."

13. Epstein (1996), 56; Curran (1983).

14. Guinan et al. (1984).

15. Polly Thomas to David Sencer, November 3, 1982, NYCDOH, box K-228, folder: "Preventable Diseases II"; Stephen Friedman to David Sencer, November 3, 1982, NYCDOH, box K-228, folder: "Preventable Diseases II"; Polly Thomas to Lyle Conrad, December 3, 1982, NYCDOH, box K-228, folder: "Preventable IV"; Thomas et al. (1984).

16. Centers for Disease Control and Prevention (1982b).

17. Larry Zyla to John Miles, October 26, 1983, NYCDOH, box L-191, folder: "Acquired Immune Deficiency Syndrome"; Sam Roberts, "Medical Detectives Hunt Clues to AIDS Outbreak," *New York Times*, June 4, 1983, 25.

18. Chamberland et al. (1985).

19. Pauline Thomas interview.

20. Rebecca Reiss to David Sencer (n.d. [July 1983]), NYCDOH, box K-192, folder: "AIDS July 1983."

21. Lawrence Mass, "Disease Rumors Largely Unfounded," *New York Native*, July 27–August 9, 1981, 7.

22. Lawrence Mass, "Cancer in the Gay Community," *New York Native*, July 27–August 9, 1981, 1.

23. Mass (1990).

24. Joseph Sonnabend to David Sencer, July 19, 1982, NYCDOH, box K-193, folder: "July-Aug."

25. Sonnabend, Witkin, and Purtilo (1984).

26. Berkowitz (2003).

27. Berkowitz (2003).

28. Silversides (2003), 20–24; Berkowitz (2003).

29. Etheridge (1992); Neustadt and Feinberg (1983).

30. Ronald Sullivan, "Ex-Head of Federal Disease Center Named City Health Commissioner," *New York Times*, November 29, 1981, 1.

31. Sencer (1983).

32. City of New York (1983).

33. Alan Kristal interview; Mary Ann Chiasson interview; Wendy Chavkin interview.

34. Office of the State Comptroller, "District Health Centers, New York City Department of Health, Audit Report NYC-12-82," typescript, December 1982, NYCDOH, box K-229, folder: "Management Audits."

35. United States Conference of Mayors (1982b).

36. United States Conference of Mayors (1982a).

37. Hatch (1982).

38. "Testimony of David Axelrod, Public Hearings on Preventive Health and

Health Services Block Grant, August 4, 1982," NYCDOH, box K-138, folder: "Block Grants."

39. Altman and Morgan (1983).
40. David Sencer to supervisory staff, January 21, 1982, NYCDOH, box K-231, folder: "December."
41. Ellen Rautenberg interview.
42. David Sencer to Alair Townsend, February 16, 1982, NYCDOH, box K-231, folder: "February."
43. "Impact of Reduced Federal Funding on the Bureau of Venereal Disease Control," typescript (n.d. [1983]), NYCDOH, box K-245, folder: "VD 1983."
44. Colgrove (2006).
45. Sencer (1983).
46. "Department of Health Consolidation Plan," February 10, 1983, NYCDOH, box K-236, folder: "Long-Range Planning"; David Sencer to Victor Botnick, March 15, 1984, NYCDOH, box K-143, folder: "March"; David Sencer to Manfred Ohrenstein, February 15, 1983, NYCDOH, box K-236, folder: "Long-Range Planning."
47. David W. Dunlap, "City Defers Plan to Close Ten Pediatric Centers," *New York Times*, March 27, 1983, 48.
48. David Sencer to James Wyngaarden, May 17, 1982, NYCDOH, box K-193, folder: "Mar-June."
49. David Sencer to Merle Gibson, July 9, 1982, NYCDOH, box K-231, folder: "July"; Sencer (1983).
50. David Sencer interview.
51. See, for example, David Sencer to Nathaniel Leventhal, April 20, 1983, and "Minutes of Meeting 4/28/82," both in NYCDOH, box K-231, folder: "May."
52. Clifford (1992).
53. David Sencer to Robert Wagner, January 13, 1983, NYCDOH, box K-192, folder: "AIDS January 1983."
54. Bayer (1995).
55. Chambre (2006); Clifford (1992).
56. Clifford (1992), 83–84; Lambright and O'Gorman (1992).
57. Stephen Friedman to deputy commissioners, May 26, 1983, NYCDOH, box K-192, folder: "AIDS May 1983."
58. Oleske et al. (1983), 2345.
59. Mass (1990).
60. Larry Kramer, "1,112 and Counting," *New York Native*, March 14, 1983, 1.
61. Clifford (1992).
62. David Sencer, typescript, March 19, 1985, NYCDOH, box K-194, folder: "March 1985."
63. Clifford (1992); Mass (1990).
64. Berkowitz (2003).
65. Yehudi Felman interview.
66. Bruce Lambert, "Koch's Record on AIDS: Fighting a Battle Without Precedent," *New York Times*, August 27, 1989, 1.
67. Clifford (1992).
68. David Sencer interview.
69. Michael VerMeulen, "The Gay Plague," *New York*, May 31, 1982, 52–62.

70. Fauci (1983).
71. See, for example, Epstein (1996); Gross (2002), 94–99; Shilts (1987), 320–23.
72. Minutes of the Inter-Agency Task Force on AIDS, June 13, 1983, NYCDOH, box K-195, folder: "AIDS June 1983."
73. "AIDS Q&A," NYCDOH, box K-192, folder: "AIDS May 1983" (emphasis in original).
74. Cited in Rushing (1995), 171.
75. Matthews and Neslund (1987).
76. Stephen Friedman interview.
77. Mayor's Inter-Agency Task Force on AIDS, April 3, 1984, NYCDOH, box K-195, folder: "April '84."
78. David Sencer to William Curran (n.d. [October 1983]), NYCDOH, box K-237, folder: "October."
79. Mary Ann Giordano, "AIDS Fear Infects Docs, He Says," *New York Daily News*, June 15, 1983.
80. Bruce Lambert, "Two Councilmen Want Quarantine on AIDS; Health Chief Says No," *Newsday*, June 15, 1983.
81. Rodger McFarlane to David Sencer, September 21, 1984, NYCDOH, box K-196, folder: "September '84."
82. Bayer (1989), 103–5.
83. Carol Bellamy to David Sencer, March 8, 1985, NYCDOH, box K-144, folder: "March"; Carol Bellamy to David Sencer, April 17, 1985, NYCDOH, box K-133, folder: "Legal."
84. Bayer (1989).
85. "Dear Doctor," April 1, 1985, NYCDOH, box K-144, folder: "April."
86. "AIDS Forum, Minutes," typescript, NYCDOH, box K-144, folder: "November"; Steven C. Arvanette, "NYC Sets Up HTLV-III Hotline," *New York Native*, April 6–21, 1985, 15; Glenn Collins, "AIDS Hotline Is Busy in the City," *New York Times*, October 7, 1985, B12.
87. Caiazza (1985).
88. Bayer (1989).
89. Bayer (1989), 110–12.
90. King Holmes to David Sencer, May 29, 1985, NYCDOH, box K-194, folder: "June 1985."
91. Wendy Chavkin interview.
92. Erik Eckholm, "Screening for Blood for AIDS Raises Civil Liberties Issues," *New York Times*, September 30, 1985, A1.
93. Mary Ann Chiasson interview.
94. Irwin Davison interview.
95. Roger Enlow to Neil Schram, September 6, 1983, NYCDOH, box K-244, folder: "Gay Men's Health Crisis Center"; Dennis Passer to David Sencer, September 9, 1983, NYCDOH, box K-191, folder: "Sept 1983."
96. Roger Enlow to Neil Schram, September 6, 1983, NYCDOH, box K-244, folder: "Gay Men's Health Crisis Center."
97. Cited in Bayer (1989), 51.
98. Martin (1987).
99. Bayer (1989).

100. Marcia Kramer and Don Singleton, "Gov: May Close Some Gay Baths," *New York Daily News*, August 27, 1983.

101. Dennis Passer to David Sencer, September 9, 1983, NCYDOH, box K-191, folder: "September 1983."

102. Chambre (2006), 54–55.

103. Chambre (2006), 55; Bayer (1989), 57.

104. Michael Callen, "Controlling the Baths and Backroom Bars," *Village Voice*, March 12, 1985, 35.

105. Bayer (1989).

106. Joyce Purnick, "AIDS and the State," *New York Times*, October 30, 1985, B4.

107. Edward Koch to David Sencer (n.d. [October 1985]), NYCDOH, box K-144, folder: "October."

108. David Sencer to Edward Koch, October 24, 1985, NYCDOH, box K-144, folder: "October."

109. Bayer (1989).

110. *City of New York v. New St. Mark's Baths*, 497 N.Y.S.2d 979 (1986).

111. Joyce Purnick, "City Closes Bar Frequented by Homosexuals, Citing Sexual Activity Linked to AIDS," *New York Times*, November 8, 1985, B3; Jeffrey Schmalz, "City Shuts Heterosexual Club for Prostitution," *New York Times*, November 23, 1985, 34.

112. *City of New York v. New St. Mark's Baths*, 497 N.Y.S.2d 979 (1986).

113. Eleanor Murphy to Pauline Thomas, July 14, 1983, NYCDOH, box K-192, folder: "AIDS July 1983."

114. Kirp (1989).

115. Jilian Mincer, "Move of AIDS Patients Raises Fear," *New York Times*, July 21, 1985, 26.

116. Brier (2006).

117. Brier (2006).

118. Kirp (1989); Brier (2006).

119. Nelkin and Hilgartner (1986).

120. Kirp (1989); Brier (2006).

121. Nelkin and Hilgartner (1986).

122. Joseph P. Fried, "Few Answers in AIDS Suit," *New York Times*, September 23, 1985, B5.

123. Brier (2006).

124. Kirp (1989).

125. Nelkin and Hilgartner (1986).

126. Brown (1987).

127. Nelkin and Hilgartner (1986), 132.

128. Kirp (1989), 109.

129. Frank Lynn, "McGrath Proposes Closing Homosexuals' Bathhouses," *New York Times*, October 2, 1985, B1.

130. Joyce Purnick, "A Protest Erupts Outside Hearing on an AIDS Bill," *New York Times*, November 16, 1985, 31; Kirp (1989).

131. *District 27 Community School Board v. Board of Education of the City of New York*, 502 N.Y.S.2d 325 (1986).

132. Hirsch and Enlow (1984).

133. Guttman and Salmon (2004).

Chapter 5

1. "Statement of Stephen Joseph, MD, MPH, Commissioner of Health, May 28, 1986," typescript, NYCDOH, box K-123, folder: "New York City Dept of Health Budget Hearing Briefing Book, March 5, 1987."
2. Joseph (1992), 69.
3. Stephen Joseph interview; Lynn Rosellini, "Two Who Quit over Baby Formula Have No Regrets," *New York Times*, June 30, 1981, 25; Philipp, Merewood, and O'Brien (2001).
4. Hopper (1990).
5. Alperstein, Rappaport, and Flanigan (1988).
6. Alperstein, Rappaport, and Flanigan (1988).
7. Anthony Gliedman to Edward Koch, June 11, 1985, NYCDOH, box K-134.
8. "Report on the Health Needs of Residents of the New York City Family Shelters and Hotels," typescript, December 1982, NYCDOH, box K-244, folder: "Family Shelter"; "Briefing on Homeless Families," typescript, September 23, 1983, NYCDOH, box K-245, folder: "Welfare Hotels"; Ellen Rautenberg to Distribution, January 27, 1984, NYCDOH, box K-143, folder: "March"; Ellen Rautenberg to David Sencer, February 21, 1984, NYCDOH, box K-257, folder: "New Needs."
9. Ellen Rautenberg interview.
10. Brecher and Horton (1993).
11. David Sencer to Edward Koch, September 26, 1983, NYCDOH, box K-245, folder: "Welfare Hotels"; "Report on Health Survey of Welfare Hotels," typescript (n.d. [1983]), NYCDOH, box K-237, folder: "September."
12. Chavkin et al. (1987).
13. Wendy Chavkin interview; Alan Kristal interview.
14. Rapoport (1987); Barbara Basler, "City Announces Program to Curb Infant Deaths Among the Homeless," *New York Times*, June 11, 1986, B10.
15. Gina Kolata, "Many with AIDS Said to Live in Shelters," *New York Times*, April 4, 1988, B1.
16. "Managing the Empire of Misfortune," *New York Times*, November 5, 1986, A30.
17. Stephen Schultz to Stephen Joseph, May 9, 1986, NYCDOH, box K-183, folder: "Shelters."
18. Norman Scherzer interview.
19. Nardell and Brickner (1996), 1260.
20. Brown (1990).
21. David Sencer to Carol Bellamy, May 15, 1984, NYCDOH, box K-143, folder: "May"; Karen Nelis, "City Launches $2.4 Million Drive to Reduce Infant Deaths," *New York Tribune*, August 24, 1984, 12.
22. Wendy Chavkin interview.
23. Wendy Chavkin interview; Stephen Joseph to Stanley Brezenoff, November 14, 1986, NYCDOH, box K-217, folder: "Infant Mortality Initiative"; Karen Nelis, "City Launches $2.4 Million Drive to Reduce Infant Deaths," *New York Tribune*, August 24, 1984, 5.
24. Stephen Joseph to Edward Koch, August 12, 1998, NYCDOH, box K-062, folder: "Aug-Oct 88."

25. "Future Plans and Direction for the Bureau of Child Health," typescript, October 1987, NYCDOH, box K-102, folder: "Child Health."
26. Katherine Lobach interview.
27. Katherine Lobach interview.
28. Melinda Henneberger, "Plan to Shift Clinics Raises Fears over Survival," *New York Times*, October 6, 1994, B3.
29. Berney (1993).
30. "Lead Poisoning Control Program Proposal to Increase Lead Screening," typescript (n.d.), NYCDOH, box K-229, folder: "Lead Poisoning."
31. "Lead Poisoning Control Program," typescript (n.d. [1982]), NYCDOH, box K-229, folder: "Lead Poisoning."
32. Marvin Rosenberg to Edward I. Koch, February 25, 1982, and Olive Pitkin to Marvin Rosenberg, May 26, 1982, both in NYCDOH, box K-229, folder: "Lead Poisoning."
33. David Sencer to Stanley Brezenoff, September 4, 1984, NYCDOH, box K-247, folder: "Lead Poisoning."
34. Tom Kaiser to Mike Bogdan, March 8, 1984, NYCDOH, box K-247, folder: "Lead Poisoning."
35. David Sencer to Stanley Brezenoff, August 23, 1985, NYCDOH, box K-144, folder: "August."
36. Stephen Joseph to Harrison Goldin, March 17, 1988, NYCDOH, box K-085, folder: "March Outgoing."
37. Coalition to End Lead Poisoning to Stanley Brezenoff, February 21, 1989, NYCDOH, box K-220, folder: "March 89."
38. Stephen Joseph to Stanley Brezenoff, April 12, 1989, NYCDPH, box K-220, folder: "April 89."
39. Brendan Sexton to David Sencer, November 2, 1983, NYCDOH, box K-148, folder: "Welfare Hotels."
40. Tom Kaiser to Mark Rapoport, January 10, 1984, NYCDOH, box K-247, folder: "Lead Poisoning"; David Sencer to Nathan Leventhal, November 1, 1983, NYCDOH, box K-245, folder: "Welfare Hotels."
41. Alperstein, Rappaport, and Flanigan (1988).
42. Brendan Sexton to David Sencer, November 2, 1983, NYCDOH, box K-148, folder: "Welfare Hotels."
43. Mark Rapoport interview; Barbara Basler, "Lead Hazards Are Cited in Shelter for Homeless," *New York Times*, March 11, 1986, B3; Ronald Smothers, "Shelter Paint Hazards Confirmed," *New York Times*, March 22, 1986, 30.
44. Robert O. Boorstin, "Families' Relocation Ordered at Shelter with Paint Hazard," *New York Times*, April 18, 1986, D19; "Shelter Is Allowed to Reopen," *New York Times*, August 31, 1986, A47.
45. Mark Rapoport interview.
46. Kenneth R. Daniel to Mark Rapoport, August 19, 1988, MCDOH, Box K.088, Folder : August Outgoing.
47. Inciardi (1987).
48. Chiasson et al. (1991); Edlin et al. (1994); Peter Kerr, "Syphilis Surge with Crack Use Raises Fears on Spread of AIDS," *New York Times*, June 29, 1988, B1.
49. Chavkin (1990).

50. Chavkin, Driver, and Forman (1989).
51. Bateman et al. (1993).
52. Chavkin and Kandall (1990).
53. Chavkin, Driver, and Forman (1989).
54. Hegarty et al. (1988).
55. Kelly Henning to Stephen Schultz, February 9, 1989, NYCDOH, box K-109; Karen Benker, "Basic Barracks for Lost Babies," *Newsday*, February 28, 1989, 60.
56. Ellen Rautenberg to Distribution, September 15, 1985, NYCDOH, box K-199, folder: "AIDS Sept 85."
57. Rowe and Ryan (1988).
58. Joseph (1988).
59. Joseph (1988); Joseph (1992), 44–45.
60. Stephen Joseph to Edward Koch, August 22, 1986, NYCDOH, box K-114.
61. Clifford (1992).
62. Joseph (1992), 44–45.
63. Joseph (1988).
64. Ellen Rautenberg to Distribution, September 15, 1985, NYCDOH, box K-199, folder: "AIDS Sept 85."
65. Brandt (1987).
66. Jane Gross, "Explicit AIDS Ads Expected to Spark Debate in New York," *New York Times*, May 11, 1987, B1.
67. James Barron, "Media Executives Hesitant to Run Explicit AIDS Ads," *New York Times*, May 12, 1987, B3.
68. Crimp (1987).
69. Crimp (1987).
70. Mark Rapoport to Stephen Joseph, April 25, 1988, NYCDOH, box K-097, folder: "AIDS."
71. James Barron, "In Condom Ads, Focus Is on Women," *New York Times*, June 3, 1987, C1.
72. Des Jarlais and Friedman (1987); Thomas, Williams, and Chiasson (1988).
73. Epstein (1996), 49–50.
74. Stoneburner et al. (1988).
75. Ronald Sullivan, "In City, AIDS Affecting Drug Users More Often," *New York Times*, October 21, 1984, 42.
76. Shilts (1987), 261.
77. Joseph (1992), 121.
78. "Blacks Are Dying from AIDS, Too," *The City Sun*, April 21–27, 1985, 5.
79. Chambre (2006), 79–81.
80. Bateman (1991).
81. Cohen (1999), 96.
82. Dalton (1989).
83. Cited in Quimby and Friedman (1989).
84. Friedman, Sotheran, et al. (1987).
85. Quimby and Friedman (1989).
86. See, for example, Dalton (1989).
87. Ravinia Hayes-Cozier interview; Freudenberg, Lee, and Silver (1989); Freudenberg and Trinidad (1992).

88. Michelle Mindlin to Nancy Bridger, September 21, 1987, NYCDOH, box K-063, folder: "October."

89. Oppenheimer (1992).

90. Musto (1999).

91. David Sencer to William Siroty, March 14, 1985, NYCDOH, box K-144, folder: "March."

92. Friedman, Des Jarlais, et al. (1987).

93. Des Jarlais, Friedman, and Hopkins (1985).

94. David Sencer interview.

95. David J. Sencer to Edward I. Koch, August 13, 1985, NYCDOH, box K-144, folder: "August."

96. Ron Morrison to Jeffrey Friedlander, September 23, 1985, NYCDOH, box K-199, folder: "AIDS Sept 85."

97. Sterling Johnson to Edward Koch, September 10, 1985, NYCDOH, box K-134.

98. "Choosing Between Two Killers," New York Times, September 15, 1985, E20.

99. "Eyes on the Needle," Staten Island Advance, September 10, 1985, 10.

100. Noach Dear to David Sencer, September 9, 1985, NYCDOH, box K-199, folder: "Sept 85."

101. Josh Barbanel, "Candidates Trade Barbs at Last Mayoral Debate," New York Times, September 6, 1985, B3.

102. Joyce Purnick, "Koch Bars Easing of Syringe Sales in AIDS Fight," New York Times, October 4, 1985.

103. Anderson (1991).

104. Joseph (1992), 193.

105. Edward Koch to Stephen Joseph, July 27, 1987, NYCDOH, box K-067, folder: "May & June 1987."

106. Stephen Joseph to Stephen Schultz, September 5, 1986, NYCDOH, box K-114.

107. Margaret Grossi to Edward Koch, July 31, 1987, NYCDOH, box K-067, folder: "May & June 1987."

108. Stephen Joseph to Paul Dickstein, April 25, 1988, NYCDOH, box K-126, folder: "April 88"; Joseph (1992), 229.

109. Stephen Joseph to Stanley Brezenoff, November 4, 1987, NYCDOH, box K-112.

110. Enoch Williams to Stephen Joseph, April 20, 1989, NYCDOH, box K-112.

111. Joseph (1992), 227.

112. Anderson (1991); Joseph (1992).

113. Gina Kolata, "Black Groups Assail Giving Bleach to Addicts," New York Times, June 17, 1990, 20; Anderson (1991).

114. Stephen Joseph to Stephen Schultz, September 24, 1987, NYCDOH, box K-063, folder: "October" (emphasis in original).

115. Anderson (1991).

116. Stephen Joseph interview.

117. "Fighting AIDS and Addiction: A Start," New York Times, February 5, 1988, A30.

118. "Halt Needle Madness Before It Kills," Daily News, October 6, 1988.

119. Dalton (1989), 219.

120. Bruce Lambert, "The Free-Needle Program Is Under Way and Under Fire," *New York Times*, November 13, 1988, E6.
121. Chambre (2006), 81.
122. Wilbert A. Tatum, "Koch Must Resign," *Amsterdam News*, November 5, 1988, 1.
123. Bruce Lambert, "The Free-Needle Program Is Under Way and Under Fire," *New York Times*, November 13, 1988, E6.
124. See letters to Stephen Joseph from, among others, State Assembly member Catherine Nolan, U.S. representative Thomas Manton, Community Board chair Vincent Arcuri, City Council member Carol Greitzer, State Assembly member Vito Lopez, and State Assembly member Franz Leichter, all in NYCDOH, box K-124, folder: "Officials '88 (anti)."
125. Anderson (1991).
126. Edward Koch to Stephen Joseph, August 15, 1988, NYCDOH, box K-120, folder: "August 88 City Hall Incoming."
127. Joseph (1992); Anderson (1991).
128. Suzanne Daley, "Two Addicts Seek Needles on First Day," *New York Times*, November 8, 1988, B1.
129. "Council Calls for End to Free-Needles Plan," *New York Times*, December 7, 1988, B10.
130. Joseph (1992).
131. Margaret Hamburg to David Dinkins, November 1, 1991, Dinkins Papers, box 13, folder 182.
132. Margaret Hamburg interview; Mireya Navarro, "Needle Swaps to Be Revived to Curb AIDS," *New York Times*, May 14, 1992, A1.
133. Fairchild, Bayer, and Colgrove (2007).
134. Phillip Boffey, "Laws Urged to Protect Identities in AIDS Testing," *New York Times*, February 25, 1987, A18.
135. William F. Buckley Jr., "Identify All the Carriers," *New York Times*, March 18, 1986, A27. In 2005 Buckley wrote that his proposal deserved "reconsideration." William F. Buckley Jr., "Killers at Large: AIDS Carriers and Their Victims," *National Review Online*, February 19, 2005. Available at: http://www.nationalreview.com/buckley/wfb200502191155.asp (accessed July 1, 2009).
136. Bayer (1989), 148–53.
137. Stephen Joseph to Irwin Davison, October 1, 1987, NYCDOH, box K-063, folder: "October"; Joseph (1992); Ronald Sullivan, "Warn AIDS Patients' Partners, Health Official Urges," *New York Times*, October 15, 1987, B1.
138. Stephen Joseph to Edward Koch, January 11, 1988, NYCDOH, box K-068, folder: "January meetings."
139. *Tarasoff v. Regents of the University of California*, 17 Cal.3d 425 (1976).
140. Ronald Sullivan, "Warn AIDS Patients' Partners, Health Official Urges," *New York Times*, October 15, 1987, B1.
141. Joseph (1992), 108–11.
142. On ACT UP, see, inter alia, Chambre (2006), 120–34; Epstein (1996), passim; Cohen (1998); Elbaz (1992); Crimp (1990).
143. Gerry Smith to Stephen Joseph, December 4, 1987, NYCDOH, box K-064, folder: "November Outgoing."

144. Stephen Joseph to Edward Koch, August 3, 1988, NYCDOH, box K-097, folder: "AIDS."

145. "New York City Department of Health, Working Paper, July 1988, Estimate of HIV-Infected New Yorkers," typescript, NYCDOH, box K-097, folder: "AIDS."

146. Stephen Joseph to Stanley Brezenoff, July 18, 1988, NYCDOH, box K-120, folder: "July '88."

147. Richard Dunne to Stephen Joseph, August 18, 1988, NYCDOH, box K-120, folder: "September 88 City Hall Incoming."

148. Mary Ann Chiasson interview.

149. Clifford (1992).

150. Interview with Steve Quester, ACT UP Oral History Project, January 17, 2004. Available at: http://www.actuporalhistory.org/interviews/images/quester.pdf (accessed June 6, 2008); Joseph (1992).

151. Mary Ann Chiasson interview; Isaac Weisfuse interview.

152. Edward Koch to Stephen Joseph, August 8, 1988, NYCDOH, box K-120, folder: "August 88."

153. Bayer (1989), 118–20.

154. Joseph (1992).

155. Ellen Rautenberg interview.

156. Bruce Lambert, "3,000 Assailing Policy on AIDS Ring City Hall," *New York Times*, March 29, 1989, B1.

157. Joseph (1992).

158. Fairchild, Bayer, and Colgrove (2007).

159. Joseph (1992), 185.

160. See letters in NYCDOH, box K-172.

161. "Dr. Joseph and AIDS Testing," *New York Times*, November 16, 1989, A30.

Chapter 6

1. "TB Timebomb," *New York Post*, October 16, 1990, 4. Leo Maker was a pseudonym.

2. Friedman et al. (1996).

3. Reichman (1991).

4. Fairchild, Bayer, and Colgrove (2007).

5. The reasons for the decline in tuberculosis and other infectious diseases in the nineteenth and twentieth centuries remain subject to debate. Historians and demographers disagree about whether targeted public health and medical interventions played a prominent role or whether declines were mostly due to improvements in the standard of living. Thomas McKeown (1979) attributed the decline in tuberculosis mortality to improved nutrition brought about by greater economic well-being rather than to any specific health interventions. For alternative views giving greater weight to public health interventions, see Szreter (1988) and Fairchild and Oppenheimer (1998).

6. Lowell (1956).

7. Duffy (1968), 547–48; New York Tuberculosis and Health Association (1954).

8. Alje Vennema to Margaret Grossi, August 18, 1981, NYCDOH, box 142361, folder: "Tuberculosis Bureau."

9. New York Lung Association (1968).

10. Council of Lung Associations (1980).

11. Alje Vennema to Reinaldo Ferrer, October 19, 1978, NYCDOH, box 142298, folder: "Tuberculosis."

12. Alje Vennema to Margaret Grossi, August 18, 1981, NYCDOH, box 142361, folder: "Tuberculosis Bureau"; Ilene Rubin to David Sencer, January 11, 1982, NYCDOH, box K-227, folder: "Tuberculosis Control"; Ronald Sullivan, "Tuberculosis in City Reported on Rise," *New York Times*, March 3, 1980, B3.

13. "New York City Tuberculosis Program Review," typescript (September 21, 1982), NYCDOH, box 227, folder: "Tuberculosis Control."

14. Mechanic (1990).

15. Alje Vennema, "Tuberculosis Control, an Impending Crisis," typescript, October 19, 1978, NYCDOH, box 142298, folder: "Tuberculosis."

16. Alje Vennema to Ellen Rautenberg, February 18, 1982, NYCDOH, box K-227, folder: Tuberculosis Control."

17. Vennema (1982).

18. New York Lung Association (1981).

19. Bureau of Health Statistics and Analysis (1981).

20. Ilene Rubin to David Sencer, January 11, 1982, NYCDOH, box K-227, folder: "Tuberculosis Control."

21. Council of Lung Associations (1980).

22. Council of Lung Associations (1980).

23. See letters in NYCDOH, box 142271, folder: "Tuberculosis."

24. Charles Felton to Reinaldo Ferrer, July 10, 1978, NYCDOH, box 142298, folder: "Tuberculosis."

25. Robert Garcia to Edward Koch, August 3, 1978, NYCDOH, box 142298, folder: "Tuberculosis. "

26. Norma Miranda to Alje Vennema, December 9, 1980, NYCDOH, box 142361, folder: "Tuberculosis Bureau."

27. Alje Vennema to David Sencer, September 21, 1982, NYCDOH, box K-227, folder: "Tuberculosis Control."

28. "New York City Tuberculosis Program Review," typescript (September 21, 1982), NYCDOH, box K-227, folder: "Tuberculosis Control."

29. Untitled typescript, March 19, 1984, NYCDOH, box K-251, folder: "Tuberculosis Control."

30. Alje Vennema to Margaret Grossi, August 18, 1981, NYCDOH, box 142361, folder: "Tuberculosis Bureau."

31. Ilene Rubin to David Sencer, January 11, 1982, NYCDOH, box K-227, folder: "Tuberculosis Control"; Alje Vennema to Ellen Rautenberg, December 31, 1981, NYCDOH, box K-234, folder: "Mayor's Office of Management and Budget"; Brudney and Dobkin (1991b).

32. David Sencer to Harrison Goldin, June 4, 1982, NYCDOH, box 227, folder: "Tuberculosis Control."

33. Gittler (1994).

34. Stephen C. Joseph to Paul Dickstein, December 3, 1986, NYCDOH, box K-098, folder: "Program Prioritization '86."

35. Edward Koch to Stephen Joseph, October 28, 1987, NYCDOH, box K-064, folder: "November Outgoing."
36. Stephen Joseph to Edward Koch, November 8, 1987, NYCDOH, box K-064, folder: "November Outgoing" (emphasis in original).
37. Chaves, Robins, and Abeles (1961); Lerner (1998).
38. "Tuberculosis, New York City and the Homeless," typescript, March 1987, NYCDOH, box K-061, folder: "July Outgoing."
39. Nardell et al. (1986).
40. Stephen Joseph to Mary Keegan, June 24, 1986, NYCDOH, box K-222, folder: "June 1986."
41. Brudney (1993); Brudney and Dobkin (1991a); City of New York (1988); Stephen Joseph to Edward Koch, November 9, 1987, NYCDOH, box K-098, folder: "November Outgoing."
42. New York Lung Association (1985).
43. Centers for Disease Control and Prevention (1987), 795; Paolo and Nosanchuk (2004).
44. Brudney (1993).
45. Brudney and Dobkin (1991a).
46. William Grinker to Stephen Joseph, July 22, 1987, NYCDOH, box K-062, folder: "August Outgoing"; Stephen Joseph to William Grinker, August 7, 1987; NYCDOH, box K-098, folder: "TB 1987"; William Grinker to Stanley Brezenoff, April 7, 1988, NYCDOH, box K-086, folder: "April Incoming."
47. William Grinker to Stanley Brezenoff, April 7, 1988, NYCDOH, box K-086, folder: "April Incoming."
48. Brudney (1993).
49. Joseph (1993); Constance L. Hays, "Shelter to Aid Homeless Men Who Have TB," *New York Times*, October 24, 1988, B1.
50. Stephen Joseph to Caryn Schwab, August 22, 1988, NYCDOH, box K-120, folder: "August 88 City Hall Outgoing."
51. *Mixon v. Grinker*, 157 Misc.2d 68 (1993).
52. Safyer et al. (1993); *Vega v. Sielaff*, 82 Civ. 6475 (1991).
53. Stephen Joseph to Edward Koch, August 10, 1988, NYCDOH, box K-120, folder: "August 88 City Hall Outgoing."
54. Stanley Brezenoff to Stephen Joseph, April 28, 1988, NYCDOH, box K-126, folder: "May 88 City Hall Outgoing."
55. Stephen Joseph to Stanley Brezenoff, May 9, 1988, NYCDOH, box K-126, folder: "May 88 City Hall Outgoing."
56. "CDC Review of Tuberculosis Control Program," typescript, 13, NYCDOH, box K-068, folder: "January Meetings."
57. Katherine Lobach interview.
58. Susan Alter to Stephen Joseph, April 6, 1987, NYCDOH, box K-041, folder: "May Outgoing."
59. Stanley Michels to Stephen Joseph, November 17, 1987, and Olga Mendez, November 19, 1987, both in NYCDOH, box K-064, folder: "November Outgoing."
60. Edward I. Koch to Stephen Joseph, February 1, 1988, Koch Papers, microfilm 41075, image 878.
61. Brecher and Horton (1993).

62. Dirk Johnson, "A Commissioner Who Knows Strife," *New York Times*, January 20, 1990, A29.
63. Woodrow Myers to Murray Blander, March 22, 1990, NYCDOH, box K-115, folder: "March 1990 Outgoing."
64. Todd S. Purdum, "Dinkins Searches for a Health Chief, but Finds a Dilemma," *New York Times*, January 18, 1990, B1.
65. Bruce Lambert, "Backers Defend Top Contender for Health Post," *New York Times*, January 12, 1990, B4; Bruce Lambert, "Dinkins Again Delays Picking a New Health Commissioner," *New York Times*, January 17, 1990, B6; Todd S. Purdum, "Leading Backers Turn Away from Applicant for Health Post," *New York Times*, January 19, 1990, B1.
66. Woodrow Myers to David Dinkins, January 18, 1990, NYCDOH, box K-105, folder: "January 1990 City Hall Outgoing."
67. Todd S. Purdum, "Dinkins Appoints Health Chief Over Objections of Gay Groups," *New York Times*, January 20, 1990, A1.
68. Woodrow Myers to Distribution, April 17, 1990, NYCDOH, box K-115, folder: "April 1990."
69. Mireya Navarro, "Health Chief Under Fire for Low-Profile Style," *New York Times*, April 9, 1991, B1.
70. Bruce Lambert, "Myers Opposes Needle Projects to Curb AIDS," *New York Times*, April 10, 1990, B4.
71. Woodrow Myers Jr. interview.
72. Woodrow Myers Jr. to David Dinkins, May 19, 1990, NYCDOH, box K-105, folder: "May 1990 Outgoing City Hall."
73. Bruce Lambert, "Health Chief Is Criticized on AIDS Shift," *New York Times*, May 10, 1990, B1.
74. Gina Kolata, "Black Group Assails Giving Bleach to Addicts," *New York Times*, June 17, 1990, 20.
75. Carmen Rivera to Norman Steisel, May 11, 1990, NYCDOH, box K-114.
76. "Transcript of the Stenographic Record (Excerpt) of the Discussion on Calendar Number 641, Held at the Meeting of the Board of Estimate on June 7, 1990," typescript, NYCDOH, box K-105, folder: "June 1990 Incoming City Hall."
77. Bruce Lambert, "The Free-Needle Program Is Under Way and Under Fire," *New York Times*, November 13, 1988, E6; Fairchild and Bayer (1999).
78. Heidi Evans, "Cancer Outrage," *Daily News*, May 6, 1990, 1, 2, 44.
79. This account is drawn from "Report of the Pap Smear Review Panel to the Commissioner of Health, New York City Department of Health, July 13, 1990," typescript, NYCDOH, box K-117, folder: "July 1990."
80. Josh Barbanel, "Health Chief Scolds Agency on Pap Tests," *New York Times*, July 24, 1990, B1.
81. Frieden et al. (1995).
82. Ronald Bogard to Woodrow Myers, November 20, 1990, NYCDOH, box K-108, folder: "November 1990 Incoming."
83. "Health Commissioner Myers Sets the Record Straight on Tuberculosis in New York City," news release, November 15, 1990, NYCDPH, box K-158.
84. Woodrow Myers to Philip Michael, December 5, 1990, NYCDOH, box K-108, folder: "December 1990 Outgoing."

85. J. Emilio Carrillo to Woodrow Myers, January 24, 1991, NYCDOH, box K-158.

86. Josh Barbanel, "Why Did New York Hire 49,000 Workers in 7 Years?" *New York Times*, October 7, 1990, E5.

87. David Dinkins to all agency heads, March 19, 1990, NYCDOH, box K-105, folder: "January 1990"; "Directive to All Heads of Agencies and Departments, October 21, 1990," NYCDOH, box K-108, folder: "November 1990."

88. Woodrow Myers to Philip Michael, April 27, 1990, NYCDOH, box K-115, folder: "April 1990 Outgoing."

89. "Testimony of Woodrow A. Myers, Jr., MD, MBA, Commissioner, New York City Department of Health, Before the Joint Committees of Finance and Health of the New York City Council, May 29, 1991," typescript, NYCDOH, box K-173.

90. Cahill (1991a).

91. Woodrow Myers to David Dinkins, May 28, 1991, NYCDOH, box K-155, folder: "May 1991 Outgoing City Hall."

92. Mireya Navarro, "Departing Health Chief Cites Maze of Problems," *New York Times*, June 10, 1991, B3.

93. Cahill (1991b).

94. Ronald Bogard to Ellen Lovitz, September 6, 1991, NYCDOH, box K-155, folder: "October 1991 Outgoing."

95. Margaret Hamburg to Norman Steisel, June 22, 1991, NYCDOH, box K-155, folder: "June 1991 Incoming City Hall"; Cahill (1991a).

96. Corman and Mocan (2000).

97. Joelle Attinger, "The Decline of New York," *Time*, September 17, 1990, 36–44.

98. Andy Logan, "The Horribles," *The New Yorker*, May 27, 1991, 95–99.

99. Safyer et al. (1993); Robert D. McFadden, "A Drug-Resistant TB Results in Thirteen Deaths in New York Prisons," *New York Times*, November 16, 1991, 1.

100. Centers for Disease Control and Prevention (1991); Coronado et al. (1993).

101. Bloom and Murray (1992).

102. Frieden et al. (1993).

103. Bloch et al. (1994).

104. U.S. Congress (1991).

105. U.S. Congress (1954), 5.

106. U.S. Congress (1991), 27.

107. Thomas Frieden interview.

108. Nivin et al. (1998).

109. Edlin et al. (1992).

110. United Hospital Fund of New York (1992).

111. Nivin et al. (1998).

112. Thomas Frieden interview.

113. Ronald Sullivan, "Federal Judge Orders Rush on Prison Tuberculosis Unit," *New York Times*, January 25, 1992, 9; Coker (2000), 97.

114. Frieden et al. (1995), 232.

115. Coker (2000), 94–95; Thomas Frieden interview.
116. Sbarbaro (1979), 751.
117. Bayer and Wilkinson (1995).
118. Chaulk et al. (1995).
119. Pablos-Mendez et al. (1997).
120. Rothman (1995), 191–92, and passim.
121. Lerner (1998).
122. *Greene v. Edwards*, 263 S.E.2d 661 (1980).
123. Markovitz and Goodman (1994); Ball and Barnes (1994).
124. Ball and Barnes (1994).
125. Bayer and Dupuis (1995).
126. Mark Barnes interview.
127. Thomas Frieden interview.
128. Coker (2000), 102.
129. Coker (2000), 102.
130. Coker (2000), 102–3.
131. Mark Barnes interview.
132. As cited in Coker (2000), 108.
133. Markovitz and Goodman (1994).
134. New York City Health Code, §11.47(f)(1)(iii), as cited in Ball and Barnes (1994, emphasis added).
135. Frieden et al. (1995), 231.
136. Fujiwara, Larkin, and Frieden (1997).
137. Fujiwara, Larkin, and Frieden (1997).
138. Thomas Frieden interview.
139. Mireya Navarro, "Confining Tuberculosis Patients: Weighing Rights vs. Health Risks," *New York Times*, November 21, 1993, 1.
140. Coker (2000), 100; Gasner et al. (1999).
141. Gasner et al. (1999).
142. Dan Ruggiero to Sharol Riley, June 8, 1984, NYCDOH, box K-251, folder: "Tuberculosis Control."
143. Gasner et al. (1999).
144. Thomas Frieden interview.
145. Thomas Frieden interview.
146. Frieden et al. (1995).
147. Frieden et al. (1995); Fujiwara, Larkin, and Frieden (1997).
148. Coker (2000), 136–39; Fiscal Policy Institute (2008); Coalition for the Homeless (2008).
149. Aaron Chaves to Harold Fuerst, November 22, 1967, NYCDOH, box 142273, folder: "10-Year Plan."
150. Michael Specter, "Tougher Measures to Fight TB Urged by New York Panel," *New York Times*, November 30, 1992, A1.

Chapter 7

1. This account of the West Nile virus outbreak and the city's responses in the fall of 1999 is drawn from the following sources: Marcelle Layton interview;

Sandra Mullin interview; Neal Cohen interview; Nash et al. (2001); Fine and Layton (2001); Asnis et al. (2002); Mullin (2003); Asnis et al. (2001); and articles in the *New York Times*, *New York Post*, and *New York Daily News*, September 4–October 31, 1999.

2. See, for example, Stephenson (1996); Garrett (1995); Preston (1995).
3. Margaret Hamburg interview; Hamburg (1998); Layton (2004).
4. Steven Lee Myers, "Aides Say Giuliani Plans to Cut 14,000 to 18,000 Jobs by 1995," *New York Times*, January 29, 1994, 1.
5. Giuliani (1996), 63, 65.
6. Lawrence K. Altman, "Plans Drawn to Help Fight Poison Attack," *New York Times*, March 26, 1995, 9.
7. Kit R. Roane, "It's Only a Test: City Agencies Practice Responding to Attacks by Terrorists," *New York Times*, November 9, 1997, 39.
8. Neal Cohen interview.
9. Somini Sengupta, "Giuliani Calls for a Merger of Two Agencies," *New York Times*, January 15, 1998, B5.
10. "The Queens of Nile Denial," *New York Post*, October 1, 1999, 34.
11. Lopez (2002); Lopez and Miller (2002).
12. *No Spray Coalition v. City of New York*, 2000 U.S.Dist. LEXIS 13919 (2000).
13. See the No Spray Coalition website at: http://www.nospray.org/index.shtml (accessed April 30, 2010).
14. Lopez and Miller (2002).
15. Centers for Disease Control and Prevention (2000).
16. Neal Cohen interview; Isaac Weisfuse interview; Sandra Mullin interview; Centers for Disease Control and Prevention (2001a).
17. Neal Cohen interview; Richard Pérez-Peña, "Trying to Command an Emergency When the Emergency Command Center Is Gone," *New York Times*, September 12, 2001, A7.
18. Rosner and Markowitz (2006).
19. Sandra Mullin interview.
20. Cole (2003).
21. Centers for Disease Control and Prevention (2001a); Lucette Lagnado, "It's Trying Time for Health Chief in New York City," *Wall Street Journal*, October 21, 2001, B1.
22. Neal Cohen interview; Isaac Weisfuse interview; Centers for Disease Control and Prevention (2001a).
23. Rosner and Markowitz (2006), 14–16.
24. Centers for Disease Control and Prevention (2003).
25. Rosner and Markowitz (2006).
26. Katz (2002); Rosner and Markowitz (2006), 24–30; Sandra Mullin interview.
27. Susan Saulny and Andrew C. Revkin, "EPA Says Air Is Safe, but Public Is Doubtful," *New York Times*, October 6, 2001, B9.
28. Centers for Disease Control and Prevention (2001a).
29. Centers for Disease Control and Prevention (2001a); Neal Cohen interview.
30. Sandra Mullin interview; Rachel Zimmerman and Ron Winslow, "Health Systems on Alert: Emergency Rooms Watch for Symptoms of Biological Attack," *Wall Street Journal*, October 9, 2001, A6.
31. Cole (2003); Centers for Disease Control and Prevention (2001b); Eric Lipton,

"Missteps Cited in Responding to NBC Scare," *New York Times*, October 15, 2001, B1.

32. Cole (2003).

33. Mirta Ojito, "Doctors Are Told to Watch for Symptoms Linked to Biological Attacks," *New York Times*, October 10, 2001, B12; Rachel Zimmerman and Ron Winslow, "Health Systems on Alert: Emergency Rooms Watch for Symptoms of Biological Attack," *Wall Street Journal*, October 9, 2001, A6.

34. Neal Cohen interview; Marcelle Layton interview; Cole (2003).

35. Blank, Moskin, and Zucker (2003); Neal Cohen interview; David Barstow, "Anthrax Found in NBC News Aide," *New York Times*, October 13, 2001, A1.

36. Blank, Muskin, and Zucker (2003).

37. Eric Lipton, "Missteps Cited in Responding to NBC Scare," *New York Times*, October 15, 2001, B1.

38. Cole (2003); Rosner and Markowitz (2006), 16–19; Centers for Disease Control and Prevention (2001c).

39. Dave Goldiner, "Anthrax Scare Hits New York," *New York Daily News*, October 13, 2001, 2; Douglas Wight and Kirsten Danis, "Hosp ERs Swamped as Test Panic Rises," *New York Post*, October 19, 2001, 5.

40. Mullin (2003).

41. Jennifer Steinhauer, "Flu Shots Are Encouraged to Reduce Anthrax Fear," *New York Times*, October 25, 2001, B7.

42. Heller et al. (2002).

43. Neal Cohen interview.

44. Heller et al. (2002).

45. Centers for Disease Control and Prevention (2001d).

46. Centers for Disease Control and Prevention (2001c); Steven Greenhouse and Eric Lipton, "Anthrax Case Shuts a New York Hospital," *New York Times*, October 30, 2001, A1.

47. Holtz et al. (2003).

48. Felton (2002); Frank et al. (2006); New York State Office of Mental Health (2006).

49. Brackbill et al. (2006).

50. Brackbill et al. (2009).

51. New York City Department of Health and Mental Hygiene (2007).

52. Judith Miller, "City and FBI Reach Agreement on Bioterror Investigations," *New York Times*, November 21, 2004, N39.

53. New York City Department of Health and Mental Hygiene, "Notice of Adoption of Amendments to Sections 11.01 and 11.55 of the New York City Health Code." Available at: http://www.nyc.gov/html/doh/downloads/pdf/public/notice-adoption.pdf (accessed January 15, 2004).

54. Cited in Rosner and Markowitz (2006), 56.

55. Centers for Disease Control and Prevention (2005).

56. See, for example, Layton (2004).

57. Avery and Zabriskie-Timmerman (2002).

58. Public Health Association of New York City (2002), 2.

59. Colgrove (2006).

60. Mullin (2003); Jennifer Steinhauer, "Hoping to Set an Example, Mayor Gets Smallpox Vaccination," *New York Times*, February 20, 2003, 4.

Chapter 8

1. Purnick (2009).
2. Michael Hill, "Hopkins Hails Top Donor by Renaming Health School," *Baltimore Sun*, April 23, 2001.
3. Khatri and Frieden (2002).
4. Jennifer Steinhauer, "Commissioner Calls Smoking Public Health Enemy No. 1 and Asks Drug Firms for Ammunition," *New York Times*, February 15, 2002, B1.
5. See, for example, Richard Pérez-Peña, "Health Chief Is a Doctor Comfortable with Orders," *New York Times*, April 30, 2003, B1; Ben Smith, "Meet Mayor's 'Mind-Meld'—Doc Frieden," *New York Observer*, May 2, 2004; Jennifer Steinhauer, "Gladly Taking the Blame for Health in the City," *New York Times*, February 14, 2004, B1.
6. Jim Rutenberg, "While Aides Get Free Hand, Bloomberg Measures Results," *New York Times*, October 18, 2005, A1.
7. Mandavilli (2006).
8. David Sencer to Nathan Leventhal, March 5, 1982, NYCDOH, box K-231, folder: "March."
9. Fielding and Frieden (2004).
10. See Community Health Survey at the New York City Department of Health and Mental Hygiene website. Available at: http://www.nyc.gov/html/doh/html/survey/survey.shtml (accessed February 23, 2010).
11. Gwynn, Garg, and Kerker (2009).
12. Thorpe et al. (2006).
13. As cited in Fairchild et al. (2007), 5.
14. Frieden et al. (2008).
15. Perrott (1945), 21.
16. Brownson and Bright (2004).
17. Foege (1978).
18. Jennifer Steinhauer, "Gladly Taking the Blame for Health in the City," *New York Times*, February 14, 2004, B1.
19. Duffy (1968), 407, 421, 449.
20. Singman et al. (1980).
21. Duffy (1968), 433; "Dr. Hess Resigning City Health Post; Led Aid to Addicts," *New York Times*, September 8, 1965, 48.
22. David Sencer to Lloyd F. Menczer, April 29, 1985, NYCDOH, box K-144, folder: "April"; Stephen Joseph to Paul Dickstein, April 25, 1988, NYCDOH, box K-126, folder: "April 88 City Hall Incoming."
23. Brownson and Bright (2004).
24. Georgeson et al. (2005).
25. Frieden (2004a), 2059.
26. Frieden et al. (2008).
27. Mary Bassett interview.
28. Colgrove and Bayer (2005).
29. New York City Department of Health and Mental Hygiene, "Mayor Bloomberg Addresses the Centers for Disease Control and Prevention's 'The Public's Health and the Law in the Twenty-First Century' Fifth Annual Partner-

ship Conference,'" June 14, 2006. Available at: http://www.nyc.gov/html/doh/html/pr2006/mr203-06.shtml (accessed January 15, 2007).

30. Jennifer Steinhauer, "Commissioner Calls Smoking Public Health Enemy No. 1 and Asks Drug Firms for Ammunition," *New York Times*, February 15, 2002, B1.

31. Brandt (2007).

32. Bayer and Colgrove (2004).

33. Duffy (1968), 434–35, 449; "Smoking Control Program Quarterly Report, January–April 1968," typescript, NYCDOH, box 142032, folder: "Smoking"; "New York Health Unit Links Smoking to City's Lung Cancer Deaths," *Wall Street Journal*, January 2, 1964; Thomas Buckley, "300 Give Up Habit at Smoking Clinic," *New York Times*, January 17, 1964, 14.

34. David Bird, "TV Heroes' Smoking Scored by City Aide," *New York Times*, October 2, 1967, 1; "Entertainers Asked to Open Antismoking Drive," *New York Times*, October 16, 1967, 55.

35. James E. Roper, "The Man Behind the Ban on Cigarette Commercials," *Reader's Digest*, March 1971, 213–18.

36. Bayer and Colgrove (2004).

37. Edward O'Rourke to Donald Fredrickson, January 31, 1968; Stanley Kreutzer to Donald Fredrickson, February 26, 1968; and Donald Fredrickson to Stanley Kreutzer, March 26, 1968, all in NYCDOH, box 142032, folder: "Smoking."

38. Max H. Siegel, "Smoking Is Banned in Supermarkets," *New York Times*, June 21, 1974, 41.

39. Nathanson (1999).

40. Bayer and Colgrove (2004); Nathanson (1999).

41. Nathanson (1999).

42. Jesus Rangel, "Antismoking Bill Prompts Debate," *New York Times*, April 14, 1985, 36.

43. Ed Koch to Bernard Bucove, July 10, 1968, NYCDOH, box 142032, folder: "Smoking."

44. David Sencer to restaurant owner, June 17, 1985, NYCDOH, box K-133, folder: "Legislation"; "Eateries to Have Non-Smoking," *Amsterdam News*, June 29, 1985, 4.

45. Jonathan Friendly, "Koch Calls for Antismoking Law; Terms It Nation's Most Stringent," *New York Times*, March 22, 1986, 1.

46. Nathanson (1999).

47. Stephen Joseph interview.

48. David E. Pitt, "Smoking Curbs Divide Hearings in City Council," *New York Times*, October 29, 1987, B3.

49. Michael Marriott, "New York Council Enacts Tough Law Against Smoking," *New York Times*, December 24, 1987, A1.

50. James Bennet, "Anti-Smoker Presses Shea Billboard Battle," *New York Times*, April 26, 1993, B3; Andrew Jacobs, "Take That, Tobacco! A Crusader Fights On," *New York Times*, August 29, 2002, B2.

51. Clarke et al. (1999).

52. Jonathan P. Hicks, "Tobacco Industry Fights New York over Smoking Bill," *New York Times*, September 26, 1994, A1.

53. Clarke et al. (1999).
54. Clarke et al. (1999).
55. Douglas Martin, "Businesses Face the Facts of Curbs on Smoking," *New York Times*, January 11, 1995, B1.
56. Centers for Disease Control and Prevention (2001e, 2002).
57. Fleenor (2003).
58. Timothy Starks, "A Potent, if Tardy, Ally to Smokers," *New York Sun*, July 5, 2002, 3; Hendrik Hertzberg, "Bloomberg Butts In," *The New Yorker*, September 9, 2002, 77.
59. Michael Cooper, "Bloomberg Seeks Cuts in Spending at Most Agencies," *New York Times*, February 14, 2002, A1.
60. Kessler (1995).
61. Lisa L. Colangelo, "Commish Is Kicking Butts," *New York Daily News*, March 6, 2002, 3.
62. Bayer and Colgrove (2004).
63. Donald T. Fredrickson to Joseph Cimino, November 1, 1973, NYCDOH, box 142283, folder: "Smoking"; Maurice Carroll, "Mayor Discloses Tax Plan for Added $880 Million," *New York Times*, March 10, 1971, 1; Emanuel Perlmutter, "State Plans Stronger Campaign to Curb Cigarette Bootlegging," *New York Times*, September 4, 1972, 19.
64. Michael Cooper, "Cigarettes Up to $7 a Pack with New Tax," *New York Times*, July 1, 2002, B1.
65. Shelley et al. (2007).
66. Sandra Mullin interview.
67. Purnick (2009), 127.
68. Sandra Mullin interview.
69. Chang et al. (2004).
70. Jennifer Steinhauer, "Bloomberg Seeks to Ban Smoking in Every City Restaurant and Bar," *New York Times*, August 9, 2002, A1.
71. Chang et al. (2004).
72. Greg Sargent, "Mayor to Kick Elected Butts on Smoking," *New York Observer*, September 30, 2002, 1.
73. Diane Cardwell, "Antismoking Bill's Chances May Hinge on Personalities," *New York Times*, October 2, 2002, B2; Jennifer Steinhauer, "Fighting Mayor's Proposed Smoking Ban Not on the Basis of Health, but of Economics," *New York Times*, October 10, 2002, B1.
74. Jennifer Steinhauer, "Bloomberg, Heckled, Presses Smoking Curbs," *New York Times*, October 11, 2002, A1.
75. Mostashari et al. (2005).
76. Cited in *NYC CLASH v. City of New York*, 315 F.Supp.2d 461 (2004).
77. See, for example, E. R. Shipp, "Bloomberg Has Taken His Puritanism Too Far," *New York Daily News*, August 13, 2002, 23; Walter Olson, "Nanny Bloomberg," *Wall Street Journal*, October 22, 2002, 43.
78. *New York Post*, December 2, 2002, 1.
79. James M. Odato, "Smoking Foes Move to Clear the Air," *Albany Times-Union*, January 16, 2003, A1; Joel Stashenko, "Smoking Ban Bill Approved by Legislature," Associated Press State and Local Wire, March 26, 2003.

80. See the NYC CLASH website at http://www.nycclash.com (accessed April 2, 2010).

81. *NYC CLASH v. City of New York*, 315 F.Supp.2d 461 (2004), 483.

82. New York City Departments of Finance, Health and Mental Hygiene, and Small Business Services, and New York City Economic Development Corporation, "The State of Smoke-Free New York City: A One-Year Review" (March 2004). Available at: http://www.nyc.gov/html/doh/downloads/pdf/smoke/sfaa-2004report.pdf (accessed April 7, 2010).

83. Miller et al. (2005).

84. New York City Department of Health and Mental Hygiene, "NYC Health Department Distributes over 45,000 Nicotine Patch Kits" (news release), July 13, 2005. Available at: http://www.nyc.gov/html/doh/html/pr/pr073-05.shtml (accessed April 10, 2010).

85. Centers for Disease Control and Prevention (2007); Claire Atkinson, "Missing a Larynx, He's Become the Voice of Anti-Smoking Efforts," *New York Times*, July 17, 2007.

86. Centers for Disease Control and Prevention (2007).

87. Frieden et al. (2005).

88. Gwynn, Garg, and Kerker (2009).

89. Van Wye et al. (2008).

90. Wallach and Rey (2009); Kim, Berger, and Matte (2006).

91. Chamany et al. (2009).

92. Steinbrook (2006).

93. Chamany et al. (2009).

94. Fairchild (2006).

95. Goldman et al. (2008); Krent et al. (2008).

96. Mariner (2007), 123.

97. Fairchild and Alkon (2007).

98. Chamany et al. (2009).

99. Chamany et al. (2009).

100. Nestle and Jacobson (2000).

101. Mary Bassett interview.

102. Guthrie, Lin, and Frazao (2002).

103. Okie (2007); Angell et al. (2009).

104. See, for example, Ascherio et al. (1999).

105. Okie (2007), 2018.

106. Bill Hoffman, "Grease and Desist: City Eateries Told to Upgrade Oils," *New York Post*, August 11, 2005, 2.

107. Angell et al. (2009).

108. McColl (2008).

109. New York City Department of Health and Mental Hygiene, "Notice of Adoption of an Amendment (§81.50) to Article 81 of the New York City Health Code." Available at: http://www.nyc.gov/html/doh/downloads/pdf/public/notice-adoption-hc-art81-50.pdf (accessed April 2, 2010).

110. Farley et al. (2009).

111. Russell Berman, "New Yorkers Like Bloomberg at City Hall, Not the White House," *New York Sun*, July 13, 2006, 4.

112. *New York State Restaurant Association v. New York City Department of Health and Mental Hygiene*, 2004 Slip. Op. 5129OU (2004).

113. Purnick (2009).

114. See, for example, "Fat Chance," *Washington Times*, September 30, 2006, A12; "No Pain, Some Gain," *The Economist*, November 25, 2006, 32; "Trans Fats: Unhealthy, but a Lifestyle Choice," *Globe and Mail*, November 1, 2006, A24.

115. See, for example, John Tierney, "One Cook Too Many," *New York Times*, September 30, 2006, 15; "Fat City," *Investor's Business Daily*, October 3, 2006, A12.

116. New York City Department of Health and Mental Hygiene (2006), 101.

117. New York City Department of Health and Mental Hygiene (2006), 96.

118. New York City Department of Health and Mental Hygiene (2006), 40.

119. New York City Department of Health and Mental Hygiene, "Notice of Adoption of an Amendment (§81.50) to Article 81 of the New York City Health Code." Available at: http://www.nyc.gov/html/doh/downloads/pdf/public/notice-adoption-hc-art81-50.pdf (accessed April 2, 2010).

120. Farley et al. (2009).

121. Mello (2009).

122. Farley et al. (2009).

123. Mello (2009).

124. A Lexis-Nexis search of U.S. newspapers and wires retrieves 8 instances of "epidemic of obesity" or "obesity epidemic" from 1985 through 1989, 23 between 1990 and 1994, 323 from 1995 through 1999, and more than 3,000 (the upper search limit) from 2000 through 2004. These figures must be interpreted cautiously, of course, because the overall number of newspaper articles indexed in the database also increased during those years. In the Proquest Historical Newspapers database, the earliest reference to an "epidemic of obesity" in the United States occurs in a *New York Times* article of August 27, 1973, by health writer Jane Brody.

125. Thomas J. Lueck, "City Plans to Place Sharp Limits on Restaurants' Use of Trans Fats," *New York Times*, September 27, 2006, A1.

126. Silver and Bassett (2008).

127. The White House, "President Obama Appoints Dr. Thomas Frieden as CDC Director" (news release), May 15, 2009. Available at: http://www.whitehouse.gov/the-press-office/president-obama-appoints-dr-thomas-frieden-cdc-director (accessed April 3, 2010). The administration also named Margaret Hamburg, the commissioner from 1991 through 1997 and Frieden's former boss, to serve as the head of the Food and Drug Administration.

128. Frieden (2004b); Richard Pérez-Peña, "City Sets Goals for the Health of New Yorkers," *New York Times*, March 24, 2004, A1.

129. New York City Department of Health and Mental Hygiene, "Mayor Bloomberg Addresses the Centers for Disease Control and Prevention's 'The Public's Health and the Law in the Twenty-First Century' Fifth Annual Partnership Conference," June 14, 2006. Available at: http://www.nyc.gov/html/doh/html/pr2006/mr203-06.shtml (accessed January 20, 2007).

130. Novak (1996).

131. Mary Bassett interview.

132. City of New York (2008).

Conclusion

1. Stephen Joseph interview.
2. Epstein (2003).
3. See, for example, Gordis (1996).
4. Mark Barnes interview.
5. Lynn Silver and Sonia Angell to Thomas Frieden, "For the Attention of the Board of Health," December 6, 2004. Available at: http://www.nyc.gov/html/doh/downloads/pdf/cardio/cardio-transfat-comments-response.pdf (accessed April 2, 2010).
6. On this point, see Nathanson (2007); Stearns and Almeida (2004).
7. Glendon (1991).
8. Farley and Cohen (2005), 235.
9. Wallack and Lawrence (2005).
10. Oliver (2006).
11. Edward I. Koch to Stephen Joseph, December 9, 1988, Koch Papers, microfilm 41076, image 9.
12. Woodrow Myers Jr. interview.
13. Cited in Coker (2000), 85.
14. See, inter alia, Shah (2001); Leavitt (1996); Brandt (1987).
15. Wegman (1977), 913.
16. Henig (1989–1990).
17. Dallek (1999), 63.
18. Freeman (2000).
19. Kirtzman (2001).
20. Sommer (1995), 657.
21. McGinnis, Williams-Russo, and Knickman (2002).
22. See, inter alia, Wilkinson and Marmot (2003); Marmot (2004); Davey Smith, Dorling, and Shaw (2001); Daniels, Kennedy, and Kawachi (2000).
23. McCord and Freeman (1990).
24. Karpati et al. (2004).
25. For contrasting views on this issue, see, for example, Krieger (1994) and Rothman, Adami, and Tichopoulos (1998).
26. Schlesinger (1967).

References

Archival Sources

LaGuardia and Wagner Archives, LaGuardia Community College, City University of New York

Abraham Beame Collection

Edward I. Koch Collection

ACT UP Oral History Project (http://www.actuporalhistory.org/)

Columbia University Oral History Research Office

Koch Administration Oral History Project

Municipal Archives, New York City Department of Records and Information Services

New York City Department of Health Papers (NYCDOH)

David Dinkins Papers

Sophia Smith Collection, Smith College

Population and Reproductive Health Oral History Project

Author Interviews

Mark Barnes, March 31, 2005, New York, N.Y.

Mary Bassett, April 23 and 29, 2010, New York, N.Y.

Eleanor Bell, May 12, 2005, New York, N.Y.

Patricia Caruso, October 11, 2005, Fort Lee, N.J.

Wendy Chavkin, April 11, 2005, New York, N.Y.

Mary Ann Chiasson, July 18, 2005, New York, N.Y.

Joseph Cimino, August 22, 2005, Valhalla, N.Y.

Neal Cohen, March 10, 2005, New York, N.Y.

Irwin Davison, August 2, 2005, New York, N.Y.

Jack Elinson, September 9, 2005, New York, N.Y.

Yehudi Felman, May 5, 2005, New York, N.Y.

Thomas Frieden, October 28, 2005, New York, N.Y.

Stephen Friedman, March 21, 2005, New York, N.Y.

Marvin Gewirtz, September 15, 2005, New York, N.Y.

Frank Grad, November 9, 2005, New York, N.Y.

Margaret Grossi, August 16, 2005, New York, N.Y.

Margaret Hamburg, March 20, 2006, New York, N.Y.

David Harris, December 6, 2005, New York, N.Y.

Ravinia Hayes-Cozier, July 24, 2009, Washington, D.C. (telephone)

Kelly Henning, February 10, 2005, New York, N.Y.

Pascal James Imperato, March 23, 2005, New York, N.Y.

Stephen Joseph, March 16 and 17, 2005, Santa Fe, N.M.

Alan Kristal, August 4, 2009, Seattle, Wa. (telephone)

Marcelle Layton, February 18 and March 9, 2005, New York, N.Y.

Peter Levin, October 20, 2005, New York, N.Y.

Katherine Lobach, March 11 and 30, 2005, New York, N.Y.

Wilfredo Lopez, February 8, 2006, New York, N.Y.

Ellen Lovitz, September 15, 2005, New York, N.Y.

Ruth Markowitz, August 30, 2005, Mineola, N.Y.

John Marr, October 10, 2005, Richmond, Va.

Mary McLaughlin, February 23, 2005, Manhassat, N.Y.

Sandra Mullin, April 20, 2010, New York, N.Y.

Woodrow Myers Jr., April 28, 2005, New York, N.Y.

Robert Newman, May 3, 2005, New York, N.Y.

Lloyd Novick, July 23 and September 14, 2009, Greenville, N.C. (telephone)

Donna O'Hare, October 12, 2005, New York, N.Y.

Jean Pakter, July 17, 2005, New York, N.Y.

Mark Rapoport, August 24, 2009, Bangkok, Thailand (telephone)

Ellen Rautenberg, April 27, 2005, New York, N.Y.

Lucille Rosenbluth, September 1, 2005, New York, N.Y.

Murray Rosenthal, October 6, 2005, New York, N.Y.

Norman Scherzer, October 28, 2005, New York, N.Y.

David Sencer, March 14, 2005, Atlanta, Ga.

Pauline Thomas, September 2, 2009, Newark, N.J.

Isaac Weisfuse, March 25, 2005, New York, N.Y.

Legal Decisions

Baden v. Koch, 799 F.2d 825 (1986)

City of New York v. New St. Mark's Baths, 497 N.Y.S.2d 979 (1986)

District 27 Community School Board v. Board of Education of the City of New York, 502 N.Y.S.2d 325 (1986)

Greene v. Edwards, 263 S.E.2d 661 (1980)

Griswold v. Connecticut, 381 U.S. 479 (1965)

Mixon v. Grinker, 157 Misc.2d 68 (1993)

New York State Restaurant Association v. New York City Department of Health and Mental Hygiene, 2004 Slip. Op. 5129OU (2004)

No Spray Coalition v. City of New York, 2000 U.S.Dist. LEXIS 13919 (2000)

NYC C.L.A.S.H. v. City of New York, 315 F.Supp.2d 461 (2004)

Robinson v. California, 370 U.S. 660 (1962)

Roe v. Wade, 410 U.S. 113 (1973)

Sorbonne Apartments Co. v. Board of Health of the City of New York, 390 N.Y.S.2d 358 (1976)

Tarasoff v. Regents of the University of California, 17 Cal.3d 425 (1976)

Vega v. Sielaff, 82 Civ. 6475 (1991)

Secondary Sources

Alford, Robert. 1975. *Health Care Politics: Ideological and Interest Group Barriers to Reform.* Chicago: University of Chicago Press.

Alperstein, Garth, Claire Rappaport, and Joan M. Flanigan. 1988. "Health Problems of Homeless Children in New York City." *American Journal of Public Health* 78(9): 1232–33.

Altman, Drew E., and Douglas H. Morgan. 1983. "The Role of State and Local Government in Health." *Health Affairs* 2(4): 7–31.

Anderson, Warwick. 1991. "The New York Needle Trial: The Politics of Public Health in the Age of AIDS." *American Journal of Public Health* 81(11): 1506–17.

Andrews, Kenneth T., and Bob Edwards. 2004. "Advocacy Organizations in the U.S. Political Process." *Annual Review of Sociology* 30: 479–506.

Angell, Sonia Y., Lynn Dee Silver, Gail P. Goldstein, Christine M. Johnson, Deborah R. Deitcher, Thomas R. Frieden, and Mary T. Bassett. 2009. "Cholesterol Control Beyond the Clinic: New York City's Trans Fat Restriction." *Annals of Internal Medicine* 151(2): 129–34.

Ascherio, Alberto, Martijn B. Katan, Peter L. Zock, Meir J. Stampfer, and Walter C. Willett. 1999. "Trans Fatty Acids and Coronary Heart Disease." *New England Journal of Medicine* 340(25): 1994–98.

Asnis, Deborah S., Rick Conetta, Alex A. Teixeira, Glenn Waldman, and Barbara

A. Sampson. 2002. "The West Nile Virus Outbreak of 1999 in New York: The Flushing Hospital Experience." *Clinical Infectious Diseases* 30(5): 413–18.

Asnis, Deborah S., Rick Conetta, Glenn Waldman, and Alex A. Teixeira. 2001. "The West Nile Virus Encephalitis Outbreak in the United States (1999–2000): From Flushing, New York, to Beyond Its Borders." *Annals of the New York Academy of Sciences* 951: 161–71.

Austin, Joe. 2001. *Taking the Train: How Graffiti Art Became an Urban Crisis in New York City.* New York: Columbia University Press.

Avery, George H., and Jennifer Zabriskie-Timmerman. 2002. "The Impact of Federal Bioterrorism Funding Programs on Local Health Department Preparedness Activities." *Evaluation and the Health Professions* 32(2): 95–127.

Ball, Carlos A., and Mark Barnes. 1994. "Public Health and Individual Rights: Tuberculosis Control and Detention Procedures in New York City." *Yale Law and Policy Review* 12(1): 38–67.

Bateman, David A. 1991. "Infant Morbidity in Harlem: A Status Report." *Journal of Health Care for the Poor and Underserved* 2(1): 41–50.

Bateman, David A., Stephen K. C. Ng, Catherine Hansen, and Margaret C. Heagarty. 1993. "The Effects of Intrauterine Cocaine Exposure in Newborns." *American Journal of Public Health* 83(2): 190–93.

Baumgartner, Leona. 1969. "One Hundred Years of Health: New York City, 1866–1966." *Bulletin of the New York Academy of Medicine* 45(6): 555–86.

Bayer, Ronald. 1978. "Methadone Under Attack: An Analysis of Popular Literature." *Contemporary Drug Problems* 7(fall): 367–400.

———. 1989. *Private Acts, Social Consequences: AIDS and the Politics of Public Health.* New York: Free Press.

———. 1995. "The Dependent Center: The First Decade of the AIDS Epidemic in New York City." In *Hives of Sickness: Public Health and Epidemics in New York City*, edited by David Rosner. New Brunswick, N.J.: Rutgers University Press.

Bayer, Ronald, and James Colgrove. 2004. "Children and Bystanders First: The Ethics and Politics of Tobacco Control in the United States." In *Unfiltered: Conflicts over Tobacco Policy and Public Health*, edited by Eric A. Feldman and Ronald Bayer. Cambridge, Mass.: Harvard University Press.

Bayer, Ronald, and Lawrence Dupuis. 1995. "Tuberculosis, Public Health, and Civil Liberties." *Annual Review of Public Health* 16: 307–26.

Bayer, Ronald, and Gerald Oppenheimer. 2000. *AIDS Doctors: Voices from the Epidemic.* New York: Oxford University Press.

Bayer, Ronald, and David Wilkinson. 1995. "Directly Observed Therapy for Tuberculosis: History of an Idea." *The Lancet* 345(8964): 1545–48.

Bellin, Lowell E. 1969. "*Realpolitik* in the Health Care Arena: Standard Setting of Professional Services." *American Journal of Public Health* 59(5): 820–25.

———. 1977. "Local Health Departments: A Prescription Against Obsolescence." *Proceedings of the Academy of Political Science* 32(3): 42–52.

Bellin, Lowell E., and Florence Kavaler. 1970. "Policing Publicly Funded Health Care for Poor Quality, Overutilization, and Fraud—The New York City Medicaid Experience." *American Journal of Public Health* 60(5): 811–20.

———. 1971. "Medicaid Practitioner Abuses and Excuses Versus Counterstrategy of the New York City Health Department." *American Journal of Public Health* 61(11): 2201–10.

Bellin, Lowell E., Florence Kavaler, and Al Schwarz. 1972. "Phase One of Consumer Participation in Policies of Twenty-two Voluntary Hospitals in New York City." *American Journal of Public Health* 62(10): 1370–78.

Bergner, Lawrence, Shirley Mayer, and David Harris. 1971. "Falls from Heights: A Childhood Epidemic in an Urban Area." *American Journal of Public Health* 61(1): 90–96.

Berkowitz, Richard. 2003. *Stayin' Alive: The Invention of Safe Sex*. Cambridge, Mass.: Westview Press.

Berney, Barbara. 1993. "Round and Round It Goes: The Epidemiology of Childhood Lead Poisoning, 1950–1990." *Milbank Quarterly* 71(1): 3–39.

Bernstein, Betty J. 1970. "Public Health—Inside or Outside the Mainstream of the Political Process? Lessons from the Passage of Medicaid." *American Journal of Public Health* 60(9): 1690–1700.

———. 1971. "What Happened to 'Ghetto Medicine' in New York State?" *American Journal of Public Health* 61(7): 1287–93.

Biggs, Hermann. 1897. *Preventive Medicine in the City of New York*. New York: Health Department.

Blank, Susan, Linda C. Moskin, and Jane R. Zucker. 2003. "An Ounce of Prevention Is a Ton of Work: Mass Antibiotic Prophylaxis for Anthrax, New York City, 2001." *Emerging Infectious Diseases* 9(6): 615–22.

Blanksma, Larry A., Henrietta K. Sachs, Edward F. Murray, and Morgan J. O'Connell. 1969. "Incidence of High Blood Lead Levels in Chicago Children." *Pediatrics* 44(5): 661–67.

Bloch, Alan B., George M. Cauthen, Ida M. Onorato, Kenneth G. Dansbury, Gloria D. Kelly, Cynthia R. Driver, and Dixie E. Snider, Jr. 1994. "Nationwide Survey of Drug-Resistant Tuberculosis in the United States." *Journal of the American Medical Association* 271(9): 665–71.

Bloom, Barry R., and Christopher J. L. Murray. 1992. "Tuberculosis: Commentary on a Reemergent Killer." *Science* 257(5073): 1055–64.

Bluestone, Naomi. 1976. "The Role of the Public Agency in the Control of Hypertension." *Bulletin of the New York Academy of Medicine* 52(6): 724–31.

Blum, John Morton. 1991. *Years of Discord: American Politics and Society, 1961–1974*. New York: Norton.

Bornfriend, A. O. 1969. "Political Parties and Pressure Groups." In *Governing the City: Challenges and Options for New York*, edited by Robert H. Connery and Demetrios Caraley. New York: Academy of Political Science.

Brackbill, Robert M., James L. Hadler, Laura DiGrande, Christine C. Ekenga, Mark R. Farfel, Stephen Friedman, Sharon E. Perlman, Steven D. Stellman, Deborah J. Walker, David Wu, Shengchao Yu, and Lorna E. Thorpe. 2009. "Asthma and Posttraumatic Stress Symptoms Five to Six Years Following Exposure to the World Trade Center Terrorist Attack." *Journal of the American Medical Association* 302(5): 502–16.

Brackbill, Robert M., Lorna E. Thorpe, Laura DiGrande, Megan Perrin, James H. Sapp II, David Wu, Sharon Campolucci, and Deborah J. Walker. 2006. "Surveillance for World Trade Center Disaster Health Effects Among Survivors of

Collapsed and Damaged Buildings." *Morbidity and Mortality Weekly Report* 55(SS-2): 1–18.

Brandt, Allan. 1987. *No Magic Bullet: A Social History of Venereal Disease in the United States Since 1880*. New York: Oxford University Press.

———. 2007. *The Cigarette Century: The Rise, Fall, and Deadly Persistence of the Product That Defined America*. New York: Basic Books.

Brandt, Allan, and Martha Gardner. 2000. "Antagonism and Accommodation: Interpreting the Relationship Between Public Health and Medicine in the United States During the Twentieth Century." *American Journal of Public Health* 90(5): 707–15.

Brash, Julian. 2003. "Invoking Fiscal Crisis: Moral Discourse and Politics in New York City." *Social Text* 21(3): 59–83.

Brauer, Carl M. 1982. "Kennedy, Johnson, and the War on Poverty." *Journal of American History* 69(1): 98–119.

Brecher, Charles, and Raymond D. Horton. 1993. *Power Failure: New York City Politics and Policy Since 1960*. New York: Oxford University Press.

Brier, Jennifer. 2006. "'Save Our Kids, Keep AIDS Out': Anti-AIDS Activism and the Legacy of Community Control in Queens, New York." *Journal of Social History* 39(4): 965–87.

Brill, Franklin E. 1966. "The Health Research Council of New York City." *Public Health Reports* 81(1): 17–20.

Brown, Howard J. 1967. "Municipal Hospitals." *Bulletin of the New York Academy of Medicine* 43(6): 450–55.

———. 1968. "Changes in the Delivery of Health Care." *American Journal of Nursing* 68(11): 2362–64.

———. 1976. *Familiar Faces, Hidden Lives: The Story of Homosexual Men in America Today*. New York: Harcourt Brace Jovanovich.

Brown, Lawrence D. 1990. "The New Activism: Federal Health Politics Revisited." *Bulletin of the New York Academy of Medicine* 66(4): 293–318.

———. 1998. "Urban Health Policy." *Journal of Urban Health* 75(2): 273–80.

Brown, Phil. 1987. "Popular Epidemiology: Community Response to Toxic Waste-Induced Disease in Woburn, Massachusetts." *Science, Technology, and Human Values* 12(3–4): 78–85.

Brownson, Ross C., and Frank S. Bright. 2004. "Chronic Disease Control in Public Health Practice: Looking Back and Moving Forward." *Public Health Reports* 119(3): 230–38.

Brudney, Karen. 1993. "Homelessness and TB: A Study in Failure." *Journal of Law, Medicine, and Ethics* 21(3–4): 360–67.

Brudney, Karen, and Jay Dobkin. 1991a. "A Tale of Two Cities: Tuberculosis Control in Nicaragua and New York City." *Seminars in Respiratory Infections* 6(4): 261–72.

———. 1991b. "Resurgent Tuberculosis in New York City: Human Immunodeficiency Virus, Homelessness, and the Decline of Tuberculosis Control Programs." *American Review of Respiratory Disease* 144(4): 745–49.

Bureau of Health Statistics and Analysis. 1981. *Service and Vital Statistics by Health Center Districts, 1980*. New York: New York City Department of Health.

Burlage, Robb. 1968. "The Municipal Hospital Affiliation Plan in New York City." *Milbank Memorial Fund Quarterly* 46(1): 171–201.

Cahill, Kevin. 1991a. "Averting Disaster: A New York City Case Study." In *Imminent Peril: Public Health in a Declining Economy*, edited by Kevin Cahill. New York: Twentieth Century Press.

———, ed. 1991b. *Imminent Peril: Public Health in a Declining Economy.* New York: Twentieth Century Press.

Caiazza, Stephen S. 1985. "Alternative Sites for Screening Blood for Antibodies to AIDS Virus." *New England Journal of Medicine* 313(18): 1158.

Cannato, Vincent. 2001. *The Ungovernable City: John Lindsay and His Struggle to Save New York.* New York: Basic Books.

Caron, Simone. 1998. "Birth Control in the Black Community in the 1960s: Genocide or Power Politics?" *Journal of Social History* 31(3): 545–69.

Centers for Disease Control and Prevention. 1981. "Pneumocystis Pneumonia—Los Angeles." *Morbidity and Mortality Weekly Report* 30(21): 250–52.

———. 1982a. "Persistent, Generalized Lymphadenopathy Among Homosexual Males." *Morbidity and Mortality Weekly Report* 31(19): 249–51.

———. 1982b. "Current Trends Update on Acquired Immune Deficiency Syndrome (AIDS)—United States." *Morbidity and Mortality Weekly Report* 31(37): 513–14.

———. 1987. "Tuberculosis and Acquired Immunodeficiency Syndrome—New York City." *Morbidity and Mortality Weekly Report* 36(48): 785–90.

———. 1991. "Nosocomial Transmission of Multidrug-Resistant Tuberculosis Among HIV-Infected Persons—Florida and New York, 1998–1991." *Morbidity and Mortality Weekly Report* 40(34): 585–91.

———. 2000. "Update: West Nile Virus Activity—Eastern United States, 2000." *Morbidity and Mortality Weekly Report* 49(46): 1044–47.

———. 2001a. "New York City Department of Health Response to Terrorist Attack, September 11, 2001." *Morbidity and Mortality Weekly Report* 50(38): 821–22.

———. 2001b. "Update: Investigation of Anthrax Associated with Intentional Exposure and Interim Public Health Guidelines." *Morbidity and Mortality Weekly Report* 50(41): 889–93.

———. 2001c. "Update: Investigation of Bioterrorism-Related Anthrax and Interim Guidelines for Clinical Evaluation of Persons with Possible Anthrax." *Morbidity and Mortality Weekly Report* 50(43): 941–48.

———. 2001d. "Update: Investigation of Bioterrorism-Related Anthrax and Adverse Events from Antimicrobial Prophylaxis." *Morbidity and Mortality Weekly Report* 50(44): 973–76.

———. 2001e. "Cigarette Smoking in 99 Metropolitan Areas—United States, 2000." *Morbidity and Mortality Weekly Report* 50(49): 1107–13.

———. 2002. "Cigarette Smoking Among Adults—United States, 2000." *Morbidity and Mortality Weekly Report* 51(29): 642–45.

———. 2003. "Potential Exposures to Airborne and Settled Surface Dust in Residential Areas of Lower Manhattan Following the Collapse of the World Trade Center—New York City, November 4–December 11, 2001." *Morbidity and Mortality Weekly Report* 52(7): 131–36.

———. 2005. "Brief Report: Terrorism and Emergency Preparedness in State and Territorial Public Health Departments—United States, 2004." *Morbidity and Mortality Weekly Report* 54(18): 459–60.

Centers for Disease Control and Prevention. 2007. "Decline in Smoking Prevalence—New York City, 2002–2006." *Morbidity and Mortality Weekly Report* 56(24): 604–8.

Chamany, Shadi, Lynn D. Silver, Mary T. Bassett, Cynthia R. Driver, Diana K. Berger, Charlotte E. Neuhaus, Namrata Kumar, and Thomas R. Frieden. 2009. "Tracking Diabetes: New York City's A1C Registry." *Milbank Quarterly* 87(3): 547–70.

Chamberland, Mary E., James R. Allen, James M. Monroe, Nelson Garcia, Carl Morgan, Rebecca Reiss, Harvard Stephens, Juliette Walker, and Stephen M. Friedman. 1985. "Acquired Immunodeficiency Syndrome in New York City: Evaluation of an Active Surveillance System." *Journal of the American Medical Association* 254(3): 383–87.

Chambre, Susan M. 2006. *Fighting for Our Lives: New York's AIDS Community and the Politics of Disease.* New Brunswick, N.J.: Rutgers University Press.

Chang, Christina, Jessica Leighton, Farzad Mostashari, Colin McCord, and Thomas R. Frieden. 2004. "The New York City Smoke-Free Air Act: Second-Hand Smoke as a Worker Health and Safety Issue." *American Journal of Industrial Medicine* 46(2): 188–95.

Chartock, Alan. 1974. "Narcotics Addiction: The Politics of Frustration." *Proceedings of the Academy of Political Science* 31(3): 239–49.

Chaulk, C. Patrick, Kristina Moore-Rice, Rosetta Rizzo, and Richard E. Chaisson. 1995. "Eleven Years of Community-Based Directly Observed Therapy for Tuberculosis." *Journal of the American Medical Association* 274(12): 945–51.

Chaves, Aaron B., Arthur B. Robins, and Hans Abeles. 1961. "Tuberculosis Case Finding Among Homeless Men in New York City." *American Review of Respiratory Disease* 84: 900–901.

Chavkin, Wendy. 1990. "Drug Addiction and Pregnancy: Policy Crossroads." *American Journal of Public Health* 80(4): 483–87.

Chavkin, Wendy, Cynthia R. Driver, and Pat Forman. 1989. "The Crisis in New York City's Perinatal Services." *New York State Journal of Medicine* 89(12): 658–63.

Chavkin, Wendy, and Stephen Kandall. 1990. "Between a 'Rock' and a Hard Place: Perinatal Drug Abuse." *Pediatrics* 85(2): 223–25.

Chavkin, Wendy, Alan Kristal, Cheryl Seaborn, and Pamela E. Guigli. 1987. "The Reproductive Experience of Women Living in Hotels for the Homeless in New York City." *New York State Journal of Medicine* 87(1): 10–13.

Cherkasky, Martin. 1967. "Voluntary Hospitals." *Bulletin of the New York Academy of Medicine* 43(6): 456–62.

Chiasson, Mary Ann, Rand L. Stoneburner, Deborah S. Hildebrandt, William E. Ewing, Edward E. Telzak, and Harold W. Jaffe. 1991. "Heterosexual Transmission of HIV-1 Associated with the Use of Smokable Freebase Cocaine (Crack)." *AIDS* 5: 1121–26.

Chowkwanyun, Merlin. 2010. "Social Justice and Public Health: Community Mobilization and Health Care in New York City, 1961–1975." Oral presentation to the annual meeting of the American Association for the History of Medicine. Rochester, Minn. (May 1).

Christian, Joseph R., Bohdan Celewycz, and Samuel L. Andelman. 1964. "A

Three-Year Study of Lead Poisoning in Chicago." *American Journal of Public Health* 54(8): 1241–45.

City of New York. 1977a. *The Mayor's Management Report*. New York: City of New York (February).

———. 1977b. *The Mayor's Management Report*. New York: City of New York (August).

———. 1978. *The Mayor's Management Report*. New York: City of New York (August).

———. 1979. *The Mayor's Management Report*. New York: City of New York (August).

———. 1980. *The Mayor's Management Report*. New York: City of New York (January).

———. 1983. *The Mayor's Management Report*. New York: City of New York (September).

———. 1988. *The Mayor's Management Report*. New York: City of New York (February).

———. 2008. *The Mayor's Management Report, 2002–2008*. New York: City of New York, Mayor's Office of Operations. Available at: http://www.nyc.gov/html/ops/html/mmr/mmr_archive.shtml (accessed April 2, 2010).

Clarke, Hillary, Michael P. Wilson, K. Michael Cummings, and Andrew Hyland. 1999. "The Campaign to Enact New York City's Smoke-Free Air Act." *Journal of Public Health Management and Practice* 5(1): 1–13.

Clifford, George W. 1992. "The AIDS Epidemic in New York City: The Responses of Community-Based Organizations, Political Action Groups, and Government from 1981 to 1990." Ph.D. diss., State University of New York at Albany.

Coalition for the Homeless. 2008. Briefing paper (December 23). Available at: http://coalitionforthehomelessorg.siteprotect.net/FileLib/PDFs/Briefing%20Paper%20--%20Record%20Number%20of%20NYC%20Homeless%20Families%2012-23-2008.pdf (accessed December 23, 2009).

Cochrane, A. L. 1972. *Effectiveness and Efficiency: Random Reflections on Health Services*. London: Nuffield Provincial Hospitals Trust.

Cohen, Cathy. 1999. *The Boundaries of Blackness: AIDS and the Breakdown of Black Politics*. Chicago: University of Chicago Press.

Cohen, Lizabeth. 2004. *A Consumer's Republic: The Politics of Mass Consumption in Post-War America*. New York: Vintage Books.

Cohen, Peter F. 1998. *Love and Anger: Essays on AIDS, Activism, and Politics*. Binghamton, N.Y.: Haworth Press.

Coker, Richard. 2000. *From Chaos to Coercion: Detention and the Control of Tuberculosis*. New York: St. Martin's Press.

Cole, Leonard. 2003. *The Anthrax Letters: A Medical Detective Story*. Washington: National Academies Press.

Colgrove, James. 2006. *State of Immunity: The Politics of Vaccination in Twentieth-Century America*. Berkeley: University of California Press.

Colgrove, James, and Ronald Bayer. 2005. "Manifold Restraints: Liberty, Public Health, and the Legacy of *Jacobson v. Massachusetts*." *American Journal of Public Health* 95(4): 571–76.

Colgrove, James, Gerald Markowitz, and David Rosner. 2008. *The Contested*

Boundaries of American Public Health, New Brunswick, N.J.: Rutgers University Press.

Colombo, Theodore J., Donald K. Freeborn, John P. Mullooly, and Vicky R. Burnham. 1979. "The Effect of Outreach Workers' Educational Efforts on Disadvantaged Preschool Children's Use of Preventive Services." *American Journal of Public Health* 69(5): 465–68.

Commission on the Delivery of Personal Health Services. 1968. *Comprehensive Community Health Services for New York City.* New York: Commission on the Delivery of Personal Health Services.

Committee on Public Health. 1985. "Statement and Recommendations Concerning the Office of the Chief Medical Examiner." *Bulletin of the New York Academy of Medicine* 61(6): 585–98.

Corman, Hope, and H. Naci Mocan. 2000. "A Time-Series Analysis of Crime, Deterrence, and Drug Abuse in New York City." *American Economic Review* 90(3): 584–604.

Cornely, Paul B. 1971. "The Hidden Enemies of Health and the American Public Health Association." *American Journal of Public Health* 61(1): 7–18.

Coronado, Victor G., Consuelo M. Beck-Sague, Mary D. Hutton, Barry J. Davis, Peter Nicholas, Carmelita Villareal, Charles L. Woodley, James O. Kilburn, Jack T. Crawford, Thomas R. Frieden, Ronda L. Sinkowitz, and William K. Jarvis. 1993. "Transmission of Multidrug-Resistant Mycobacterium Tuberculosis Among Persons with Human Immunodeficiency Virus Infection in an Urban Hospital: Epidemiologic and Restriction Fragment Length Polymorphism Analysis." *Journal of Infectious Diseases* 168: 1052–55.

Council of Lung Associations. 1980. *New Approaches to a Resurging Crisis: Report of the Task Force on Tuberculosis in New York, 1980.* New York: Council of Lung Associations.

Craddock, Susan. 2000. *City of Plagues: Disease, Poverty, and Deviance in San Francisco.* Minneapolis: University of Minnesota Press.

Crimp, Douglas. 1987. "How to Have Promiscuity in an Epidemic." *October* 43 (winter): 237–71.

———. 1990. *AIDS Demo Graphics.* Seattle: Bay Press.

Curran, James. 1983. "AIDS—Two Years Later." *New England Journal of Medicine* 309(10): 609–11.

Dallek, Robert. 1999. *Ronald Reagan: The Politics of Symbolism.* Cambridge, Mass.: Harvard University Press.

Dalton, Harlan. 1989. "AIDS in Blackface." *Daedalus* 118(3): 205–27.

Daniels, Norman, Bruce Kennedy, and Ichiro Kawachi. 2000. *Is Inequality Bad for Our Health?* New York: Beacon Press.

Davey Smith, George, Daniel Dorling, and Mary Shaw. 2001. *Poverty, Inequality, and Health in Britain, 1800–2000: A Reader.* Bristol: Policy Press.

Davis, Karen, and Cathy Schoen. 1978. *Health and the War on Poverty: A Ten-Year Appraisal.* Washington, D.C.: Brookings Institution.

Denerstein, Daniel, Lloyd F. Novick, Regina Lowenstein, and James G. Bianco. 1976. "Converting Child Health Stations to Pediatric Treatment Centers: Utilization Patterns of Children Using Three Upper Manhattan Facilities Offering Treatment Services." *American Journal of Public Health* 66(6): 579–81.

Des Jarlais, Don, and Samuel R. Friedman. 1987. "HIV Infection Among Intravenous Drug Users: Epidemiology and Risk Reduction." *AIDS* 1(2): 67–76.

Des Jarlais, Don, Samuel R. Friedman, and William Hopkins. 1985. "Risk Reduction for Acquired Immunodeficiency Syndrome Among Intravenous Drug Users." *Annals of Internal Medicine* 103(5): 755–59.

Des Jarlais, Don, Denise Paone, and Samuel R. Friedman. 1995. "Regulating Controversial Programs for Unpopular People: Methadone Maintenance and Syringe Exchange Programs." *American Journal of Public Health* 85(11): 1577–84.

Dole, Vincent P., and Marie Nyswander. 1965. "A Medical Treatment for Diacetylmorphine (Heroin) Addiction." *Journal of the American Medical Association* 193(8): 646–50.

———. 1967a. "Rehabilitation of the Street Addict." *Archives of Environmental Health* 14(3): 477–80.

———. 1967b. "Heroin Addiction—A Metabolic Disease." *Archives of Internal Medicine* 120(1): 19–24.

Dole, Vincent P., Marie E. Nyswander, and Mary Jane Kreek. 1966. "Narcotic Blockade—A Medical Technique for Stopping Heroin Use by Addicts." *Transactions of the Association of American Physicians* 79: 122–36.

Dole, Vincent P., Marie E. Nyswander, and Alan Warner. 1968. "Successful Treatment of 750 Criminal Addicts." *Journal of the American Medical Association* 206(12): 2708–11.

Domke, Herbert, and Gladys Coffey. 1966. "The Neighborhood-Based Public Health Worker: Additional Manpower for Community Health Services." *American Journal of Public Health* 56(4): 603–8.

Donovan, Ronald. 1990. *Administering the Taylor Law: Public Employee Relations in New York.* Ithaca, N.Y.: ILR Press.

Drusin, Lewis M., John S. Marr, Eleanor C. Lambertson, and Barbara Topff Olstein. 1977. "The New York City Nurse-Epidemiology Program." *Bulletin of the New York Academy of Medicine* 53(6): 569–85.

Duffy, John. 1968. *A History of Public Health in New York City, 1866–1966.* Vol. 2. New York: Russell Sage Foundation.

———. 1979. "The American Medical Profession and Public Health: From Support to Ambivalence." *Bulletin of the History of Medicine* 53(1): 1–15.

———. 1990. *The Sanitarians: A History of American Public Health.* Urbana: University of Illinois Press.

Edlin, Brian R., Kathleeen L. Irwin, Sairus Faruque, Clyde B. McCoy, Carl Word, Yolanda Serrano, James A. Inciardi, Benjamin P. Bowser, Robert F. Schilling, Scott D. Holmberg, and the Multicenter Crack Cocaine and HIV Infection Study Team. 1994. "Intersecting Epidemics—Crack Cocaine Use and HIV Infection Among Inner-City Young Adults." *New England Journal of Medicine* 331(21): 1422–27.

Edlin, Brian R., Jerome I. Tokars, Michael H. Grieco, Jack T. Crawford, Julie Williams, Emelia M. Sordillo, Kenneth R. Ong, James O. Kilburn, Samuel W. Dooley, Kenneth G. Castro, William R. Jarvis, and Scott D. Holmberg. 1992. "An Outbreak of Multidrug-Resistant Tuberculosis Among Hospitalized Patients with the Acquired Immunodeficiency Syndrome." *New England Journal of Medicine* 326(23): 1514–21.

Eidsvold, Gary, Anthony Mustalish, and Lloyd F. Novick. 1974. "The New York City Department of Health: Lessons in a Lead Poisoning Control Program." *American Journal of Public Health* 64(10): 956–62.

Elbaz, Gilbert. 1992. "The Sociology of AIDS Activism: The Case of ACT UP/ New York, 1987–1992." Ph.D. diss., City University of New York.

Emerson, Haven, and Martha Luginbuhl. 1945. *Local Health Units for the Nation.* New York: Commonwealth Fund.

Ensminger, Barry. 1980. "Political Commitment to Immunization Programs at the Local Level." In U.S. Department of Health, Education, and Welfare, *Fifteenth Immunization Conference Proceedings.* Atlanta: Centers for Disease Control.

Epstein, Richard. 2003. "Let the Shoemaker Stick to His Last: In Defense of the 'Old' Public Health." *Perspectives in Biology and Medicine* 46(3 Suppl): 138–59.

Epstein, Steven. 1996. *Impure Science: AIDS, Activism, and the Politics of Knowledge.* Berkeley: University of California Press.

Etheridge, Elizabeth. 1992. *Sentinel for Health: A History of the Centers for Disease Control.* Berkeley: University of California Press.

Fairchild, Amy L. 2006. "Diabetes and Disease Surveillance." *Science* 313(5784): 175–76.

Fairchild, Amy L., and Ava Alkon. 2007. "Back to the Future? Diabetes, HIV, and the Boundaries of Public Health." *Journal of Health Politics, Policy, and Law* 32(4): 561–93.

Fairchild, Amy L., and Ronald Bayer. 1999. "Uses and Abuses of Tuskegee." *Science* 248(5416): 919–21.

Fairchild, Amy L., Ronald Bayer, and James Colgrove. 2007. *Searching Eyes: Privacy, the State, and Disease Surveillance in America.* Berkeley: University of California Press.

Fairchild, Amy L., and Gerald O. Oppenheimer. 1998. "Public Health Nihilism Versus Pragmatism: History, Politics, and the Control of Tuberculosis." *American Journal of Public Health* 88(7): 1105–17.

Fairchild, Amy L., David Rosner, James Colgrove, Ronald Bayer, and Linda P. Fried. 2010. "The Exodus of Public Health: What History Can Tell Us About Its Future." *American Journal of Public Health* 100(1): 54–63.

Farley, Thomas A., Anna Caffarelli, Mary T. Bassett, Lynn Silver, and Thomas R. Frieden. 2009. "New York City's Fight over Calorie Labeling." *Health Affairs* 28(6): w1098–1109.

Farley, Tom, and Deborah A. Cohen. 2005. *Prescription for a Healthy Nation.* Boston: Beacon Press.

Fauci, Anthony S. 1983. "The Acquired Immune Deficiency Syndrome: The Ever-Broadening Clinical Spectrum." *Journal of the American Medical Association* 249(17): 2375–76.

Fee, Elizabeth. 1988. *Disease and Discovery: A History of the Johns Hopkins School of Hygiene and Public Health, 1916–1939.* Baltimore: Johns Hopkins University Press.

Fee, Elizabeth, and Evelynn M. Hammonds. 1995. "Science, Politics, and the Art of Persuasion: Promoting the New Scientific Medicine in New York City." In *Hives of Sickness: Public Health and Epidemics in New York City,* edited by David Rosner. New Brunswick, N.J.: Rutgers University Press.

Felton, Chip J. 2002. "Project Liberty: A Public Health Response to New Yorkers' Mental Health Needs Arising from the World Trade Center Attacks." *Journal of Urban Health* 79(3): 429–33.

Fielding, Jonathan E., and Thomas R. Frieden. 2004. "Local Knowledge to Enable Local Action." *American Journal of Preventive Medicine* 27(2): 183–84.

Fine, Annie, and Marcelle Layton. 2001. "Lessons from the West Nile Virus Encephalitis Outbreak in New York City, 1999: Implications for Bioterrorism Preparedness." *Clinical Infectious Diseases* 32: 277–82.

Fiscal Policy Institute. 2008. *Pulling Apart in New York: An Analysis of Income Trends in New York State.* New York: Fiscal Policy Institute. Available at: www.fiscalpolicy.org (accessed December 20, 2009).

Fleenor, Patrick. 2003. "Cigarette Taxes, Black Markets, and Crime: Lessons from New York's Fifty-Year Losing Battle." Cato Institute policy analysis 468 (February 6). Available at: http://www.cato.org/pub_display.php?pub_id=1327 (accessed April 6, 2010).

Foege, William H. 1978. "The Changing Priorities of the Center for Disease Control." *Public Health Reports* 93(6): 616–21.

Fox, Daniel M. 1995. "The Politics of Public Health in New York City: Contrasting Styles Since 1920." In *Hives of Sickness: Public Health and Epidemics in New York City,* edited by David Rosner. New Brunswick, N.J.: Rutgers University Press.

Frank, Richard G., Talia Pindyck, Sheila A. Donahue, Elizabeth A. Pease, M. Jameson Foster, Chip J. Felton, and Susan M. Essock. 2006. "Impact of a Media Campaign for Disaster Mental Health Counseling in Post–September 11 New York." *Psychiatric Services* 57(9): 1304–8.

Freeman, Joshua B. 2000. *Working-Class New York: Life and Labor Since World War II.* New York: New Press.

Freudenberg, Nicholas, Jacalyn Lee, and Diana Silver. 1989. "How Black and Latino Community Organizations Respond to the AIDS Epidemic: A Case Study in One New York City Neighborhood." *AIDS Education and Prevention* 1(1): 12–21.

Freudenberg, Nicholas, and Urayoana Trinidad. 1992. "The Role of Community Organizations in AIDS Prevention in Two Latino Communities in New York City." *Health Education Quarterly* 19(2): 219–32.

Frieden, Thomas R. 2004a. "Asleep at the Switch: Local Public Health and Chronic Disease." *American Journal of Public Health* 94(12): 2059–61.

———. 2004b. "Take Care New York: A Focused Health Policy." *Journal of Urban Health* 81(3): 314–16.

Frieden, Thomas R., Mary T. Bassett, Lorna E. Thorpe, and Thomas A. Farley. 2008. "Public Health in New York City, 2002–2007: Confronting Epidemics of the Modern Era." *International Journal of Epidemiology* 37(5): 966–77.

Frieden, Thomas R., Paula I. Fujiwara, Rita M. Washko, and Margaret A. Hamburg. 1995. "Tuberculosis in New York City—Turning the Tide." *New England Journal of Medicine* 333(4): 229–33.

Frieden, Thomas R., Farzad Mostashari, Bonnie D. Kerker, Nancy Miller, Anjum Hajat, and Martin Frankel.. 2005. "Adult Tobacco Use Levels After Intensive Tobacco Control Measures: New York City, 2002–2003." *American Journal of Public Health* 95(6): 1016–23.

Frieden, Thomas R., Timothy Sterling, Ariel Palos-Mendez, James O. Kilburn, George M. Cauther, and Samuel W. Dooley. 1993. "The Emergence of Drug-Resistant Tuberculosis in New York City." *New England Journal of Medicine* 328(8): 521–26.

Friedman, Lloyd, Michael T. Williams, Tejinder P. Singh, and Thomas R. Frieden. 1996. "Tuberculosis, AIDS, and Death Among Substance Users on Welfare in New York City." *New England Journal of Medicine* 334(13): 828–33.

Friedman, Samuel R., Don C. Des Jarlais, Jo L. Sotheran, Jonathan Garber, Henry Cohen, and Donald Smith. 1987. "AIDS and Self Organization Among Intravenous Drug Users." *International Journal of the Addictions* 22(3): 201–20.

Friedman, Samuel R., Jo L. Sotheran, Abu Abdul-Quader, Beny J. Primm, Don C. Des Jarlais, Paula Kleinman, Conrad Maugé, Douglas S. Goldsith, Wafaa El-Sadr, and Robert Maslansky. 1987. "The AIDS Epidemic Among Blacks and Hispanics." *Milbank Quarterly* 65(2 Suppl): 455–99.

Fuchs, Victor R. 1983. *Who Shall Live? Health, Economics, and Social Choice.* New York: Basic Books.

Fujiwara, Paula, Christine Larkin, and Thomas R. Frieden. 1997. "Directly Observed Therapy in New York City: History, Implementation, Results, and Challenges." *Clinics in Chest Medicine* 18(1): 135–48.

Galishoff, Stuart. 1975. *Safeguarding the Public Health: Newark, 1895–1918.* Westport, Conn.: Greenwood.

Garrett, Charles. 1961. *The La Guardia Years: Machine and Reform Politics in New York City.* New Brunswick, N.J.: Rutgers University Press.

Garrett, Laurie. 1995. *The Coming Plague.* New York: Penguin Books.

Gasner, M. Rose, Khin Lay Maw, Gabriel E. Feldman, Paula I. Fujiwara, and Thomas R. Frieden. 1999. "The Use of Legal Action in New York City to Ensure Treatment of Tuberculosis." *New England Journal of Medicine* 340(5): 359–66.

Georgeson, Mari, Lorna E. Thorpe, Mario Merlino, Thomas R. Frieden, Jonathan E. Fielding, and the Big Cities Health Coalition. 2005. "Shortchanged? An Assessment of Chronic Disease Programming in Major U.S. City Health Departments." *Journal of Urban Health* 82(2): 183–90.

Ginzberg, Eli. 1971. *Urban Health Services: The Case of New York.* New York: Columbia University Press.

Gittler, Josephine. 1994. "Controlling Resurgent Tuberculosis: Public Health Agencies, Public Policy, and the Law." *Journal of Health Politics, Policy and Law* 19(1): 107–47.

Giuliani, Rudolph. 1996. "The Role of Government in Combating Urban Health Problems." *Bulletin of the New York Academy of Medicine* 73(1): 60–69.

Glaser, Edward L., and Matthew E. Kahn. 1999. "From John Lindsay to Rudy Giuliani: The Decline of the Local Safety Net?" *Federal Reserve Bank of New York Economic Policy Review* 1999(September): 117–32.

Glendon, Mary Ann. 1991. *Rights Talk: The Impoverishment of Political Discourse.* New York: Free Press.

Goldman, Janlori, Sydney Kinnear, Jeannie Chung, and David J. Rothman. 2008. "New York City's Initiatives on Diabetes and HIV/AIDS: Implications for Patient Care, Public Health, and Medical Professionalism." *American Journal of Public Health* 98(5): 807–13.

Gordis, Leon. 1996. *Epidemiology.* Philadelphia: W. B. Saunders.

Gordon, Diana R. 1973. *City Limits: Barriers to Change in Urban Government.* New York: Charterhouse.

Gordon, Jeoffrey B. 1969. "The Politics of Community Medicine Projects: A Conflict Analysis." *Medical Care* 7(6): 419–28.

Greenberg, Morris, Harold Jacobziner, Mary C. McLaughlin, Harold T. Fuerst, and Ottavio Pellitteri. 1958. "A Study of Pica in Relation to Lead Poisoning." *Pediatrics* 22(4): 756–60.

Gross, Larry P. 2002. *Up from Invisibility: Lesbians, Gay Men, and the Media in America.* New York: Columbia University Press.

Guinan, Mary E., Pauline A. Thomas, Paul F. Pinsky, James T. Goodrich, Richard M. Selik, Harold W. Jaffe, Harry W. Haverkos, Gary Noble, and James W. Curran. 1984. "Heterosexual and Homosexual Patients with the Acquired Immune Deficiency Syndrome." *Annals of Internal Medicine* 100(2): 213–18.

Gusfield, Joseph. 1981. *The Culture of Public Problems: Drinking-Driving and the Symbolic Order.* Chicago: University of Chicago Press.

Guthrie, Joanne F., Biing-Hwan Lin, and Elizabeth Frazao. 2002. "Role of Food Prepared Away from Home in the American Diet, 1977–1978 Versus 1994–1996: Changes and Consequences." *Journal of Nutrition Education and Behavior* 34(3): 140–50.

Guttman, Nurit, and Charles T. Salmon. 2004. "Guilt, Fear, Stigma, and Knowledge Gaps: Ethical Issues in Public Health Communication Interventions." *Bioethics* 18(6): 531–52.

Gwynn, R. Charon, Renu K. Garg, and Bonnie D. Kerker. 2009. "Contributions of a Local Health Examination Survey to the Surveillance of Chronic and Infectious Diseases in New York City." *American Journal of Public Health* 99(1): 152–59.

Hamburg, Margaret. 1998. "Emerging and Resurgent Pathogens in New York City." *Journal of Urban Health* 75(3): 471–79.

Hammonds, Evelynn Maxine. 1999. *Childhood's Deadly Scourge: The Campaign to Control Diphtheria in New York City, 1880–1930.* Baltimore: Johns Hopkins University Press.

Hanlon, John J. 1973. "Is There a Future for Local Health Departments?" *Health Services Reports* 88(10): 898–901.

Harris, David, Donna O'Hare, Jean Pakter, and Frieda G. Nelson. 1973. "Legal Abortion 1970–1971—The New York City Experience." *American Journal of Public Health* 63(5): 409–18.

Hatch, Orrin. 1982. "Health and the New Federalism." In *Local Public Health Programs.* Washington, D.C.: United States Conference of Mayors (December).

Hegarty, James D., Elaine J. Abrams, Vincent E. Hutchinson, Stephen W. Nicholas, Maria S. Suarez, and Margaret C. Heagarty. 1988. "The Medical Care Costs of Human Immunodeficiency Virus–Infected Children in Harlem." *Journal of the American Medical Association* 260(13): 1901–5.

Heller, Michael B., Michel L. Bunning, Martin E. B. France, Debra M. Niemeyer, Leonard Peruski, Tim Naimi, Phillip M. Talboy, Patrick H. Murray, Harald W. Pietz, John Kornblum, William Oleszko, Sara T. Beatrice, Joint Microbiological Rapid Response Team, and New York City Anthrax Investigation Working Group. 2002. "Laboratory Response to Anthrax Bioterrorism, New York City, 2001." *Emerging Infectious Diseases* 8(10): 1096–1102.

Henig, Jeffrey R. 1989–1990. "Privatization in the United States: Theory and Practice." *Political Science Quarterly* 104(4): 649–70.

Hirsch, Dan Alan, and Roger Enlow. 1984. "The Effects of Acquired Immune Deficiency Syndrome on Gay Lifestyle and the Gay Individual." *Annals of the New York Academy of Sciences* 437: 273–82.

Hollister, Robert M., Bernard M. Kramer, and Seymour S. Bellin. 1974. *Neighborhood Health Centers.* Lexington, Mass.: Lexington Books.

Holtz, Timothy H., Joel Ackelsberg, Jacob L. Kool, Richard Rosselli, Anthony Marfin, Thomas Matte, Sara T. Beatrice, Michael B. Heller, Dan Hewett, Linda C. Moskin, Michel L. Bunning, Marcelle Layton, and the New York City Anthrax Investigation Working Group. 2003. "Isolated Case of Bioterrorism-Related Inhalational Anthrax, New York City, 2001." *Emerging Infectious Diseases* 9(6): 689–96.

Hopper, Kim. 1990. "The New Urban Niche of Homelessness: New York City in the Late 1980s." *Bulletin of the New York Academy of Medicine* 66(5): 435–50.

Horton, Raymond Daniel. 1971. "The Municipal Labor Relations System in New York City: 1954–1970." Ph.D. diss., Columbia University.

Hyman, Herbert. 1973. "The Unfulfilled Health Hopes in New York City." in *The Politics of Health Care: Nine Case Studies of Innovative Planning in New York City*, edited by Herbert Hyman. New York: Praeger.

Illich, Ivan. 1976. *Medical Nemesis: The Expropriation of Health.* New York: Pantheon Books.

Imperato, Pascal James. 1978. "The Effect of New York City's Fiscal Crisis on the Department of Health." *Bulletin of the New York Academy of Medicine* 54(3): 276–89.

———. 1979. "Current Problems of Some New York City Health Agencies." *Bulletin of the New York Academy of Medicine* 55(5): 463–76.

———. 1983. *The Administration of a Public Health Agency: A Case Study of the New York City Department of Health.* New York: Human Sciences Press.

Inciardi, James A. 1987. "Beyond Cocaine: Basuco, Crack, and Other Coca Products." *Contemporary Drug Problems* 14(3): 461–91.

Institute of Medicine. 1988. *The Future of Public Health.* Washington, D.C.: National Academies Press.

———. 1995. *Federal Regulation of Methadone Treatment.* Washington, D.C.: National Academies Press.

———. 2003. *The Future of the Public's Health in the Twenty-First Century.* Washington, D.C.: National Academies Press.

Jackson, Kenneth T. 1985. *Crabgrass Frontier: The Suburbanization of the United States.* New York: Oxford University Press.

Jacobziner, Harold. 1965. "A Pediatric Treatment Clinic in a Health Department." *Bulletin of the New York Academy of Medicine* 41(1): 107–116.

———. 1966. "Lead Poisoning in Childhood: Epidemiology, Manifestations, and Prevention." *Clinical Pediatrics* 5(5): 277–86.

Jacobziner, Harold, and H. W. Raybin. 1958. "Lead Poisoning in Infancy and Young Children." *New York State Journal of Medicine* 58(6): 897–99.

Jaffe, Harold W., Keehwan Choi, Pauline A. Thomas, Harry W. Haverkos, David M. Auerbach, Mary E. Guinan, Martha F. Rogers, Thomas J. Spira, William W. Darrow, Mark A. Kramer, Stephen J. Friedman, James M. Monroe, Alvin E. Friedman-Kien, Linda J. Laubnstein, Michael Marmor, Bijan Safai, Selma K. Dritz, Salvatore J. Crispi, and Shirley L. Fannin. 1983. "National Case Control Study of Kaposi's Sarcoma and *Pneumocystis carinii* Pneumonia in Homosexual Men: Part 1, Epidemiologic Results." *Annals of Internal Medicine* 99(2): 145–51.

James, George. 1966. "Family Planning and the Department of Health of the City of New York." *Bulletin of the New York Academy of Medicine* 42(1): 54–60.

Johnson, Ralph J. 1952. "Health Departments and the Housing Problem." *Public Health Reports* 67(1): 65–72.

Jonas, Steven. 1977a. *Quality Control of Ambulatory Care: A Task for Health Departments*. New York: Springer.

———. 1977b. "Organized Ambulatory Services and the Enforcement of Health Care Quality Standards in New York State." In *The Impact of National Health Insurance on New York*, edited by Marvin Lieberman. New York: Prodist.

Jones, Marian Moser. 2005. *Protecting Public Health in New York City: Two Hundred Years of Leadership*. New York: Department of Health and Mental Hygiene.

Joseph, Stephen C. 1988. "Current Issues Concerning AIDS in New York City." *New York State Journal of Medicine* 88(5): 253–58.

———. 1992. *Dragon Within the Gates: The Once and Future AIDS Epidemic*. New York: Carroll & Graf.

———. 1993. "New York City, Tuberculosis, and the Public Health Infrastructure." *Journal of Law, Medicine, and Ethics* 21(3–4): 372–75.

Kahneman, Daniel, Paul Slovic, and Amos Tversky. 1982. *Judgment Under Uncertainty: Heuristics and Biases*. Cambridge: Cambridge University Press.

Kaplan, Emanuel, and Robert Shaull. 1961. "Determination of Lead in Paint Scrapings as an Aid in the Control of Lead Pain Poisoning in Young Children." *American Journal of Public Health* 51(1): 65–69.

Karpati, Adam, Bonnie Kerker, Farzad Mostashari, Tejinder Singh, Anjum Hajat, Lorna Thorpe, Mary T. Bassett, Kelly Henning, and Thomas R. Frieden. 2004. *Health Disparities in New York City*. New York: New York City Department of Health and Mental Hygiene.

Katz, Alyssa. 2002. "Toxic Haste: New York's Media Rush to Judgment on New York's Air." *The American Prospect* (February 25): 13.

Katz, Michael B. 1986. *In the Shadow of the Poorhouse: A Social History of Welfare in America*. New York: Basic Books.

Kaufman, Herbert. 1959. *The New York City Health Centers*. Tuscaloosa: University of Alabama Press.

———. 1969. "Bureaucrats and Organized Civil Servants." In *Governing the City: Challenges and Options for New York*, edited by Robert H. Connery and Demetrios Caraley. New York: Praeger.

Kessler, David A. 1995. "Nicotine Addiction in Young People." *New England Journal of Medicine* 333(15): 186–89.

Khatri, G. R., and Thomas Frieden. 2002. "Rapid DOTS Expansion in India." *Bulletin of the World Health Organization* 80(6): 457–63.

Kilcoyne, Margaret M. 1973. "Hypertension and Heart Disease in the Urban Community." *Bulletin of the New York Academy of Medicine* 49(6): 501–9.

———. 1976. "Techniques of Screening." *Bulletin of the New York Academy of Medicine* 52(6): 657–64.

Kim, M., D. Berger, and T. Matte. 2006. *Diabetes in New York City: Public Health Burden and Disparities*. New York: New York City Department of Health and Mental Hygiene.

Kingdon, John W. 1984. *Agendas, Alternatives, and Public Policy*. Boston: Little, Brown.

Kirp, David, with Steven Epstein. 1989. *Learning by Heart: AIDS and Schoolchildren in America's Communities*. New Brunswick, N.J.: Rutgers University Press.

Kirtzman, Andrew. 2001. *Rudy Giuliani: Emperor of the City.* New York: Harper-Collins.

Klein, Woody. 1970. *Lindsay's Promise: The Dream That Failed.* New York: Macmillan.

Knowles, John H., ed. 1977a. *Doing Better and Feeling Worse: Health in the United States.* New York: Norton.

———. 1977b. "The Responsibility of the Individual." *Daedalus* 106(1): 57–80.

Kotchian, S. 1997. "Perspectives on the Place of Environmental Health and Protection in Public Health and Public Health Agencies." *Annual Review of Public Health* 18: 245–59.

Krent, Harold J., Nicholas Gingo, Monica Kapp, Rachel Moran, Mary Neal, Meghan Paulas, Punect Sarna, and Sarah Suma. 2008. "Whose Business Is Your Pancreas? Potential Privacy Problems in New York City's Mandatory Diabetes Registry." *Annals of Health Law* 17(1): 1–37.

Krieger, Nancy. 1994. "Epidemiology and the Web of Causation: Has Anyone Seen the Spider?" *Social Science and Medicine* 39(7): 887–903.

Lalonde, Marc. 1974. *A New Perspective on the Health of Canadians.* Ottawa: Canada Department of National Health and Welfare.

Lambright, W. Henry, and Mark O'Gorman. 1992. "New York State's Response to AIDS: Evolution of an Advocacy Agency." *Journal of Public Administration Research and Theory* 2(2): 175–98.

Lander, Byron G. 1971. "Group Theory and Individuals: The Origin of Poverty as a Political Issue in 1964." *Western Political Quarterly* 24(3): 514–26.

Layton, Marcelle. 2004. "Interview with Marcelle C. Layton, MD, Assistant Commissioner, Bureau of Communicable Disease, New York City Department of Health and Mental Hygiene." *Biosecurity and Bioterrorism* 2(4): 245–50.

Leavitt, Judith Walzer. 1982. *The Healthiest City: Milwaukee and the Politics of Health Reform.* Princeton, N.J.: Princeton University Press.

———. 1996. *Typhoid Mary: Captive to the Public's Health.* Boston: Beacon Press.

Lefkowitz, Bonnie. 2007. *Community Health Centers: A Movement and the People Who Made It Happen.* New Brunswick, N.J.: Rutgers University Press.

Lerner, Barron. 1998. *Contagion and Confinement: Controlling Tuberculosis Along the Skid Road.* Baltimore: Johns Hopkins University Press.

Lerner, Raymond C., Judith Bruce, Joyce R. Ochs, Sylvia Wassertheil-Smoller, and Charles B. Arnold. 1974. "Abortion Programs in New York City: Services, Policies, and Potential Health Hazards." *Milbank Memorial Fund Quarterly* 52(1): 15–38.

Levenson, Irving, and Jeffrey H. Weiss. 1976. *Analysis of Urban Health Problems.* New York: Spectrum Publications.

Levitan, Sar. 1974. "Healing the Poor in Their Own Back Yards." In *Neighborhood Health Centers,* edited by Robert M. Hollister, Bernard M. Kramer, and Seymour S. Bellin. Lexington, Mass.: Lexington Books.

Lopez, Wilfredo. 2002. "West Nile Virus in New York City." *American Journal of Public Health* 92(8): 1218–21.

Lopez, Wilfredo, and James R. Miller. 2002. "The Legal Context of Mosquito Control for West Nile Virus in New York City." *Journal of Law, Medicine and Ethics* 30(3): 135–38.

Lowell, Anthony M. 1956. *Socio-Economic Conditions and Tuberculosis Prevalence,*

New York City, 1949–1951. New York: New York Tuberculosis and Health Association.

Luckham, Jane, and David W. Swift. 1969. "Community Health Aides in the Ghetto: The Contra Costa Project." *Medical Care* 7(4): 332–39.

MacLeod, Kenneth I. E. 1967. "Providing Adequate Public Health Services: A Tale of Two Cities." *Public Health Reports* 82(10): 933–37.

MacMahon, E. J., and Fred Siegel. 2005. "Gotham's Fiscal Crisis: Lessons Unlearned." *Public Interest* 158(winter): 96–110.

Mahler, Jonathan. 2005. *Ladies and Gentlemen, The Bronx Is Burning: 1977, Baseball, Politics, and the Battle for the Soul of a City.* New York: Farrar, Straus & Giroux.

Mandavilli, Apoorva. 2006. "Profile: Thomas Frieden." *Nature Medicine* 12(4): 378.

Mann, Jonathan M. 1999. "Medicine and Public Health, Ethics, and Human Rights." In *Health and Human Rights: A Reader,* edited by Jonathan M. Mann, Sofia Gruskin, Michael A. Grodin, and George J. Annas. New York: Routledge.

Mariner, Wendy K. 2007. "Medicine and Public Health: Crossing Legal Boundaries." *Journal of Health Care Law and Policy* 10(1): 121–51.

Markovitz, Ruth, and Olivia Goodman. 1994. "Tuberculosis Amendments to the New York City Health Code." *Infectious Diseases in Clinical Practice* 3(5): 327–33.

Markowitz, Gerald, and David Rosner. 1996. *Children, Race, and Power: Kenneth and Mamie Clark's Northside Center.* Charlottesville: University Press of Virginia.

———. 2002. *Deceit and Denial: The Deadly Politics of Industrial Pollution.* Berkeley: University of California Press.

Marmot, Michael. 2004. *The Status Syndrome: How Social Standing Affects Our Health and Longevity.* New York: Henry Holt.

Martin, John L. 1987. "The Impact of AIDS on Gay Male Sexual Behavior Patterns in New York City." *American Journal of Public Health* 77(5): 578–81.

Mass, Lawrence. 1990. *Dialogues of the Sexual Revolution,* vol. 1: *Homosexuality and Sexuality.* New York: Haworth Press.

Masur, Henry, Mary Ann Michelis, Jeffrey B. Greene, Ida Onorato, Robert A. Vande Stouwe, Robert S. Holzman, Gary Wormser, Lee Brettman, Michael Lange, Henry W. Murray, and Susanna Cunningham-Rundles. 1981. "An Outbreak of Community-Acquired *Pneumocystis Carinii* Pneumonia: Initial Manifestation of Cellular Immune Dysfunction." *New England Journal of Medicine* 305(24): 1431–37.

Matthews, Gene W., and Verna Neslund. 1987. "The Initial Impact of AIDS on Public Health Law in the United States–1986." *Journal of the American Medical Association* 257(3): 344–52.

Matusow, Allan. 1984. *The Unraveling of America: A History of Liberalism in the 1960s.* New York: Harper & Row.

Mazur, Allan. 1977. "Public Confidence in Science." *Social Studies of Science* 7(1): 123–25.

McColl, Karen. 2008. "The Fattening Truth About Restaurant Food." *BMJ* 337: a2229.

McCord, Colin, and Harold P. Freeman. 1990. "Excess Mortality in Harlem." *New England Journal of Medicine* 322(3): 173–77.

McGinnis, J. Michael, Pamela Williams-Russo, and James R. Knickman. 2002. "The Case for More Active Policy Attention to Health Promotion," *Health Affairs* 21(2): 78–93.

McKeown, Thomas. 1979. *The Role of Medicine: Dream, Mirage or Nemesis?* Princeton, N.J.: Princeton University Press.

McLaughlin, Mary C. 1968a. "Issues and Problems Associated with the Initiation of the Large-Scale Ambulatory Care Program in New York City." *American Journal of Public Health* 58(7): 1181–87.

———. 1968b. "Present Status and Problems of New York City's Comprehensive Neighborhood Family Care Health Centers." *Bulletin of the New York Academy of Medicine* 44(11): 1390–95.

———. 1971. "Transmutation into Protector of Consumer Health Services." *American Journal of Public Health* 61(10): 1996–2004.

McLaughlin, Mary C., Florence Kavaler, and James Stiles. 1971. "Ghetto Medicine Program in New York City." *New York State Journal of Medicine* 71(19): 2321–25.

Mechanic, David. 1990. "Deinstitutionalization: An Appraisal of Reform." *Annual Review of Sociology* 16: 301–27.

Meckel, Richard. 1998. *Save the Babies: American Public Health Reform and the Prevention of Infant Mortality, 1850–1929.* Ann Arbor: University of Michigan Press.

Mello, Michelle M. 2009. "New York City's War on Fat." *New England Journal of Medicine* 360(19): 2015–20.

Melosi, Martin. 2000. *The Sanitary City: Urban Infrastructure in America from Colonial Times to the Present.* Baltimore: Johns Hopkins University Press.

Miles, Rufus E., Jr. 1974. *The Department of HEW.* New York: Praeger.

Miller, C. Arden, Edward F. Brooks, Gordon H. DeFriese, Benjamin Gilbert, Sagar C. Jain, and Florence Kavaler. 1977. "A Survey of Local Public Health Departments and Their Directors." *American Journal of Public Health* 67(10): 931–39.

Miller, C. Arden, and Merry-K Moos. 1981. *Local Health Departments: Fifteen Case Studies.* Chapel Hill, N.C.: American Public Health Association.

Miller, Bess, Sally K. Stansfield, Matthew M. Zack, James W. Curran, Jonathan E. Kaplan, Lawrence B. Schonberger, Henry Falk, Thomas J. Spira, and Donna Mildvan. 1984. "The Syndrome of Unexplained Generalized Lymphadenopathy in Young Men in New York City." *Journal of the American Medical Association* 251(2): 242–46.

Miller, Nancy, Thomas R. Frieden, Sze Yan Liu, Thomas D. Matte, Farzad Mostashan, Deborah R. Deitcher, K. Michael Cummings, Christina Chang, Ursula Bauer, and Mary T. Bassett. 2005. "Effectiveness of a Large-Scale Distribution Program of Free Nicotine Patches: A Prospective Evaluation." *The Lancet* 365(9474): 1849–54.

Mindlin, Rowland L., and Paul M. Densen. 1969. "Medical Care of Urban Infants: Continuity of Care." *American Journal of Public Health* 59(8): 1294–1301.

Morris, Charles R. 1980. *The Cost of Good Intentions: New York City and the Liberal Experiment, 1960–1975.* New York: Norton.

Mostashari, Farzad, Bonnie D. Kerker, Anjum Hajat, Nancy Miller, and Thomas R. Frieden. 2005. "Smoking Practices in New York City: The Use of a Population-Based Survey to Guide Policy-Making and Programming." *Journal of Urban Health* 82(1): 58–70.

Mullin, Sandra. 2003. "New York City's Communication Trials by Fire, from West Nile to SARS." *Biosecurity and Bioterrorism* 1(4): 267–72.

Mustalish, Anthony C., Gary Eidsvold, and Lloyd F. Novick. 1976. "Decentralization in the New York City Department of Health: Reorganization of a Public Health Agency." *American Journal of Public Health* 66(12): 1149–54.

Musto, David. 1999. *The American Disease: Origins of Narcotic Control.* New York: Oxford University Press.

Nardell, Edward A., and Philip W. Brickner. 1996. "Tuberculosis in New York City: Focal Transmission of an Often Fatal Disease." *Journal of the American Medical Association* 276(15): 1259–60.

Nardell, E., B. McInnis, B. Thomas, and S. Weidhaas. 1986. "Exogenous Reinfection with Tuberculosis in a Shelter for the Homeless." *New England Journal of Medicine* 315(25): 1570–75.

Nash, Denis, Farzad Mostashari, Annie Fine, James Miller, Daniel O'Leary, Kristy Murray, Ada Huang, Amy Rosenberg, Abby Grenberg, Margaret Sherman, Susan Wong, Grant L. Campbell, John T. Roehrig, Duane J. Gubber, Wun-Ju Shieh, Sherif Zaki, Perry Smith, and Marcelle Layton. 2001. "The Outbreak of West Nile Virus Infection in the New York City Area in 1999." *New England Journal of Medicine* 344(24): 1807–14.

Nathanson, Constance A. 1999. "Social Movements as Catalysts for Policy Change: The Case of Smoking and Guns." *Journal of Health Politics, Policy, and Law* 24(3): 421–88.

———. 2007. *Disease Prevention as Social Change: The State, Society, and Public Health in the United States, France, Great Britain, and Canada.* New York: Russell Sage Foundation.

Nelkin, Dorothy, and Stephen Hilgartner. 1986. "Disputed Dimensions of Risk: A Public School Controversy over AIDS." *Milbank Quarterly* 64(1 Suppl): 118–42.

Nelson, Jennifer A. 2001. "'Abortions Under Community Control': Feminism, Nationalism, and the Politics of Reproduction Among New York City's Young Lords." *Journal of Women's History* 13(1): 157–80.

Nestle, Marion, and Michael F. Jacobson. 2000. "Halting the Obesity Epidemic: A Public Health Policy Approach." *Public Health Reports* 115(1): 12–24.

Nestlebaum, Zamir. 1979. "The Fall and Fall of the N.Y.C DOH." *Health/PAC Bulletin* 83–85: 5–16.

Neustadt, Richard E., and Harvey V. Feinberg. 1983. *The Epidemic That Never Was: Policy-Making and the Swine Flu Scare.* New York: Vintage Books.

New York City Department of Health. 1981. *Promoting Health in Schools: A Review and Plan for Action for New York City.* New York: New York City Department of Health.

———. AIDS Surveillance. 1986. "The AIDS Epidemic in New York City, 1981–1984." *American Journal of Epidemiology* 123(6): 1013–25.

New York City Department of Health and Mental Hygiene. 2006. "Public Hearing on Trans Fat and Calorie Labeling Proposals Health Codes 81.08 and 81.50" (October 30). Available at: http://www.nyc.gov/html/doh/downloads/pdf/public/notice-intention-hc-art81-minutes.pdf (accessed March 2, 2010).

New York City Department of Health and Mental Hygiene. 2007. *Public Health in New York City, 2004–2006*. New York: New York City Department of Health and Mental Hygiene.

New York Lung Association. 1968. *Report of the Task Force on Tuberculosis in New York City, 1968*. New York: New York Lung Association.

———. 1981. *Tuberculosis in New York City, 1980*. New York: New York Lung Association.

———. 1985. *Tuberculosis in New York City, 1979–1984*. New York: New York Lung Association.

New York State Office of Mental Health. 2006. "Psychiatric Services Features Fifteen Articles on New York's Project Liberty" (September 11). Available at: http://www.omh.state.ny.us/omhweb/news/pr_psych_services.html (accessed May 2, 2010).

Newfield, Jack, and Paul DuBrul. 1977. *The Abuse of Power: The Permanent Government and the Fall of New York*. New York: Viking Press.

Newman, Robert. 1977. *Methadone Treatment in Narcotic Addiction: Program Management, Findings, and Prospects for the Future*. New York: Academic Press.

Newman, Robert, and Margot S. Cates. 1974, "The New York City Narcotics Register: A Case Study." *American Journal of Public Health* 64(12 Suppl): 24–28.

Newman, Robert, and Nina Peyser. 1991. "Methadone Treatment: Experiment and Experience." *Journal of Psychoactive Drugs* 23(2): 115–21.

Nivin, Beth, Peter Nicholas, Mitchell Gayer, Thomas R. Frieden, and Paula I. Fujiwara. 1998. "A Continuing Outbreak of Multidrug-Resistant Tuberculosis, with Transmission in a Hospital Nursery." *Clinical Infectious Diseases* 26(2): 303–7.

Nossiff, Rosemary. 2001. *Before Roe: Abortion Policy in the States*. Philadelphia: Temple University Press.

Novak, William. 1996. *The People's Welfare: Law and Regulation in Nineteenth-Century America*. Chapel Hill: University of North Carolina Press.

Novick, Lloyd F., Anthony Mustalish, and Gary Eidsvold. 1975. "Converting Child Health Stations to Pediatric Treatment Centers." *Medical Care* 13(9): 744–52.

Nutt, Paul C. 1976. "The Merits of Using Experts or Consumers as Members of Planning Groups: A Field Experiment in Health Planning." *Academy of Management Journal* 19(3): 378–94.

Nyswander, Marie, and Vincent P. Dole. 1967. "The Present Status of Methadone Blockade Treatment." *American Journal of Psychiatry* 123: 1441–42.

Okie, Susan. 2007. "New York to Trans Fats: You're Out!" *New England Journal of Medicine* 356(20): 2017–21.

Oleske, James, Anthony Minnefor, Roger Cooper, Kathleen Thomas, Antonio dela Cruz, Houman Ahdieh, Isabel Guerrero, Vijay V. Joshi, and Franklin Desposito. 1983. "Immune Deficiency Syndrome in Children." *Journal of the American Medical Association* 249(17): 2345–49.

Oliver, Thomas R. 2006. "The Politics of Public Health Policy." *Annual Review of Public Health* 27: 195–233.

Opdycke, Sandra. 2000. *No One Was Turned Away: The Role of Public Hospitals in New York City Since 1900*. New York: Oxford University Press.

Oppenheimer, Gerald M. 1992. "To Build a Bridge: The Use of Foreign Models by Domestic Critics of U.S. Drug Policy." *Milbank Quarterly* 69(3): 495–526.

Oppenheimer, Gerald M., Ronald Bayer, and James Colgrove. 2002. "Health and Human Rights: Old Wine in New Bottles?" *Journal of Law, Medicine, and Ethics* 30(4): 522–32.

O'Rourke, Edward. 1969. "Medicaid in New York: Utopianism and Bare Knuckles in Public Health." *American Journal of Public Health* 59(5): 814–15.

Pablos-Mendez, Ariel, Charles A. Knirsch, R. Graham Barr, Barron H. Lerner, and Thomas R. Frieden. 1997. "Nonadherence in Tuberculosis Treatment: Predictors and Consequences in New York City." *American Journal of Medicine* 102(2): 164–70.

Paolo, William F., and Joshua D. Nosanchuk. 2004. "Tuberculosis in New York City: Recent Lessons and a Look Ahead." *Lancet Infectious Diseases* 4(12): 287–93.

Parker, R. Andrew. 1973. "The Case of Ghetto Medicine." In *The Politics of Health Care: Nine Case Studies of Innovative Planning in New York City*, edited by Herbert Hyman. New York: Praeger.

Payte, J. Thomas. 1997. "Methadone Maintenance Treatment: The First Thirty Years." *Journal of Psychoactive Drugs* 29(2): 149–53.

Pearl, Arthur, and Frank Riessman. 1965. *New Careers for the Poor: The Nonprofessional in Human Service*. New York: Free Press.

Perrott, George St. J. 1945. "The Problem of Chronic Disease." *Psychosomatic Medicine* 7(1): 21–27.

Philipp, Barbara L., Anne Merewood, and Susan O'Brien. 2001. "Physicians and Breastfeeding Promotion in the United States: A Call for Action." *Pediatrics* 107(3): 584–87.

Pierson, Paul, and Theda Skocpol. 2007. "American Politics in the Long Run." In *The Transformation of American Politics: Activist Government and the Rise of Conservatism*, edited by Paul Pierson and Theda Skocpol. Princeton, N.J.: Princeton University Press.

Piore, Nora, Purlaine Lieberman, and James Linnane. 1977. "Public Expenditures and Private Control? Health Care Dilemmas in New York City." *Milbank Memorial Fund Quarterly* 55(1): 79–116.

Poen, Monte M. 1979. *Harry S. Truman Versus the Medical Lobby: The Genesis of Medicare*. Columbia: University of Missouri Press.

Preston, Richard. 1995. *The Hot Zone*. New York: Anchor Press.

Public Health Association of New York City. 2001. *Strengthening New York City's Public Health Infrastructure*. New York: Public Health Association of New York City.

———. 2002. *Public Health at a Crossroads: Proposals for Protecting and Strengthening New York City's Public Health System*. New York: Public Health Association of New York City.

Purnick, Joyce. 2009. *Mike Bloomberg: Money, Power, Politics*. New York: Public Affairs.

Quimby, Ernest, and Samuel R. Friedman. 1989. "Dynamics of Black Mobilization Against AIDS in New York City." *Social Problems* 36(4): 403–15.

Rapoport, Mark. 1987. "Dr. Mark Rapoport on the Homeless Health Initiative." *Health Matrix* 5(1): 56–60.

Rappleye, Willard C. 1961. "The Hospitals of New York City." *Bulletin of the New York Academy of Medicine* 37(8): 525–30.

Ravitch, Diane. 2000. *The Great School Wars: A History of the New York City Public Schools*. Baltimore: Johns Hopkins University Press.

Reagan, Leslie J. 1997. *When Abortion Was a Crime: Women, Medicine, and Law in the United States, 1867–1973*. Berkeley: University of California Press.

Reichman, Lee. 1991. "The U-Shaped Curve of Concern." *American Review of Respiratory Disease* 144(4): 741–42.

Renthal, A. Gerald. 1971. "Comprehensive Health Centers in Large U.S. Cities." *American Journal of Public Health* 61(2): 324–36.

Riessman, Frank. 1964. *Mental Health for the Poor*. New York: Free Press of Glencoe.

Rodriguez, Iris. 1972. "Ghetto Medicine." *American Journal of Public Health* 62(1): 3–4.

Roemer, Milton I. 1973. "The American Public Health Association as a Force for Change in Medical Care." *Medical Care* 11(4): 338–51.

Rogers, Naomi. 2001. "'Caution: The AMA May Be Dangerous to Your Health': The Student Health Organizations (SHO) and American Medicine, 1965–1970." *Radical History Review* 2001(80): 5–34.

Rosen, George. 1971. "The First Neighborhood Health Center Movement—Its Rise and Fall." *American Journal of Public Health* 61(8): 1620–37.

Rosenbaum, Marsha. 1995. "The Demedicalization of Methadone Maintenance." *Journal of Psychoactive Drugs* 27(2): 145–49.

Rosenberg, Charles. 1962. *The Cholera Years: The United States in 1832, 1849, and 1866*. Chicago: University of Chicago Press.

Rosenkrantz, Barbara Gutmann. 1972. *Public Health and the State: Changing Views in Massachusetts, 1869–1936*. Cambridge, Mass.: Harvard University Press.

Rosner, David, and Gerald Markowitz. 2006. *Are We Ready? Public Health Since 9/11*. Berkeley: University of California Press.

Rothman, Kenneth J., Hans-Olov Adami, and Dimitrios Tichopoulos. 1998. "Should the Mission of Epidemiology Include the Eradication of Poverty?" *The Lancet* 352(9134): 810–13.

Rothman, Sheila M. 1995. *Living in the Shadow of Death: Tuberculosis and the Social Experience of Illness and American History*. Baltimore: Johns Hopkins University Press.

Rowe, Mona, and Caitlin C. Ryan. 1988. "Comparing State-Only Expenditures for AIDS." *American Journal of Public Health* 78(4): 424–29.

Rushing, William A. 1995. *The AIDS Epidemic: Social Dimensions of an Infectious Disease*. Boulder, Colo.: Westview Press.

Safyer, Steven M., Lynn Richmond, Eran Bellin, and David Fletcher. 1993. "Tuberculosis in Correctional Facilities: The Tuberculosis Control Program of the Montefiore Medical Center Rikers Island Health Services." *Journal of Law, Medicine, and Ethics* 21(3–4): 342–51.

Sardell, Alice. 1988. *The U.S. Experiment in Social Medicine: The Community Health Center Program, 1965–1986*. Pittsburgh: University of Pittsburgh Press.

Sayre, Wallace, and Herbert Kaufman. 1960. *Governing New York City: Politics in the Metropolis*. New York: Russell Sage Foundation.

Sbarbaro, John A. 1979. "Compliance: Inducements and Enforcements." *Chest* 76(6): 750–56.

Schlesinger, Jr., Arthur M. 1967. *The Bitter Heritage: Vietnam and American Democracy, 1941–1966*. Boston: Houghton Mifflin.

Schultz, Stanley K., and Clay McShane. 1978. "To Engineer the Metropolis: Sewers, Sanitation, and City Planning in Late-Nineteenth-Century America." *Journal of American History* 65(2): 389–411.

Sencer, David. 1983. "Major Urban Health Departments: The Ideal and the Real." *Health Affairs* 2(4): 88–95.

Shah, Nayan. 2001. *Contagious Divides: Epidemics and Race in San Francisco's Chinatown*. Berkeley: University of California Press.

Shalala, Donna E., and Carol Bellamy. 1976. "A State Saves a City: The New York Case." *Duke Law Journal* 1976(6): 1119–32.

Shefter, Martin. 1992. *Political Crisis, Fiscal Crisis: The Collapse and Revival of New York City*. New York: Columbia University Press.

Shelley, Donna, Jennifer Cantrell, Joyce Moon-Howard, Destiny Q. Ramjohn, and Nancy Van Devanter. 2007. "The $5 Man: The Underground Economic Response to a Large Cigarette Tax Increase in New York City." *American Journal of Public Health* 97(8): 1483–88.

Shilts, Randy. 1987. *And the Band Played On*. New York: Penguin Books.

Shonick, William, and Walter Price. 1977. "Reorganizations of Health Agencies by Local Government in American Urban Centers: What Do They Portend for 'Public Health'?" *Milbank Memorial Fund Quarterly* 55(2): 233–71.

Sieben, R. L., J. D. Leavitt, and J. H. French. 1971. "Falls as Childhood Accidents: An Increasing Urban Risk." *Pediatrics* 47(5): 886–90.

Silver, Lynn, and Mary T. Bassett. 2008. "Food Safety for the Twenty-First Century." *Journal of the American Medical Association* 300(8): 957–59.

Silversides, Ann. 2003. *AIDS Activist: Michael Lynch and the Politics of Community*. Toronto: Between the Lines.

Singman, Henry S., Sylvia N. Berman, Catherine Cowell, Ethel Maslansky, and Morton Archer. 1980. "The Anti-Coronary Club: 1957 to 1972." *American Journal of Clinical Nutrition* 33(6): 1183–91.

Skocpol, Theda. 1992. *Protecting Soldiers and Mothers: The Political Origins of Social Policy in the United States*. Cambridge, Mass.: Belknap Press of Harvard University Press.

Smillie, Wilson. 1947. *Public Health Administration in the United States*. New York: Macmillan.

Sommer, Alfred. 1995. "W(h)ither Public Health?" *Public Health Reports* 110(6): 657–61.

Sonnabend, Joseph A., Steven S. Witkin, and David T. Purtilo. 1984. "A Multifactorial Model for the Development of AIDS in Homosexual Men." *Annals of the New York Academy of Sciences* 437: 177–83.

Specter, Michael J., Vincent F. Guinee, and Bernard Davidow. 1971. "The Unsuitability of Random Urinary Delta Aminolevulinic Acid Samples as a Screening Test for Lead Poisoning." *Journal of Pediatrics* 79(5): 799–804.

Spiegel, Charlotte N., and Francis C. Lindaman. 1977. "Children Can't Fly: A Program to Prevent Childhood Morbidity and Mortality from Window Falls." *American Journal of Public Health* 67(12): 1143–47.

Starin, Irving, and Nicetas Kuo. 1966. "The Queensbridge Health Maintenance Service for the Elderly." *Public Health Reports* 81(1): 75–82.

Starin, Irving, Nicetas Kuo, and Mary McLaughlin. 1962. "Queensbridge Health Maintenance Service for the Elderly." *Public Health Reports* 77(12): 1041–47.

Starr, Paul. 1982. *The Social Transformation of American Medicine*. New York: Basic Books.

Stearns, Linda Brewster, and Paul D. Almeida. 2004. "The Formation of State Actor Social Movement Coalitions and Favorable Policy Outcomes." *Social Problems* 51(4): 478–504.

Steinbrook, Robert. 2006. "Facing the Diabetes Epidemic—Mandatory Reporting of Glycosylated Hemoglobin Values in New York City." *New England Journal of Medicine* 354(6): 545–48.

Stephenson, Joan. 1996. "Confronting a Biological Armageddon: Experts Tackle Prospect of Bioterrorism." *Journal of the American Medical Association* 276(5): 349–51.

Stevens, Robert, and Rosemary Stevens. 1974. *Welfare Medicine in America: A Case Study of Medicaid*. New York: Free Press.

Stewart, James C., and William R. Hood. 1970. "Using Workers from 'Hard-Core' Areas to Increase Immunization Levels." *Public Health Reports* 85(2): 177–85.

Stoneburner, Rand, Don C. Des Jarlais, Diane Benezra, Leo Gorelkin, Jo L. Sotheran, Samuel R. Friedman, Stephen Schultz, Michael Marmor, Donna Mildvan, and Robert Maslansky. 1988. "A Larger Spectrum of Severe HIV-1-Related Disease in Intravenous Drug Users in New York City." *Science* 242(4880): 916–19.

Sugrue, Thomas. 1996. *The Origins of the Urban Crisis: Race and Inequality in Postwar Detroit*. Princeton, N.J.: Princeton University Press.

Szreter, Simon. 1988. "The Importance of Social Intervention in Britain's Mortality Decline c. 1850–1914: A Reinterpretation of the Role of Public Health." *Social History of Medicine* 1(1): 7–10.

Tabb, William K. 1982. *The Long Default: New York City and the Urban Fiscal Crisis*. New York: Monthly Review Press.

Terry, Luther L. 1964. "The Health Officer and Medical Care Administration." *American Journal of Public Health* 54(11): 1799–1803.

Thomas, Lewis. 1983. *The Youngest Science: Notes of a Medicine Watcher*. New York: Viking Press.

Thomas, Pauline A., Harold W. Jaffe, Thomas J. Spira, Rebecca Reiss, Isabel C. Guerrero, and David Auerbach. 1984. "Unexplained Immunodeficiency in Children: A Surveillance Report." *Journal of the American Medical Association* 252(5): 639–44.

Thomas, Pauline A., Rosalind Williams, and Mary Ann Chiasson. 1988. "HIV Infection in Heterosexual Female Intravenous Drug Users in New York City, 1977–1980." *New England Journal of Medicine* 319(6): 374.

Thorpe, Lorna E., R. Charon Gwynn, Jenna Mandel-Ricci, Sarah Roberts, Benjamin Tsoi, Lew Berman, Kathryn Porter, Yechiam Ostchega, Lester R. Curtain, Jill Montaquila, Leyla Mohadjer, and Thomas R. Frieden. 2006. "Study Design and Participation Rates of the New York City Health and Nutrition Examination Survey, 2004." *Preventing Chronic Disease* 3(3): A94.

Tomes, Nancy. 2006. "Patients or Health-Care Consumers? Why the History of Contested Terms Matters." In *History and Health Policy in the United States: Putting the Past Back In*, edited by Rosemary A. Stevens, Charles E. Rosenberg, and Lawton R. Burns. New Brunswick, N.J.: Rutgers University Press.

———. 2008. "Speaking for the Public: The Ambivalent Quest of Twentieth-

Century Public Health." In *The Contested Boundaries of American Public Health*, edited by James Colgrove, David Rosner, and Gerald Markowitz. New Brunswick, N.J.: Rutgers University Press.

Traub, James. 2004. *The Devil's Playground: One Hundred Years in Times Square*. New York: Random House.

United Hospital Fund of New York. 1992. *The Tuberculosis Revival: Individual Rights and Societal Obligations in a Time of AIDS*. New York: United Hospital Fund.

United States Conference of Mayors. 1982a. *Human Services in FY '82: Shrinking Resources in Troubled Times*. Washington, D.C.: United States Conference of Mayors (October).

———. 1982b. *The Federal Budget and the Cities*. Washington, D.C.: United States Conference of Mayors (February).

U.S. Congress. 1954. *Tuberculosis in New York City, 1953*. New York: New York Tuberculosis and Health Association.

———. 1991. *Tuberculosis in New York City: An Epidemic Returns*. Hearing before the U.S. House of Representatives, Committee on Government Operations, Human Resources and Intergovernmental Relations Subcommittee. 102d Cong., 1st sess., December 18, 1991. Washington: U.S. Government Printing Office.

U.S. Senate. Committee on Finance. 1970. *Medicare and Medicaid: Problems, Issues, and Alternatives*. Washington: U.S. Government Printing Office.

Van Wye, Gretchen, Bonnie D. Kerker, Thomas Matte, Shadi Chamany, Donna Eisenhower, Thomas R. Frieden, and Lorna Thorpe. 2008. "Obesity and Diabetes in New York City, 2002 and 2004." *Preventing Chronic Disease* 5(2): 1–11.

Vennema, Alje. 1982. "The Status of Tuberculosis Control in New York City." *Public Health Reports* 97(2): 127–33.

Wallach, Jonathan B., and Mariano J. Rey. 2009. "A Socioeconomic Analysis of Obesity and Diabetes in New York City." *Preventing Chronic Disease* 6(3): A108.

Wallack, Lawrence, and Regina Lawrence. 2005. "Talking About Public Health: Developing America's 'Second Language.'" *American Journal of Public Health* 95(4): 567–70.

Waserman, Manfred. 1975. "The Quest for a National Health Department in the Progressive Era." *Bulletin of the History of Medicine* 49(3): 353–80.

Wassertheil-Smoller, Sylvia, Polly Bijur, and M. Donald Blaufox. 1978. "An Evaluation of the Utility of High Blood Pressure Detection Fairs." *American Journal of Public Health* 68(8): 768–70.

Wegman, Myron E. 1977. "Health Departments: Then and Now." *American Journal of Public Health* 67(10): 913–14.

Wilkinson, Richard, and Michael Marmot, eds. 2003. *Social Determinants of Health: The Solid Facts*. Geneva: World Health Organization.

Wooley, Mary, and Georges Benjamin. 2004. "Research! America/APHA National Poll on America's Attitudes Toward Public Health." Oral presentation to the Annual Meeting of the American Public Health Association. Washington, D.C. (November 9).

Yerby, Alonzo S. 1967. "Health Departments, Hospitals, and Health Services." *Medical Care* 5(2): 70–74.

Young Lords Party. 1971. *Palante!* New York: McGraw-Hill.

Index

Boldface numbers refer to photos and posters.